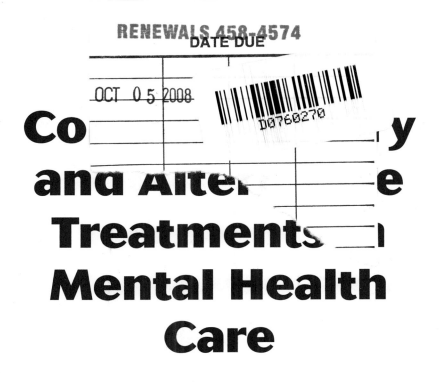

Co   y
and Alter   e
Treatments
Mental Health
Care

Complementary and Alternative Treatments in Mental Health Care

Edited by

James Lake, M.D.
David Spiegel, M.D.

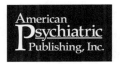

American Psychiatric Publishing, Inc.

Washington, DC
London, England

If you would like to buy between 25 and 99 copies of this or any other APPI title, you are eligible for a 20% discount; please contact APPI Customer Service at appi@psych.org or 800-368-5777. If you wish to buy 100 or more copies of the same title, please e-mail us at bulksales@psych.org for a price quote.

Copyright © 2007 American Psychiatric Publishing, Inc.
ALL RIGHTS RESERVED

Manufactured in the United States of America on acid-free paper
10   09   08   07   06   5   4   3   2   1
First Edition

Typeset in Adobe's Cosmos and Bembo.

American Psychiatric Publishing, Inc.
1000 Wilson Boulevard
Arlington, VA 22209-3901
www.appi.org

Library of Congress Cataloging-in-Publication Data
Complementary and alternative treatments in mental health care / edited by James Lake, David Spiegel. — 1st ed.
    p. ; cm.
  Includes bibliographical references and index.
  ISBN 1-58562-202-8 (pbk. : alk. paper)
  1. Psychiatry. 2. Mental health services. 3. Mental illness—Alternative treatment.   I. Lake, James, 1956–   .   II. Spiegel, David, 1945–   .
  [DNLM: 1. Mental Disorders—therapy. 2. Complementary Therapies. WM 400 C7366 2006]
  RC460.C66442 2006
  616.89'1—dc22

                                                             2006025873

British Library Cataloguing in Publication Data
A CIP record is available from the British Library.

Contents

I
Background Issues

II
Review of the Evidence and Clinical Guidelines

Nonconventional Biological Treatments

Lifestyle and Women's Issues

Spirituality, Mindfulness, and Mind–Body Practices

Contributors

Iris R. Bell, M.D., M.D.(H.), Ph.D.
Professor, Departments of Family and Community Medicine, Psychiatry, Psychology, Medicine (Program in Integrative Medicine), and Public Health, The University of Arizona Colleges of Medicine and Public Health, Tucson, Arizona, and the American Medical College of Homeopathy, Phoenix, Arizona

Richard P. Brown, M.D.
Associate Clinical Professor of Psychiatry, Department of Psychiatry, Columbia University College of Physicians and Surgeons, New York, New York

Michael H. Cohen, J.D.
Attorney-at-Law; Assistant Clinical Professor of Medicine, Harvard Medical School, and Assistant Professor at Harvard School of Public Health, Boston, Massachusetts; President, Institute for Integrative and Energy Medicine, Cambridge, Massachusetts

Brian J. Ellinoy, Pharm.D.
Integrative Pharmacist; private consultant practice, Monterey, California

Marlene P. Freeman, M.D.
Associate Professor, Departments of Psychiatry, Obstetrics and Gynecology, and Nutritional Sciences and Director, Women's Mental Health Program, Department of Psychiatry, University of Arizona College of Medicine, Tucson, Arizona

Andrew Freinkel, M.D.
Research Physician, California Pacific Medical Center Research Institute, San Francisco, California; and Staff Physician, Stanford Clinic for Integrative Medicine, Stanford, California

Patricia L. Gerbarg, M.D.
Clinical Assistant Professor, Department of Psychiatry and Behavioral Sciences, New York Medical College, Valhalla, New York

Rebecca A. Hill, M.B.B.S.(Hons.)
Staff Psychiatrist, Werribee Mercy Mental Health Program, Werribee, Victoria, Australia

Melanie Hingle, M.P.H., R.D.
Senior Research Specialist, Department of Nutritional Sciences, University of Arizona, Tucson, Arizona

Christopher Hobbs, L.Ac., A.H.G.
Writer and lecturer on herbal medicine; private practice in clinical herbalism and acupuncture, Santa Cruz, California

James Lake, M.D.
Private practice, Monterey, California; and adjunct clinical faculty, Department of Psychiatry and Behavioral Sciences, Stanford University Hospital & Clinics, Stanford, California

Roberta Lee, M.D.
Medical Director, Continuum Center for Health and Healing, and Co-Director, Program in Integrative Medicine, Beth Israel Medical Center, New York, New York

Robert B. Lutz, M.D., M.P.H.
Adjunct Assistant Professor, School of Professional Studies, Department of Nursing, Gonzaga University, Spokane, Washington

Grace Naing, M.D.
Consulting Physician in Integrative Medicine and Acupuncture, Berkshire Family Medicine, Wyomissing, Pennsylvania; and in Addiction Medicine, Caron, Wernersville, Pennsylvania

Pamela A. Pappas, M.D., M.D.(H.)
Fellow, Program in Integrative Medicine, The University of Arizona College of Medicine, Tucson, Arizona; and Clinical Faculty, American Medical College of Homeopathy, Phoenix, Arizona

Sudha Prathikanti, M.D.
Associate Clinical Professor of Psychiatry, University of California, San Francisco, California

Jeffrey D. Rediger, M.D., M.Div.
Medical Director, McLean Hospital, Harvard Medical School, Brockton, Massachusetts

Carolyn Coker Ross, M.D., M.P.H.
Chief, Eating Disorders Program, and Head, Integrative Therapies Department, Sierra Tucson, CRC Health Group, Inc., Tucson, Arizona

Ronald Schouten, M.D., J.D.
Director, Law and Psychiatry Service, Massachusetts General Hospital; and Associate Professor of Psychiatry, Harvard Medical School, Boston, Massachusetts

Janet E. Settle, M.D.
Clinical Instructor, Department of Psychiatry, School of Medicine, University of Colorado at Denver Health Sciences Center, Denver, Colorado

Priti Sinha, M.D.
Clinical Assistant, Department of Psychiatry, University of Arizona College of Medicine, Tucson, Arizona

David Spiegel, M.D.
Jack, Lulu, and Sam Willson Professor in the School of Medicine and Associate Chair, Department of Psychiatry and Behavioral Sciences, Stanford University School of Medicine, Stanford, California

Lauren Summers, M.Div. Candidate
Harvard Divinity School, Cambridge, Massachusetts

Julia Thie, L.Ac., Dipl.Ac., Dipl.C.H.
NCCAOM board-certified acupuncturist and Chinese herbalist; California and Tennessee state-licensed acupuncturist; private oriental medicine practice, Kingsport, Tennessee; and President Emeritus, Tennessee Acupuncture Council

Pamela S. Yee, M.D.
Assistant Attending in Internal Medicine, Department of Medicine, Beth Israel Medical Center, New York, New York; Consulting Physician for Meridian Medical Group, New York, New York, and The Foundation for Integrated Medicine, New York, New York

Preface

David Spiegel, M.D.

Why would one examine in detail complementary and alternative medicine (CAM) treatments in mental health care in an era when traditional psychotherapeutic and psychopharmacological treatments have never been better? There are at least two reasons: one is empirical, the other is theoretical.

First, empirical data show that public interest in CAM treatments is growing rapidly, and it is thus incumbent on physicians to follow their patients' lead and become knowledgeable about these treatments (Spiegel 2000; Spiegel et al. 1998). Each year, an additional 1% of the population in the United States asks for a CAM therapy, with comparable increases in interest in other Western countries and long-standing high levels of interest in non–Western nations (Cassileth 1999; Downer et al. 1994; Gore-Felton et al. 2003; Wetzel et al. 1998). Since the mid-1990s, patients have been making more visits to CAM practitioners and spending more money out of pocket on them than on mainstream ambulatory or hospital-based care. Patients frequently combine these nonbiomedical treatments with traditional medical care; however, they often do not disclose their use of "alternative" treatments to their physicians (Eisenberg et al. 1993, 1998). This gap in physician knowledge about patients' use of other treatments can lead to a "disintegration" of care, creating distrust between the patient and physician, preventing the physician from assessing potentially harmful interactions, and interfering with the patient's adherence to prescribed treatments.

Second, the constraints placed on medicine, psychiatry, and psychology by increasingly biotechnological treatments and the domination of Western biomedicine by managed care and insurance companies are fueling this trend toward alternative forms of care. Health care professionals are viewed as biotechnicians and saddled with demeaning titles such as *provider,* implying that one practitioner is just as good as another and that continuity of care or an ongoing relationship with a health care professional is of little importance. The amount of time available for physicians to spend with each patient is being ratcheted down. Whereas CAM practitioners generally spend 30–50 minutes with each patient, the typical medical interview with a primary care physician lasts 7 minutes and psychiatric "medication visits" are limited to 15 minutes. Psychiatrists who routinely scheduled 50-minute hours with patients decades ago are now reimbursed primarily for 15-minute medication evaluations. Patients' needs, however, are moving in the opposite direction, as they increasingly seek knowledgeable professionals who can and will form a relationship and spend time with them. This is nowhere more true than in the field of mental health care, where the complexity, sensitivity, and cognitive, emotional, and social implications of illness make the provider-patient relationship a key diagnostic and therapeutic instrument.

Furthermore, contemporary treatments in psychiatry, psychology, and medicine are far from perfect, and exploration of "alternative" approaches is often productive. Science is a great leveler. One can evaluate any treatment, no matter how unusual, nontraditional, or implausible, using the empirical methods of science, including randomized clinical trials, advanced brain imaging technologies, and other physiological measures of claimed mechanisms of action and treatment outcomes. It is not the nature of a specific treatment as much as the quality of evidence supporting its use that determines its place in the therapeutic repertoire ("Psychosocial intervention" 1989). Treatments that were once considered odd herbal interventions are now mainstream therapies. For example, foxglove, which was used centuries ago for dropsy, is the plant source of digitalis, a treatment for congestive heart failure that is highly effective because of the drug's positive inotropic effect, which enhances the contractility of cardiac muscle. The bark of the Pacific yew tree is now paclitaxel (Taxol), a cytotoxic chemotherapeutic agent widely used to treat breast cancer. Treatments are alternative until they are found to be effective for a specific medical problem and subsequently accepted into Western medicine (Lang et al. 2000). Certainly for every story of a medication's transition from alternative to mainstream, there are hundreds of examples of treatments that do not have specific efficacy and will probably remain in the alternative domain. Nonetheless, the widespread use of such treatments and the increasing evidence supporting their therapeutic benefits call for a concerted scientific effort to integrate those that work into mainstream medicine.

Nonconventional treatments are nowhere more relevant than in the domain of mental health care. They challenge our existing understanding of mind–brain–body interactions by providing a wide array of treatments with body–mind (herbal treatments, physical manipulations) and mind–brain (energy therapies, mindfulness) effects. They also challenge us to understand and better use bidirectional effects of body on mind and mind on body. Thus integrative treatments challenge us to better understand what our patients are doing and what we as mental health professionals are doing as well.

This book reviews the history and rationale for a variety of CAM treatments as well as the risks and benefits of their integration into mainstream mental health care. It covers herbal and other natural products, stress management, homeopathy, and other techniques largely developed and used in the West as well as ancient Eastern treatment systems, including the Indian holistic Ayurveda and traditional Chinese medicine. Indeed, as information becomes more widely and rapidly disseminated around the globe through the Internet and other means of electronic communication, it becomes possible to examine, better understand, and use previously exotic or unheard of treatment approaches. The very interconnectedness of the global population challenges medicine to expand its frame of reference.

The chapter authors in this volume have risen to the challenge of presenting their specialized knowledge of nonconventional treatments with a rigorous evaluation of the scientific evidence. Our goal in writing this book is to help mental health practitioners and patients become knowledgeable consumers, not true believers or inveterate skeptics. We hope to expand the repertoire of legitimate treatments in mental health care while also shedding light on limitations of approaches that are still regarded as alternative, nonconventional, or unproven. Humanity has been struggling with mental health problems for millennia. We have tried to distill a vast body of scientific information, wisdom, and experience to help mental health professionals and their patients more effectively address these problems.

REFERENCES

Cassileth BR: Complementary therapies: overview and state of the art. Cancer Nurs 22:85–90, 1999

Downer SM, Cody MM, McCluskey P, et al: Pursuit and practice of complementary therapies by cancer patients receiving conventional treatment. BMJ 309:86–89, 1994

Eisenberg DM, Kessler RC, Foster C, et al: Unconventional medicine in the United States: prevalence, costs, and patterns of use. N Engl J Med 328:246–252, 1993

Eisenberg DM, Davis RB, Ettner SL, et al: Trends in alternative medicine use in the United States, 1990–1997: results of a follow-up national survey. JAMA 280:1569–1575, 1998

Gore-Felton C, Vosvick M, Power R, et al: Alternative therapies: a common practice among men and women living with HIV. J Assoc Nurses AIDS Care 14:17–27, 2003

Lang E, Benotsch E, Fink L, et al: Adjunctive non-pharmacological analgesia for invasive medical procedures: a randomised trial. Lancet 355:1486–1490, 2000

Psychosocial intervention and the natural history of cancer (editorial). Lancet 2(8668):901, 1989

Spiegel D: Complementary medicine in North America, in Encyclopedia of Stress, Vol 1. Edited by Fink G. San Diego, CA, Academic Press, 2000, pp 512–515

Spiegel D, Stroud P, Fyfe A: Complementary medicine. West J Med 168:241–247, 1998

Wetzel MS, Eisenberg DM, Kaptchuk TJ: Courses involving complementary and alternative medicine at US medical schools. JAMA 280:784–787, 1998

Introduction

James Lake, M.D.

Complementary and Alternative Treatments in Mental Health Care is a concise overview of many complementary and alternative medicine (CAM) approaches currently used in North America and Europe to treat or self-treat mental health problems. It is intended to be a resource that provides mental health practitioners and patients with current information about effective treatments of mental illness that are not yet fully examined or endorsed by the institutions of conventional biomedicine. In so doing, it reviews nonconventional treatments for common psychiatric disorders, establishes guidelines for their appropriate use, and discusses other modalities that do not meet the necessary safety and effectiveness criteria.

Given the growing patient interest in CAM therapies, it is important for psychiatrists and other mental health professionals to develop a basic knowledge of these treatments and a familiarity regarding which ones are supported by research evidence and others that may be widely used, even in the absence of such evidence. Because many nonconventional approaches have not yet been fully validated, we have worked to assemble current information about the safety and efficacy of CAM approaches that are widely used to treat mental health problems. This book provides essential clinical information that the mental health professional can rely on in recommending appropriate nonconventional treatments or medical practitioners while keeping the patient's safety foremost in mind.

The chapter authors are psychiatrists, psychologists, pharmacists, herbalists, acupuncturists, and other health care professionals motivated by the shared vision of creating a practical, evidence-based clinical resource to be used when CAM approaches are being considered for the outpatient management of common psychiatric disorders. Many psychiatrists who contributed chapters to this book are trained in one or more complementary or alternative medical approaches. They write about the management of mental illness from the unique perspectives of their eclectic training and research and their work as mental health professionals. Conventionally trained mental health professionals, including psychiatrists, psychologists, licensed clinical social workers, and marriage and family therapists,

can refer to this book when consulting with patients about the evidence supporting CAM therapies for their particular mental or emotional problems. Herbalists,
clinical nutritionists, Chinese medical practitioners, homeopaths, Ayurvedic
physicians, and other medical practitioners trained in nonconventional methods
will find in these pages a critical and balanced review of the most widely used
nonconventional treatments of mental or emotional problems in Western countries. This book is offered as a bridge between the orthodox theories and practices of conventional biomedicine and the established theories and practices of
the world's major systems of medicine as they pertain to mental health care. The
book is not a comprehensive compendium of research findings on the range of
nonconventional approaches used in mental health care, although researchers will
find it to be a valuable resource when designing future studies.

The use of nonconventional approaches to treat mental health problems is
growing, and mental health professionals need to learn more about these approaches. In North America, Western Europe, and other industrialized regions,
an increasing number of patients are seeking out nonconventional medical practitioners for mental health care or using nonconventional approaches to self-treat
mental or emotional problems (Eisenberg 1999; Eisenberg et al. 1998; Fisher
1994). Most patients who use CAM approaches are well educated, express a
strong commitment to personal growth or spirituality, are satisfied with their
conventional medical care, and use both alternative and conventional treatments
for the same medical or psychiatric problem (Astin 1998; Astin et al. 1998). The
use of all CAM approaches is significantly greater among individuals who meet
DSM-IV (American Psychiatric Association 1994) criteria for any psychiatric
disorder than the general population (Unutzer et al. 2000). Approximately 20%
of all patients diagnosed with a depressive or anxiety disorder use relaxation techniques, 10% receive spiritual or energy treatments for their symptoms, and 7%
take herbs, vitamins, or other natural substances (Kessler et al. 2001).

As more patients embrace nonconventional therapies, conventionally trained
mental health professionals are increasingly acknowledging the validity and clinical benefits of many CAM modalities. Many conventionally trained mental health
professionals are taking courses in one or more nonconventional modalities to
provide more *integrative* care to their patients. Dually trained practitioners, including psychiatrists and psychologists, are administering conventional biomedical
treatments and nonconventional therapies to patients during a single session.
Largely at patients' requests, psychiatrists and psychologists are more frequently
referring patients to qualified nonconventional medical practitioners for the management of mental or emotional symptoms through acupuncture, Chinese herbal
formulas, Western herbal medicines, vitamins, amino acids and other nonherbal
natural substances, homeopathy, massage, and other treatments currently outside
of conventional Western biomedicine (Astin 1998; Astin et al. 1998; Ernst et al.
1995). Psychiatrists and other mental health professionals who do not yet use

nonconventional approaches are referring patients to nonconventional medical practitioners for the treatment of psychiatric disorders, including depressed mood, bipolar disorder, generalized anxiety, and other major psychiatric disorders.

A diagnosis of major depressive disorder is a strong predictor of concurrent use of antidepressants and nonprescription supplements (Druss and Rosenheck 2000). It is estimated that 67% of severely depressed or anxious patients who receive or self-administer nonconventional therapies concurrently use conventional Western treatments (Kessler et al. 2001). Because of the widely held perception that most conventionally trained physicians are critical of nonorthodox medical treatments, many patients do not disclose their use of nonconventional treatments to their primary care physician or psychiatrist. A large survey found that only 38% of individuals who use a CAM treatment for any problem disclose this fact to their physician (Eisenberg et al. 1998). This has resulted in unknown risks of treatment failures or treatment complications, including toxicities and interactions between conventional pharmacological treatments and nonconventional therapies. Incomplete information about how a patient is being treated for a mental or emotional problem by an alternative medical practitioner places significant constraints on the capacity of conventionally trained mental health professionals and nonconventionally trained medical practitioners to make informed treatment recommendations or adequately assess reasons for patient noncompliance or poor outcomes.

Many nonconventional treatments are strongly endorsed in the popular media and by the general public, and a growing popular fascination with CAM has emerged as a kind of fad in many Western countries. Most patients who use nonconventional therapies to self-treat mental health problems rate them as equally effective as conventional biomedical treatments, even in the absence of conclusive evidence to this effect (Kessler et al. 2001). Emerging research and clinical findings suggest that many nonconventional treatments are probably effective and safe. However, the quality of evidence for most nonconventional therapies used to self-treat or treat mental health problems is uneven at best. Because many patients use both conventional and nonconventional treatments, it is important to consider the case for nonconventional treatments in mental health care in the broader context of the evidence supporting conventional psychopharmacological treatments. Despite decades of concerted research, billions of dollars of research (and advertising) funding by the pharmaceutical industry, and hundreds of carefully designed, double-blind, placebo-controlled studies, a systematic review of rigorously conducted studies concluded that most conventional antidepressants have significant placebo effect components, and that risks of adverse effects associated with conventional pharmacological therapy may in some situations outweigh potential benefits (Keitner 2004; Moncrieff et al. 2004). Some patients are reluctant to take conventional psychotropic medications but are more open to CAM treatments. Systematic reviews and meta-analyses endorse certain nonconventional treatments as comparable in efficacy with contemporary biomedical treatments of psychiatric disorders while also confirming the absence of serious safety issues for most common nonconventional modalities (Birdsall 1998; Criconia et al. 1994; Linde et al. 1996). The limitations of findings supporting many conventional pharmacological treatments used in mental health care, in the context of accumulating evidence supporting claims of efficacy and safety of certain nonconventional treatments, and unresolved and in some cases increasing concerns about adverse effects, drug–drug interactions, and toxicities associated with conventional pharmacological treatments, have resulted in an increased intellectual openness among physicians, researchers, and patients to nonconventional treatments.

The comparative benefits and risks of biomedical and nonconventional treatments in mental health care have not been clearly established, and at present there are no evidence-based or expert consensus guidelines for the use of nonconventional treatments alone or in combination with conventional biomedical treatments. However, these very problems underscore the necessity for rigorous clinical trial evaluation and data review for the diverse therapies that are regarded as being alternative or complementary. Our intention in writing this book was to advance the dialogue on uses of nonconventional treatments in mental health care and to add significant new information and perspectives to the debate over conventional versus nonconventional treatments based on a critical and open-minded appraisal of the evidence.

HOW TO USE THIS BOOK

Complementary and Alternative Treatments in Mental Health Care is intended as a practical reference tool and can be used in many different ways. Part I can be used as a resource for learning about or preparing lectures on the conceptual and historical foundations, safety concerns, and medicolegal issues pertaining to the use of nonconventional treatments in mental health care. The reader who wishes to learn about the evidence for a particular CAM approach can find concise reviews of important clinical material for the most widely used nonconventional treatments in mental health care in Part II, or, when searching for evidence-based treatments addressing a specific clinical problem, can go directly to Appendix A, which ranks evidence for the various treatment modalities by major psychiatric disorder and is cross-referenced with the material in Part II. This book is focused on specific CAM treatments and is not designed as a manual for the overall practice of integrative psychiatry.

Part I: Background Issues

Part I discusses the historical and scientific foundations of complementary, alternative, and integrative medicine and provides a conceptual framework for the specific nonconventional approaches in mental health care developed in Part II. Emerging ideas and trends that are shaping the evolution of these types of medicine in general and in mental health care in particular are reviewed in Chapter 1. Chapter 2 reviews important legal and ethical considerations pertaining to CAM modalities in general and illustrates how these concepts apply to mental health care. The legal-regulatory "territory" of CAM treatments is only beginning to be formally defined. The prudent mental health professional will have a basic familiarity with ethical practices and potential liability issues when using nonconventional treatments or referring patients to nonconventional medical practitioners. Important safety considerations pertaining to alternative treatments of psychiatric disorders are reviewed in Chapter 3. Potential interactions between conventional drugs and nonconventional biological treatments are described in detail, and adverse effects sometimes encountered with somatic, mind–body, energetic, and spiritual treatments are also briefly reviewed. Chapter 4 focuses on integrative mental health care, presenting a general discussion of issues that are important to take into account when a clinician is considering the concurrent use of conventional pharmacological treatments with nonconventional treatments.

Part II: Review of the Evidence and Clinical Guidelines

Part II reviews the evidence gleaned from nonconventional modalities or alternative systems of medicine in current use in North America and Europe to treat mental or emotional problems. Chapters 5–17 provide practical clinical information on many of the most widely used nonconventional treatments of psychiatric disorders. All chapters in Part II review historical uses of the specified modality, summarize significant recent research findings, and critically analyze the evidence supporting uses of the specified approach in common psychiatric disorders (where available), including major depressive disorder, bipolar disorder, schizophrenia, anxiety disorders, dementia, alcoholism, and drug addictions. Unresolved safety issues relevant to the specified nonconventional treatment modality or alternative system of medicine are concisely presented, and clinical guidelines pertaining to the specified modality are developed on the basis of the evidence reviewed. All Part II chapters contain practical guidelines describing the clinical uses of the particular nonconventional approach discussed. Appendix A at the end of the book contains a tabular summary of the most salient clinical and research findings presented in the modality-specific chapters.

Part II consists of three sections. In the first of these, titled Nonconventional Biological Treatments, six chapters review the evidence for nonconventional biological and combined biological–energetic approaches in treating mental or emotional problems in the major world systems of medicine. Chapters 5 and 6 review the evidence for Western herbal medicines and nonherbal natural products, respectively. Chapter 7 focuses exclusively on omega-3 fatty acids; there is a growing interest in the clinical use of these natural substances in both medicine and psychiatry. Recent research findings on the central role of omega-3 fatty acids in brain functioning are reviewed, and their use in the management of specific psychiatric disorders is described.

Chapters 8–10 describe approaches to mental health problems used in three major nonbiomedical systems of medicine: Chinese medicine, homeopathy, and Ayurveda. Brief overviews of the basic medical theory are presented, clinical evidence is summarized, and the different concepts of "energy" used in the assessment and treatment of mental or emotional symptoms are introduced. The growing body of evidence supporting uses of Chinese medical treatments for mental and emotional disorders is reviewed in Chapter 8. Chapter 9 presents the theory behind homeopathic medicine and reviews research findings supporting the use of homeopathic treatments in mental health care. Although most psychiatrists have a limited understanding of basic principles of homeopathy, we believe this is an important area to address because of the widespread use of homeopathic remedies to treat mental and emotional problems in the United States and other Western countries. Chapter 10 introduces what is perhaps the most ancient and highly evolved professional system of medicine—Ayurveda—which will probably make important contributions to the future of mental health care in Western countries as conventional biomedicine becomes increasingly integrative. Ayurvedic herbal and energetic treatments addressing mental and emotional disorders are reviewed.

The second section of Part II, Lifestyle and Women's Issues, addresses lifestyle changes and women's mental health. Chapter 11 reviews the role of nutrition in the maintenance of good mental health in general and describes dietary strategies addressing specific psychiatric disorders. Chapter 12 summarizes the evidence for exercise in maintaining good mental health and treating depressed mood, anxiety, and other mental and emotional problems. Chapter 13 discusses uses of nonconventional approaches in the management of depressed mood in women, who often have a poor response to conventional biomedical treatments. Knowledge of effective nonconventional alternatives when managing premenstrual, postpartum, or menopausal mood disorders should be a high priority for psychiatrists and other mental health professionals.

In Part II's third and final section, Spirituality, Mindfulness, and Mind–Body Practices, four chapters review the evidence supporting the use of mind–body practices, mindfulness training, different energetic healing approaches in mental health care, and the role of spirituality and religion in mental health. Chapter 14 addresses the role of meditation and other mindfulness practices, and Chapter 15 examines the role of spirituality, religious beliefs and practices, and intention in maintaining or improving mental health. It is important for psychiatrists and other mental health professionals to be familiar with the research evidence supporting spiritual healing approaches in view of the widespread use of individual and group prayer in the United States (Barnes et al. 2004). Studies on the mental health benefits of two widely practiced mind–body techniques, yoga and qigong, are discussed in Chapters 16 and 17, respectively.

Appendixes

We have provided three appendixes. Appendix A is a matrix organized by major psychiatric disorder that summarizes the most significant research findings pertaining to nonconventional modalities covered in this book. Modalities are ranked according to levels of evidence supporting their use for a specific disorder. All entries are cross-referenced with the modality-specific chapters of Part II to help the busy clinician quickly locate relevant material when considering different treatment choices. This will be useful for a clinician reviewing the text of a modality-specific chapter. Appendix B is a glossary of frequently used terms in complementary and alternative medicine. Appendix C contains a list of important Web sites, textbooks, professional associations, and other resources addressing the major nonconventional modalities and non-Western systems of medicine covered in this book.

DISCLAIMER

This book is intended as a clinical introduction to the evidence-based use of CAM treatments in mental health care. Information presented in its chapters should not be interpreted as constituting specific treatment recommendations for particular patients. The authors and editors are not responsible for unfavorable or disappointing outcomes arising from the clinical application or recommendation of general concepts or guidelines contained in this book. The complex and unique history, symptoms, values, and preferences of each patient— together with the unique training and experience of the treating mental health professional and potential safety issues, costs, and availability of competent local providers—must be taken into account when advising patients about nonconventional approaches in mental health care (Eisenberg 1997). The authors strongly encourage psychiatrists, therapists, and alternative medical practitioners who treat patients with mental health problems to make responsible and informed decisions when using this book as a resource for treatment planning.

REFERENCES

American Psychiatric Association: Diagnostic and Statistical Manual of Mental Disorders, 4th Edition. Washington, DC, American Psychiatric Association, 1994

Astin J: Why patients use alternative medicine. JAMA 279:1548–1553, 1998

Astin J, Marie A, Pelletier K, et al: A review of the incorporation of complementary and alternative medicine by mainstream physicians. Arch Intern Med 158:2303–2310, 1998

Barnes PM, Powell-Griner E, McFann K, et al: Complementary and alternative medicine use among adults: United States, 2002. Adv Data (343):1–19, 2004

Birdsall TC: 5-Hydroxytryptophan: a clinically effective serotonin precursor. Altern Med Rev 3:271–280, 1998

Criconia AM, Araquistain JM, Daffina N, et al: Results of treatment with S-adenosyl-L-methionine in patients with major depression and internal illnesses. Current Therapeutic Research 55:666–674, 1994

Druss BG, Rosenheck RA: Use of practitioner-based complementary therapies by persons reporting mental conditions in the United States. Arch Gen Psychiatry 57:708–714, 2000

Eisenberg D: Advising patients who seek alternative medical therapies. Ann Intern Med 127:61–69, 1997

Eisenberg D: Complementary and alternative medicine: epidemiology and overview. Paper presented at the Siemens Medical Solutions (SMS) Health Executives Forum, Naples, FL, October 17–20, 1999

Eisenberg D, Davis R, Ettner S, et al: Trends in alternative medicine use in the United States, 1990–1997: results of a follow-up survey. JAMA 280:1569–1575, 1998

Ernst E, Resch K, White A: Complementary medicine: what physicians think of it: a meta-analysis. Arch Intern Med 155:2405–2408, 1995

Fisher P, Ward A: Complementary medicine in Europe. BMJ 309:107–111, 1994

Keitner G: Limits to the treatment of major depression. Paper presented at the annual meeting of the American Psychiatric Association, New York, May 1–6, 2004

Kessler R, Soukup J, Davis R, et al: The use of complementary and alternative therapies to treat anxiety and depression in the United States. Am J Psychiatry 158:289–294, 2001

Linde K, Ramirez G, Mulrow C, et al: St. John's wort for depression: an overview and meta-analysis of randomized clinical trials. BMJ 313:253–258, 1996

Moncrieff J, Wessely S, Hardy R: Active placebos versus antidepressants for depression. Cochrane Database Syst Rev 1:CD003012, 2004

Unutzer J, Klap R, Sturm R, et al: Mental disorders and the use of alternative medicine: results from a national survey. Am J Psychiatry 157:1851–1857, 2000

Part I

Background Issues

Complementary and Alternative Treatments in Mental Health Care

Overview and Significant Trends

James Lake, M.D.
David Spiegel, M.D.

EVOLUTION OF COMPLEMENTARY AND ALTERNATIVE MEDICINE IN INDUSTRIALIZED COUNTRIES

Resolving Ambiguity: Thinking and Speaking Clearly About Complementary and Alternative Medicine

At present there is no accepted, standardized vocabulary for describing or classifying medical treatments that lie outside of mainstream biomedicine (Kaptchuk and Eisenberg 2001b). A single term can have very different connotations depending on whether it is used in the popular media or in peer-reviewed journal articles (Eskinazi 1998; Gevitz 1995). This ambiguity often results in confusion and miscommunication when physicians and other health care professionals discuss nonconventional therapies with each other and patients.

The perceived legitimacy of any conventional or nonconventional diagnosis or treatment is heavily influenced by cultural beliefs. Therefore, any attempt to characterize nonconventional treatments must take into account the fact that fundamentally different understandings of the causes or meanings of illness are implicit in disparate cultural belief systems (Pachter 1994). Folk medicine has always been an important part of Western as well as non–Western cultures, and folk medicine beliefs and traditions significantly influence patient perceptions of nonconventional medical practices (Hufford 1997). However, folk medicine and complementary and alternative medicine (CAM) are not equivalent domains of knowledge or clinical practice. In contrast to established alternative or complementary approaches, many folk medicine traditions are transmitted orally and have not been developed into systematic or formalized medical practices. The situation is further complicated by the fact that most patients perceive CAM approaches as being more or less familiar or effective in the absence of a clear understanding of postulated mechanisms of action or the relative merits of the empirical evidence (Furnham 2000).

When examining the diverse perspectives of medicine, it is helpful to think in terms of a basic conceptual divide between conventional and nonconventional treatments. For purposes of this book, *conventional treatments* are contemporary biomedical modalities in mainstream use in North America and western Europe. At present, conventional treatments in psychiatry encompass psychopharmacology, somatic treatments (e.g., electroconvulsive therapy, transcranial magnetic stimulation, vagal nerve stimulation), and many different forms of psychotherapy, including hypnosis. It should be noted that many approaches used in contemporary Western psychiatry have not been formally validated by the rigorous standards of biomedical research recently described as "evidence-based medicine" (Geddes et al. 1996). Indeed, although most conventional nonpharmacological treatments of psychiatric disorders can be evaluated using randomized prospective clinical trial methodology, relatively few such trials have been conducted. Furthermore, it is much more difficult to propose and test a claimed mechanism of action. Nevertheless, psychotherapy, hypnosis, and other conventional nonpharmacological or somatic treatments remain in widespread use because of practice guidelines established through expert consensus.

The National Center for Complementary and Alternative Medicine (NCCAM) of the National Institutes of Health defines CAM practices as "those health care and medical practices that are not currently an integral part of conventional medicine" ("Major domains of complementary and alternative medicine," available at http://nccam.nih.gov/health/whatiscam). In other words, CAM includes all modalities that are not currently accepted as conventional medical practices. This approach defines CAM in terms of what it is not and contrasts it with the domain of conventional Western medicine, but it does not clearly demarcate the scope of conventional or nonconventional medical practices. It thus provides an ambiguous conceptual framework within which to understand the concepts and treatments of nonconventional medicine.

In lay publications, professional medical journals, and textbooks, the terms *alternative medicine* and *complementary medicine* are often treated as equivalent categories. They are not the same, however, and the gap between the treatments denoted by these terms and their actual practice has led to considerable confusion. To avoid the linguistic and conceptual muddle that has arisen in the dialogue on nonbiomedical approaches in medicine, it is important at the outset to introduce a few unambiguous terms.

A particular treatment is described as alternative or complementary with respect to approaches endorsed by the dominant system of medicine that defines the broad social and cultural context in which that nonconventional treatment is being used. In other words, the body of treatments that comprise mainstream medicine is constantly changing; by the same token, a particular treatment can be regarded as complementary or alternative depending on implicit or explicit assumptions that comprise the philosophical framework of the system of medicine within which they are regarded. Just as the whole domain of CAM modalities is defined by its exclusion from mainstream medicine, components are categorized based on whether they are used instead of (*alternative*) or along with (*complementary*) standard medical care. In view of the above, it is reasonable to describe a particular alternative or complementary approach in the broader context of the conceptual framework underlying mainstream medical theory that defines conventional practices where that treatment is used. At present in North America and western Europe, biomedicine is the dominant system of medicine; thus in these regions it makes sense to regard nonconventional treatments as complementary, alternative, or integrative with respect to the core tenets or current practices of conventional biomedicine. The nonconventional treatments used in Western industrialized countries include modalities that rest on claimed mechanisms of action that are outside of current conceptual foundations of biomedicine in the West ("Defining and describing complementary and alternative medicine" 1997). More than 100 complementary or alternative therapies are currently practiced in industrialized countries, and an unknown number of "traditional" practices are used in developing world regions (Ernst 1997).

For example, acupuncture is classified as an alternative treatment because the conceptual framework in which acupuncture is accepted as a legitimate medical treatment involves a postulated "energy" (*qi*) that is outside of the worldview of contemporary biomedicine. Using the same criterion, Chinese medicine is thus an alternative system of medicine. In contrast, a complementary treatment rests on a mechanism of action that can be explained by mainstream biomedicine but, because of social, ideological, or other nonscientific reasons, is not endorsed by orthodox medical theory. An example of a complementary treatment in mental health care is the use of St. John's wort (*Hypericum perforatum*) to treat depressed mood. Integrative approaches are combinations of alternative or complementary modalities with one or more conventional biomedical treatments.

As emerging research findings support some mainstream and nonconventional treatments while refuting others, the domain of legitimate biomedical practices will continue to change, and practices that are outside of conventional medical practice will necessarily change to accommodate the shifting landscape of Western medicine. Emerging theories in physics, the life sciences, and consciousness studies and novel methods for evaluating treatment outcomes will eventually lead to the validation of some nonconventional medical practices that are currently at odds with the paradigm of contemporary Western science and not susceptible to present methods of measurement or verification (Ernst 1996; Margolin et al. 1998; Verhoef et al. 2000). A classic example is foxglove, which contains digitalis and was used for centuries as an herbal treatment for what was then called *dropsy* (congestive heart failure). As the methods of medicine continue to evolve, certain approaches that are now regarded as alternative will be embraced as orthodox treatments, whereas other approaches that are now entrenched in conventional biomedicine will be refuted or relegated to a future alternative medicine.

Changing Conceptual Foundations of Western Medicine

Subjective experiences of mental illness are influenced by expectations and internalized meanings that reflect shared cultural attitudes and values, including beliefs about what medicine is and how medicine works to alleviate symptoms or bring about healing. In Western cultures, biomedicine is the dominant explanatory model of health and illness. According to this view, medical and psychiatric disorders are constructed on the basis of recurring patterns of observable signs or symptoms that are causally linked to identifiable stresses. In conventional biomedicine, a diagnosis requires the confirmation of subjective symptoms reported by patients and objective signs of pathology observed by physicians or other medically trained personnel. In contrast, diagnosis and assessment methods in alternative or complementary systems of medicine (e.g., Chinese medicine, Ayurveda, homeopathy) construct symptoms into disorders on the basis of criteria that are seldom congruent with core materialistic assumptions of contemporary biomedicine (Krippner 1995); many nonconventional systems of medicine are based on metaphysical assumptions about the nature of the human body in time and space, the role of consciousness in healing, and the primary influences of disparate psychological or biological factors in illness and health ("Defining and describing complementary and alternative medicine" 1997). Most CAM treatments assume the validity of one or more of the following mechanisms of action:

- *Conventional biological processes,* such as herbal medicines, aromatherapy, essential oils, and other natural substances including omega-3 essential fatty acids, minerals, vitamins, amino acids, and amino acid precursors
- *Somatic manipulation or mind–body approaches,* such as massage and exercise and mind–body approaches (e.g., yoga, qigong)

- *Scientifically validated forms of energy or information,* such as electroencephalogram biofeedback, other kinds of biofeedback using sound or light, electroconvulsive therapy, transcranial magnetic stimulation, and bright-light exposure
- *Forms of "energy" or information that are not yet scientifically validated,* such as "subtle energy" assessment and treatment methods including healing touch and reiki, homeopathy, qigong, directed intention, prayer, and some mind–body practices

Conventional biomedicine has historically borrowed concepts from physics, chemistry, and biology (Hahn 1995). Basic understandings of sickness and health are often fundamentally disparate in different cultures, and the methods used to treat sickness in a given culture are constantly changing (Conrad et al. 1995; Fabrega 1997). Contemporary biomedical models equate health and sickness with normal and abnormal biological functioning, respectively. This approach assumes that symptoms can be adequately characterized in terms of measurable changes in basic biological processes in the human body and reduces all health or illness phenomena to these processes. By extension, conventional Western medicine argues that human consciousness can be described in terms of neurophysiology. Biomedical psychiatry has endorsed this model and the corollary that normal and pathological states of consciousness are reducible to basic neurophysiological or neurochemical processes. In this broad context, it has been argued that the claims of CAM are often capricious and lack scientific rigor. It has been suggested that there is "only scientifically proven...evidence-based medicine...or unproven medicine for which scientific evidence is lacking" (Fontanarosa and Lundberg 1998, p. 1618). However, many professional systems of medicine that originated in non-Western cultures do not accept the orthodox mode of explanation that Western scientific materialism assumes to be true (Kaptchuk and Eisenberg 2001a). This has resulted in important practical problems for researchers attempting to reconcile methods and clinical evidence supporting nonconventional treatments with the basic physical or biological processes posited by Western science.

In recent decades, biomedicine has reexamined many of its core premises in response to emerging theories in physics and the life sciences that call into question some of the basic tenets of contemporary Western science (Turner 1998). Novel theories in the domain of Western science are providing conceptual frameworks that may eventually yield orthodox explanations of certain nonconventional medical treatments. These new ways of seeing reality—including human consciousness—include quantum field theory, complexity theory, and the theory of dissipative structures. Basic research on human consciousness using recent advances in functional brain imaging technologies, including quantitative electroencephalogram, functional magnetic resonance imaging, and positron emission tomography, will permit future Western researchers to design experiments capable of confirming or refuting claims of so-called energy healing methods such as qigong. In the coming decades, some "energy" treatments now regarded as being alternative will probably become empirically validated by future research methods and accepted into mainstream medicine, whereas others will be refuted and the theories on which they are based will be proven false by emerging technologies, as have conventional treatments such as the insulin coma and prefrontal lobotomy. Other nonconventional treatments will probably continue in widespread use on the basis of anecdotal evidence, despite the absence of confirmatory findings of a putative mechanism of action or a verifiable therapeutic effect in Western-style research studies.

The rapid evolution in the conceptual foundations of Western science has led to renewed openness among conventionally trained physicians who are advancing holistic models about the nature, causes, or meanings of illness, including a possible primary role of self-regulation or self-healing in physical and mental health; the interdependence of immunology, psychiatry, and neurology in symptom formation; and possibly other direct effects of stress, social support, and human consciousness on health and illness (Astin et al. 1998; Dacher 1996). The evolution in Western scientific theories has led many physicians to embrace concepts that have long been the domain of alternative medicine, including the central role of genetic and biochemical individuality in health and illness, the importance of a homeodynamic (in contrast to homeostatic) model of health as a state of dynamic balance, and the idea that most treatments do not cure illness but, more accurately, serve as catalysts for the body's innate healing capacities. For example, McEwen (1998) posited a model of *allostatic load* as affecting a variety of health outcomes. Allostasis involves a resetting of stress response mechanisms in reaction to repeated stressors. The resulting allostatic load can produce impairment in stress response systems, thus affecting stress hormones such as cortisol and prolactin, immune function, and autonomic nervous system activity, resulting in chronic hyper- or hyporeactivity to stressors. Such dysregulation can affect brain structure and function (McEwen 1999; Sapolsky 1996) and disease progression (Grippo and Johnson 2002; Sephton and Spiegel 2003; Sephton et al. 2000; Steptoe et al. 2003).

Growth of Complementary, Alternative, and Integrative Medicine in Industrialized Countries

It is estimated that 80% of the populations of Asia, Africa, and South America rely on "traditional" medicine for the treatment of all medical and psychiatric problems. Conventional biomedical treatments are not available or are unaffordable in these regions. In 2002, the World Health Organization announced a strategic initiative aimed at assisting developing countries in regulating the use of traditional medicines, improving safety and efficacy standards, and ensuring that natural product sources of medicines are sustainable in the future ("WHO launches the first global strategy on traditional and alternative medicine" 2002). Rapid growth in the acceptance of CAM treatments in industrialized countries reflects the influences of complex scientific, social, and economic factors on conventional Western biomedicine (Astin 1998; Ernst et al. 1995). For example, classifying prayer as a nonconventional treatment approach means that 25%–50% of the adult population in western Europe uses some form of CAM and that approximately 33% of adult Americans use a nonconventional treatment on a regular basis (Eisenberg 1999; Fisher and Ward 1994). When findings on the uses of prayer in healing are taken into account, the number of adults who have used any CAM treatment in the past year increases to 62% (Barnes et al. 2004). Anxiety and depression are among the most widely cited reasons for using non-conventional therapies. Approximately 26% of adults who use any nonconventional approach for a medical or mental health problem do so pursuant to the advice of a medical professional. Furthermore, 28% of U.S. adults who use any nonconventional approach believe that conventional medical treatments they have tried for the same problem are ineffective (Barnes et al. 2004).

The gradual opening of Western medicine to novel ideas and clinical methods is taking place in the context of a contentious debate between Western physicians and nonconventional medical practitioners over questions of validity, efficacy, and safety of many CAM therapies that are already in widespread use in industrialized countries. In North America, for example, physicians continue to debate the conceptual validity and practical value of many nonconventional treatments. Conventional pharmacological treatments of depression and anxiety are effective but far from perfect and have serious unresolved safety problems, including so-called discontinuation syndromes and unclear risks associated with long-term use (Coupland et al. 1996; Frost and Lal 1995; Leo 1999; Pies 1997; Schatzberg et al. 1997; "Study: SSRIs achieve remission" 2004; Thase 2002). A central goal of future mental health research should be the rigorous and systematic evaluation of promising nonconventional treatments. With that objective in mind, the American Psychiatric Association (APA) recently established the Caucus on Complementary, Alternative and Integrative Care (see www.APACAM. org). The primary goal of the caucus is to provide reliable safety and efficacy information on nonconventional treatments to psychiatrists and other mental health professionals. The caucus will formulate clinical practice guidelines for using nonconventional approaches in mental health care and advise the APA on significant emerging research findings or safety considerations pertaining to the range of CAM modalities.

NCCAM together with private and public research centers is beginning to address these issues. More than 20 federally funded centers for CAM research are exploring basic questions pertaining to mechanisms of disease and healing posed by nonorthodox medicine. Postgraduate training programs in integrative medicine have been founded in affiliation with several prominent medical schools, including Harvard Medical School, the University of California at San Francisco School of Medicine, Columbia University College of Physicians and Surgeons, and the University of Arizona College of Medicine. However, no NCCAM-endorsed center for research on nonconventional treatments specifically in mental health care has been established, due in part to unresolved issues pertaining to research methodologies for evaluating outcomes of these treatments on psychiatric symptoms. In contrast to conventional treatments, which target presumed dysfunction at the level of neurotransmitters and their receptors, many nonconventional biological, mind–body, somatic, and energy-based approaches being explored as potential treatments for mental illness rest on assumptions about consciousness that may not be susceptible to empirical investigation with contemporary scientific methods.

Future of Western Medicine Shaped by a Balance of Competing Factors

In the first years of the new millennium, Western medicine has continued to embrace a conventional biomedical framework whose conceptual origins can be traced to the ancient Greeks (Hahn 1995; Lake 2002). In the context of broad social and economic trends, biomedical research is legitimizing the claims of many nonconventional treatments for both medical and psychiatric disorders. At the same time, materialism remains the philosophical cornerstone of Western science, resulting in Western medicine's continuing exclusion of nonconventional treatments that cannot be adequately described in empirical terms according to known biological mechanisms of action (Astin 1998). This section addresses the interplay between factors and trends that favor an increasing acceptance of nonconventional medicine in North America and Europe and those that favor continuation of the status quo—the marginalization of nonconventional approaches in industrialized countries and the continued dominant role of contemporary biomedicine as an explanatory model of health and illness.

Factors Delaying Acceptance of Nonconventional Medicine in Industrialized Countries

Despite an atmosphere of increasing intellectual openness to CAM methodologies, many factors are delaying or interfering with the growth and acceptance of nonconventional medicine in North America, western Europe, and other industrialized regions of the world (Eskinazi 1998; Linde 2000). These factors are summarized below:

- Fundamental differences exist between the philosophical assumptions and conceptual frameworks underlying conventional biomedicine and nonconventional systems of medicine. These differences frequently translate into a wholesale dismissal of claims of mechanisms of action or treatment outcomes that are not susceptible to empirical verification by contemporary Western science.

- Ideological or economic competition takes place among practitioners committed to different systems of medicine. This is perpetuated by both conventionally and nonconventionally trained practitioners.
- Using currently available methods, it is difficult to formulate a hypothesis or design a rigorous experiment to test efficacy claims for many nonconventional treatments because of inherent limitations in the quality of available information. Future advances in the basic sciences will probably result in the validation or refutation of many nonconventional therapies.
- Unlike in studies of conventional biomedicine, numerous methodological approaches are used in studies of nonconventional medical treatments, leading to the absence of a unified or standardized framework of nonconventional medicine. A consequence of this is the interpretation by Western researchers of responses to CAM treatments as being sporadic, unpredictable, or idiosyncratic. In other words, contemporary biomedical research methods tend to negatively bias Western biomedical interpretations of nonconventional treatments. From a Western scientific perspective, apparently "ambiguous" findings imply the absence of a specific mechanism of action—and, by extension, the absence of specific effects on illness. This bias frequently results in biomedical researchers ascribing outcomes of nonconventional treatments to placebo effects. Designing appropriate controls and blinding protocols for many kinds of complementary, alternative, or integrative treatments is often difficult or impossible. For example, it is impossible to blind a practitioner or a patient to an acupuncture treatment protocol. There is also controversy over the meaning of a "sham" acupuncture treatment, in view of that fact that Chinese medical theory posits a range of specific or general energetic effects when acupuncture needles are inserted anywhere on the body. Furthermore, attempts to take into account the effects of the therapeutic relationship on outcomes of "patient-centered" nonconventional treatments often lead to ambiguous outcomes measures.
- Many integrative treatments, such as those in traditional Chinese medicine, are by design highly individualized, based on a detailed analysis of a given patient's pattern of energy and other complex assessments. This makes the application of standardized protocols quite difficult or, conversely, a distortion of the treatment itself if used.
- Disparities in research funding of conventional biomedical versus nonconventional treatments limit the number of large, well-designed studies on most nonconventional approaches. National Institutes of Health research funding of nonconventional treatments is negligible compared with funding for conventional biomedical treatments.
- Inadequate research skills among most CAM practitioners result in few studies being regarded as well designed by Western researchers.

- Limited or absent academic support for most CAM researchers, including university or institutional research grants and access to computer or library facilities, places constraints on the quality of study designs and the sophistication of data analysis.
- Liability and malpractice issues for medical doctors practicing a nonconventional modality or referring to a nonconventional medical practitioner are only beginning to be defined. Currently there are no accepted professional guidelines directing medical doctors who treat patients using nonconventional modalities or who refer patients to nonconventional practitioners. (See Chapter 2 for a review of important medicolegal issues pertaining to the use of nonconventional approaches in mental health care.)
- In contrast to studies on conventional biomedical treatments, the small number of patients enrolled in most studies on nonconventional treatments frequently results in statistically insignificant findings, even when outcomes are consistently positive.
- Barriers to performing rigorous systematic reviews or meta-analyses of findings in a particular research area result from disqualification of studies due to the absence of standard methodological approaches, small study size, or other design flaws. As a consequence, studies on CAM treatments are systematically excluded from standard medical informatics databases (including *PubMed*), and relatively few nonconventional modalities are appraised in systematic reviews.

Because of the above issues, relatively few large controlled studies have investigated CAM treatments in mental health care. Psychopharmacology is the dominant conceptual framework in which mental illnesses are studied and treated in industrialized countries.

A related issue is the widespread and unquestioned acceptance of the neurotransmitter theory as a sufficient explanatory model of the causes of psychiatric disorders. The scientific and ideological perspectives of contemporary biological psychiatry are based on widely accepted biological theories in genetics, molecular biology, and neurobiology. Until recent decades, few efforts were made to investigate nonorthodox conceptual frameworks as possible explanatory models of psychopathology. The pharmaceutical industry conducts internal studies or funds third-party research on psychopharmacological medications, and there is limited funding for studies on natural products or other nonconventional treatments. The consequence is the limited quality of research on putative biological, mind–body, and energetic models of mental illness causation. Advances in CAM treatments have been delayed by the poor quality of research in many areas and a priori skepticism about even clearly positive findings.

Many nonconventional approaches have been used for considerable periods, reportedly with good results. However, contemporary Western scientific standards require independent replication of reports of apparent positive outcomes despite strong anecdotal evidence of efficacy and safety or large numbers of positive case reports. Biomedical investigations of putative alternative treatments are conducted using standardized Western methodologies for research design and data analysis. This is done to clarify the presence of specific or general effects of any treatment and to determine the role (if any) of placebo (or nocebo) effects that are sometimes present because of differences in expectations in culturally diverse populations complaining of similar symptoms. Furthermore, regulations imposed on the use of alternative treatments in the United States and in other Western countries oblige researchers and clinicians to use established scientific standards to demonstrate the efficacy and safety of any treatment before that treatment is approved for widespread use.

Despite the absence of compelling biomedical evidence for many nonconventional treatments, alternative medical practitioners have argued that many treatments presently outside of orthodox Western medicine are valid, although their validity is not verifiable using available empirical methods, or that claimed outcomes can be replicated while not always fulfilling criteria required for empirical verification by contemporary biomedicine (Carlston 2004; Richardson 2002). Consequently, studies of putative "healing effects" of many alternative approaches are often critiqued or dismissed by Western medicine before basic experiments are performed to determine their efficacy or appraise the significance of reported outcomes. Proponents of nonconventional medicine have suggested that by rejecting treatments before the evidence for their efficacy and safety is reviewed, conventional biomedicine does not adhere to the rigorous standards of empirical validation that it demands of CAM. In fact, it can be argued that approximately 50% of conventional therapeutics in all areas of medicine are not supported by compelling research findings (Smith 1991). This state of affairs is complicated by the fact that many mainstream medical databases, systematic reviews, and meta-analyses cite only studies on certain biological or psychological treatments that meet specified arbitrary criteria of study size, study methodology, and duration. Published peer-reviewed articles on alternative medical research are sometimes excluded from mainstream medical literature databases and are therefore unavailable to patients or physicians who are seeking reliable information on efficacy or safety.

All of the above factors present difficulties for both physicians and patients who try to make informed choices about safe and effective nonconventional treatment approaches. It is often difficult for physicians to obtain reliable information showing which treatments work and which do not work or pose risks to patients. Thus it is not surprising that Western trained physicians and alternative medical practitioners continue to debate the validity, safety, and effectiveness of most nonconventional modalities. The gap between current popular uses of nonconventional treatments and the evidence supporting their use suggests widespread popular beliefs about healing and the possible efficacy of nonconventional biological, mind–body, or energy techniques that have not yet been empirically validated by Western science.

Factors Favoring Growth of Nonconventional Medicine in Industrialized Countries

With the above-noted factors and social trends working against the continued growth of nonconventional medicine in North America and western Europe, increasing numbers of patients are willing to pay out of pocket for CAM medical services (Eisenberg 1999; Eisenberg et al. 1998). This social trend is forcing the health insurance industry, managed care organizations, academic medical centers, and Western physicians in general to reconsider historically negative biases against nonconventional medicine in North America and Europe. Major medical conferences frequently include sessions on research findings covering a range of nonconventional treatments so that most mainstream Western physicians are increasingly conversant with the evidence in support of emerging nonconventional treatments entering into use in their medical specialties. The increased level of awareness of nonconventional treatments will ultimately benefit patients, physicians, and nonconventional medical practitioners by elevating the debate over the appropriate role of nonconventional medicine from its present level of emotionally charged, uninformed skepticism to a more reasoned dialogue that will be increasingly focused on outcomes from rigorous scientific investigations of mechanisms of action, efficacy, and safety.

Before discussing trends in the use of nonconventional medicine, it is important to comment on the limitations of surveys from which estimates are obtained. Many patient surveys of nonconventional medical practices do not use established diagnostic criteria or trained raters to confirm a formal medical or psychiatric diagnosis, resulting in ambiguous information about symptoms or disorders being treated or unreliable estimates of use rates of nonconventional treatments for a particular disorder. Furthermore, most surveys of nonconventional medical practices fail to distinguish between self-use and prescribed use of nonconventional treatments. With these limitations in mind, it is more reasonable to interpret use rates of the nonconventional modalities discussed below as estimates or trends and not as firm statistics.

Nonconventional medical modalities have played an important historical role in North America and western Europe. Recent surveys (Astin 1998; Eisenberg et al. 1998; Kaptchuk and Eisenberg 2001a) suggest that the increasing use of nonconventional medical practices is driving the industrialized regions of the world toward medical pluralism or integration. These changes are related to consumer demands for new kinds of health care in the context of cultural and demographic trends favoring increased openness to medical practices currently outside of Western biomedicine. Between 1990 and 1997, the overall use of nonconventional treatments in the United States increased from 34% to 42% of the adult population (Eisenberg 1999). This change was largely due to more individuals seeking nonconventional treatments rather than increased visits per patient. In 1997, the most recent year for which financial data are available, out-of-pocket payments for all nonconventional professional medical services and therapies were between $36 billion and $47 billion. Between $12 billion and $19 billion of this total went to nonconventional health care providers, which exceeded the total out-of-pocket costs for all conventional medical services during 1997. It is likely that annual patient visits to nonconventional medical practitioners in the United States have exceeded conventional outpatient appointments since that year. A large survey of more than 31,000 U.S. adults conducted in 2002 concluded that 62% of adults had used some form of nonconventional treatment during the previous year; 43% of respondents reported using prayer for self-healing, and 24% requested prayers from others in the hope of improving health problems (Barnes et al. 2004). Western European countries are also embracing CAM (Ernst 1997).

IMPACT OF COMPLEMENTARY AND ALTERNATIVE APPROACHES ON CONVENTIONAL PSYCHIATRY

Issues Influencing the Use of Nonconventional Treatments in Mental Health Care

Some CAM approaches are substantiated by strong empirical evidence, whereas research on other modalities has begun only recently. It is important to stress that although many nonconventional modalities in current use have not yet been validated by Western-style biomedical research, their use is supported by anecdotal reports or provisional research findings. Many nonconventional approaches are self-administered, whereas others require the skilled supervision of a professional medical practitioner. Some nonconventional treatments are inexpensive compared with conventional pharmacological treatments or psychotherapy and others are costly, are unavailable in many geographical regions, or are not covered by insurance. Additional research evidence supporting the use of nonconventional approaches alone or in combination with conventional biomedical treatments will enhance outcomes and improve safety while increasing the overall cost-effectiveness of mental health care.

The availability of many kinds of medical services reflects an underlying "medical pluralism" in which disparate traditions of healing coexist in a common cultural milieu. A strong historical tradition of medical pluralism in the United States and many western European countries will ensure continued interest in nonbiomedical treatments among both patients and physicians (Kaptchuk and Eisenberg 2001a).

Uses of Nonconventional Treatments in Mental Health Care

A higher percentage of individuals who meet criteria for any mental illness use nonconventional treatment than among the general population (Sparber and Wootton 2002; Unutzer et al. 2000). Furthermore, as in the population at large, most people who use a nonconventional treatment for a mental health problem concurrently use conventional approaches (Eisenberg et al. 1998; Unutzer et al. 2000). Patients who report severe depressed mood or anxiety symptoms use nonconventional treatments most often (Unutzer et al. 2000); 41% of severely depressed patients and 43% of patients reporting panic attacks use at least one nonconventional treatment versus 28% of the overall adult population (Eisenberg et al. 1998). These two patient populations also use conventional treatments at higher rates than the general population (Kessler et al. 2001). In fact, approximately 67% of severely depressed or acutely anxious patients who use a nonconventional treatment also consult with a conventionally trained mental health professional, and 90% of individuals see a psychiatrist while self-treating anxiety or depression with one or more nonconventional therapies. Severe depression is a strong predictor of concurrent use of antidepressants and at least one nonprescription supplement (Druss and Rosenheck 2000). Patients reporting generalized anxiety, bipolar mood swings, or psychotic symptoms use nonconventional treatments less often than severely depressed or acutely anxious patients but at rates that are comparable with those in the general population (Unutzer et al. 2000).

According to one recent patient survey (Kessler et al. 2001), relaxation techniques (20%) and "spiritual healing by others" (10%) are the most widely used nonconventional treatments for depressed mood or anxiety symptoms in the United States. In contrast, orally administered natural substances, including Western herbal medicines or Chinese herbs, homeopathy, and megavitamins, are used by approximately 7% of patients who self-report panic attacks or other acute anxiety symptoms and 9% of patients who self-report severe depressed mood. Approximately 60% of individuals who self-treated acute anxiety symptoms rated nonconventional treatments as "very helpful," compared with 68% who rated conventional pharmacological treatments as "very helpful." Over 50% of respondents who self-reported "severe depressed mood" rated nonconventional treatments as "very helpful" compared with 59% who rated conventional therapies as "very helpful." Although the Kessler et al. (2001) survey was limited by the absence of clinically trained interviewers and the fact that standardized DSM-IV (American Psychiatric Association 1994) diagnostic criteria were not used, these findings suggest widely shared beliefs that established conventional pharmacological treatments and nonconventional approaches have equivalent efficacy for the management of severe depressed mood and anxiety symptoms. These findings raise the issue of possible nonspecific or placebo effects in response to certain CAM treatments in contrast to the specific targeted effects of conventional biomedical treatments (Ernst 1996). The available survey data do not provide evidence to show that beneficial outcomes take place, nor do they clarify how individuals arrive at their beliefs about outcomes. However, on the basis of these findings, it is reasonable to infer that many nonconventional treatments used in mental health care are probably well tolerated and beneficial.

In summary, there is a trend toward increasing acceptance of nonconventional approaches in mental health care among both patients and conventionally trained psychiatrists. However, the effectiveness and safety of many nonconventional treatments have not yet been clearly established. In addition, the concurrent use of conventional biomedical treatments and nonconventional therapies is a cause for concern in view of the unknown magnitude and types of safety risks associated with the combined use of psychopharmacological drugs and many nonconventional treatments. Nondisclosure by patients of most nonconventional treatments to physicians makes this situation even more problematic. Most individuals who use any nonconventional treatment for severe depressed mood or anxiety also take a conventional pharmacological treatment for the same problem; however, less than 33% report this to their psychiatrist or family practice physician (Eisenberg et al. 1998). Severely depressed and acutely anxious individuals use both conventional and nonconventional treatments at higher rates than the adult population overall, and patients who report these symptoms believe that conventional and nonconventional treatments are equally effective. Finally, it is significant that relaxation techniques and "spiritual healing by others" (see Chapter 15 in this volume) are the most widely used nonconventional treatments for anxiety or depressed mood, followed by herbs, homeopathy, megavitamins, and naturopathy.

FUTURE ROLE OF NONCONVENTIONAL TREATMENTS IN MENTAL HEALTH CARE

Despite widespread institutionalized opposition or indifference to nonconventional medicine by the pharmaceutical industry, academic medicine, and the U.S. Food and Drug Administration, CAM approaches in mental health care are attracting increasing interest. Research protocols and clinical treatment methods used in orthodox Western biomedicine are gradually embracing the ideas and techniques of nonconventional medicine. This trend is being driven by an increasing intellectual openness among Western physicians (including psychiatrists) to novel models of illness, increased use rates of certain nonconventional modalities for diverse medical and psychiatric symptoms, and changing relationships between physicians and well-educated patients who more frequently advocate for a broad range of treatment choices, including nonconventional therapies. Findings of large physician and patient surveys have identified changing perspectives and use patterns pertaining to nonconventional approaches in mental health care and confirm that conventionally trained physicians are increasingly using nonconventional medical practices together with conventional drug treatments and psychotherapy as well as referring patients to nonconventional medical practitioners at increasing rates. Changes in the conceptual foundations and clinical methods of nonconventional medicine are both the cause and effect of an emerging integrative paradigm in Western medicine. (See Chapter 4 for a discussion of integrative approaches in mental health care.)

REFERENCES

American Psychiatric Association: Diagnostic and Statistical Manual of Mental Disorders, 4th Edition. Washington, DC, American Psychiatric Association, 1994

Astin J: Why patients use alternative medicine. JAMA 279:1548–1553, 1998

Astin J, Marie A, Pelletier K, et al: A review of the incorporation of complementary and alternative medicine by mainstream physicians. Arch Intern Med 158:2303–2310, 1998

Barnes PM, Powell-Griner E, McFann K, et al: Complementary and alternative medicine use among adults: United States, 2002. Adv Data (343):1–19, 2004

Carlston M: Review of research in homeopathy: theory and methodology. Seminars in Integrative Medicine 2:72–81, 2004

Conrad L, Neve M, Nutton V, et al: The Western Medical Tradition: 800 BC to AD 1800. Cambridge, UK, Cambridge University Press, 1995

Coupland N, Bell C, Potokar JP: Serotonin reuptake inhibitor withdrawal. J Clin Psychopharmacol 16:356–362, 1996

Dacher E: Post modern medicine. J Altern Complement Med 2:531–537, 1996

Defining and describing complementary and alternative medicine. Panel on Definition and Description, CAM Research Methodology Conference, April 1995. Altern Ther Health Med 3:49–57, 1997

Druss B, Rosenheck R: Use of practitioner-based complementary therapies by persons reporting mental conditions in the United States. Arch Gen Psychiatry 57:708–714, 2000

Eisenberg D: Complementary and alternative medicine: epidemiology and overview. Paper presented at the Siemens Medical Solutions (SMS) Health Executives Forum, Naples, FL, October 17–20, 1999

Eisenberg D, Davis R, Ettner S, et al: Trends in alternative medicine use in the United States, 1990–1997: results of a follow-up national survey. JAMA 280:1569–1575, 1998

Ernst E: Complementary medicine: patients first? Wien Klin Wochenschr 108:631–633, 1996

Ernst E: Complementary medicine: the facts. Phys Ther Rev 2:49–57, 1997

Ernst E, Resch K, White A: Complementary medicine: what physicians think of it: a meta-analysis. Arch Intern Med 155:2405–2408, 1995

Eskinazi D: Policy perspectives: factors that shape alternative medicine. JAMA 280:1621–1623, 1998

Fabrega H: Evolution of Sickness and Healing. Berkeley, University of California Press, 1997

Fisher P, Ward A: Complementary medicine in Europe. BMJ 309:107–111, 1994

Fontanarosa PB, Lundberg GD: Alternative medicine meets science. JAMA 280:1618–1619, 1998

Frost L, Lal S: Shock-like sensations after discontinuation of selective serotonin reuptake inhibitors. Am J Psychiatry 152:810, 1995

Furnham A: How the public classify complementary medicine: a factor analytic study. Complement Ther Med 8:82–87, 2000

Geddes JR, Game D, Jenkins NE, et al: What proportion of primary psychiatric interventions are based on evidence from randomized controlled trials? Qual Health Care 5:215–217, 1996

Gevitz N: Alternative medicine and the orthodox canon. Mt Sinai J Med 62:127–131, 1995

Grippo AJ, Johnson AK: Biological mechanisms in the relationship between depression and heart disease. Neurosci Biobehav Rev 26:941–962, 2002

Hahn R: Sickness and healing: an anthropological perspective. New Haven, CT, Yale University Press, 1995

Haynes BR: A warning to complementary medicine practitioners: get empirical or else. BMJ 319:1629–1632, 1999

Hufford D: Folk medicine and health culture in contemporary society. Prim Care 24:723–741, 1997

Kaptchuk T, Eisenberg D: Varieties of healing, 1: medical pluralism in the United States. Ann Intern Med 135:189–195, 2001a

Kaptchuk T, Eisenberg D: Varieties of healing, 2: a taxonomy of unconventional healing practices. Ann Intern Med 135:196–204, 2001b

Kessler R, Soukup J, Davis R, et al: The use of complementary and alternative therapies to treat anxiety and depression in the United States. Am J Psychiatry 158:289–294, 2001

Krippner S: A cross-cultural comparison of four healing models. Altern Ther Health Med 1:21–29, 1995

Lake J: Alternative, complementary, and integrative medicine, in Handbook of Mind–Body Medicine for Primary Care. Edited by Moss D, McGrady A, Davies TC, et al. Thousand Oaks, CA, Sage, 2002, pp 57–68

Leo R: Movement disorders associated with the serotonin selective reuptake inhibitors. J Clin Psychiatry 57:449–454, 1999

Linde K: How to evaluate the effectiveness of complementary therapies. J Altern Complement Med 6:253–256, 2000

Margolin A, Avants S, Kleber H: Investigating alternative medicine therapies in randomized controlled trials. JAMA 280:1626–1628, 1998

McEwen BS: Protective and damaging effects of stress mediators. N Engl J Med 338:171–179, 1998

McEwen BS: Stress and the aging hippocampus. Front Neuroendocrinol 20:49–70, 1999

Pachter L: Culture and clinical care: folk illness beliefs and behaviors and their implications for health care delivery. JAMA 271:690–694, 1994

Pies R: Must we now consider SRIs neuroleptics? J Clin Psychopharmacol 17:443–445, 1997

Richardson J: Evidence-based complementary medicine: rigor, relevance and the swampy lowlands. J Altern Complement Med 8:221–223, 2002

Sapolsky RM: Why stress is bad for your brain. Science 273:749–750, 1996

Schatzberg A, Haddad P, Kaplan E, et al: Serotonin reuptake inhibitor discontinuation syndrome: a hypothetical definition. J Clin Psychiatry 58 (suppl 7):5–10, 1997

Sephton S, Spiegel D: Circadian disruption in cancer: a neuroendocrine immune pathway from stress to disease? Brain Behav Immun 17:321–328, 2003

Sephton SE, Sapolsky RM, Kraemer HC, et al: Diurnal cortisol rhythm as a predictor of breast cancer survival. J Natl Cancer Inst 92:994–1000, 2000

Smith R: Where is the wisdom? BMJ 303:798–799, 1991

Sparber A, Wootton JC: Surveys of complementary and alternative medicine, V: use of alternative and complementary therapies for psychiatric and neurologic diseases. J Altern Complement Med 8:93–96, 2002

Steptoe A, Kunz-Ebrecht S, Owen N, et al: Socioeconomic status and stress–related biological responses over the working day. Psychosom Med 65:461–470, 2003

Study: SSRIs achieve remission in about one third of patients. CNS News, August 2004. Available at: www.central-nervous-system.com/indexpub.cfm?pubid=4. Accessed November 2005.

Thase M: Antidepressant effects: the suit may be small, but the fabric is real. Prevention and Treatment 5:32, 2002. Available at: http://content.apa.org/journals/pre/5/1/32. Accessed July 2006.

Turner RN: A proposal for classifying complementary therapies. Complement Ther Med 6:141–143, 1998

Unutzer J, Klap R, Sturm R, et al: Mental disorders and the use of alternative medicine: results from a national survey. Am J Psychiatry 157:1851–1857, 2000

Verhoef MI, Casebeer AL, Hilsdew RJ: Assessing efficacy of complementary medicine: adding qualitative research methods to the "gold standard." J Altern Complement Med 8:275–281, 2000

WHO launches the first global strategy on traditional and alternative medicine. World Health Organization Press Release No. WHO/38, May 16, 2002

2

Legal, Regulatory, and Ethical Issues

Michael H. Cohen, J.D.
Ronald Schouten, M.D., J.D.

Clinical integration of complementary and alternative medicine (CAM) therapies (e.g., acupuncture and traditional Oriental medicine, chiropractic, herbal medicine, massage therapy, mind–body therapies) into mental health care raises important legal issues for psychiatrists, clinical psychologists, licensed social workers, licensed mental health care professionals, and other counselors. Legal questions concern therapeutic recommendations regarding the use or avoidance of one or more CAM therapies, referral of a patient to a CAM practitioner for evaluation and treatment, comanagement of patients with CAM practitioners, informed consent and shared decision making, and how to respond to a patient who insists on using a CAM therapy against medical advice.

In this respect, *integrative mental health care*, in which conventional care is judiciously combined with CAM therapies, presents situations in which mental health care practitioners can find themselves caught by the competing demands of patient expectations, clinical judgment, and liability considerations. Practitioners often receive little professional guidance for how to proceed in such complex scenarios, either from their home institutions or from relevant professional groups. This chapter offers guidance for psychiatrists in particular, and mental health professionals in general, who are seeking to navigate these dilemmas.

The authors gratefully acknowledge funding through National Institutes of Health grant IG-13L-M0-7475-01, "Legal and Social Barriers to Alternative Therapies"; the National Library of Medicine; and grants from the Frederick S. Upton and Helen M. and Annetta E. Himmelfarb Foundations to the Institute for Integrative and Energy Medicine.

LAW APPLICABLE TO USE OF CAM THERAPIES

The law governing CAM practitioners and therapies (and, by extension, integrative care) grows out of and overlaps with several different areas of law governing conventional care. The major areas of law are licensure, scope of practice, malpractice, professional discipline, third-party reimbursement, and fraud (discussed under "Liability Risk Management") (Cohen 1998).

Licensure

Licensure refers to the requirement that health care practitioners maintain a current state license to practice their professional healing art. Although a few states have recently enacted statutes authorizing nonlicensed CAM practitioners to practice (Cohen 2004), in most states, licensure serves as the first requirement for professional practice. Licensure of CAM practitioners varies by state; chiropractors, for example, are licensed in every state; massage therapists and acupuncturists, in well over half the states; and naturopaths, in over a dozen states (Eisenberg et al. 2002). In many states, massage therapists are licensed at the local level (e.g., by the municipality) rather than at the state level; local massage ordinances may regulate the massage establishment itself as well as the establishment's practitioners.

Scope of Practice

Scope of practice refers to the legally authorized boundaries of care within the given profession. For example, chiropractors can give nutritional advice in some states but not others, and massage therapists are typically prohibited from mental health counseling. State licensing statutes usually define a CAM practitioner's scope of practice; regulations by the relevant state licensing board (e.g., the chiropractic board) may supplement or interpret the relevant licensing statute, and courts interpret the scope of practice provisions in statutes and administrative regulations (Cohen 1998, pp. 39–46).

Malpractice

Medical malpractice refers to negligence, which is defined as failure to use due care (or follow the standard of care) in treating a patient, thereby resulting in injury to the patient. In general, although licensed medical doctors are judged by medical standards of care within their specialties, each CAM profession (e.g., acupuncture, chiropractic, physical therapy, massage therapy) is judged by its own standard of care (Cohen 1998, pp. 64–66). In cases where the practitioner's clinical care overlaps with medical care (e.g., the chiropractor who takes and reads a patient's X ray), then the medical standard may be applied (Cohen 1998, pp. 66–67).

An in-depth discussion of the intricacies of malpractice insurance is beyond the scope of this chapter. It should be noted, however, that states vary in their requirements for malpractice coverage (American Medical Association 2004), and individual insurers vary in their coverage of CAM therapies. The individual practitioner is advised to determine the coverage available and the amount, if any, required by his or her state.

Professional Discipline

Professional discipline refers to the power of the relevant professional board—in the psychiatrist's case, the state medical board—to sanction a clinician, with the most severe penalty being revocation of the clinician's license. The concern over inappropriate disciplinary actions based on medical board antipathy to inclusion of CAM therapies has led consumer groups in many states to lobby for "health freedom" statutes—laws providing that physicians may not be disciplined solely on the basis of incorporating CAM modalities (Cohen 1998, pp. 92–95). The Federation of State Medical Boards (FSMB; 2002) has also issued Model Guidelines for Physician Use of Complementary and Alternative Therapies (see below) that reaffirm this same principle.

Third-Party Reimbursement

Third-party reimbursement involves a number of insurance policy provisions and corresponding legal rules designed to ensure that reimbursement is limited to "medically necessary" treatment; it does not, in general, cover "experimental" treatments and is not subject to fraud or abuse (Cohen 1998, pp. 96–108). In general, insurers have been slow to cover CAM therapies as core benefits, largely because of insufficient evidence of these therapies' safety, efficacy, and cost-effectiveness, although a number of insurers have offered policyholders discounted access to a network of CAM practitioners.

MALPRACTICE LIABILITY

The issue of malpractice liability is frequently the dominant concern among mental health professionals who are considering, or who have been asked by their patients to consider, inclusion of CAM therapies. Health care institutions are primarily concerned with liability issues surrounding patient requests for dietary supplements and other CAM therapies (Cohen and Ruggie 2004).

Conventional care offers several bases for malpractice liability that might apply to the inclusion of CAM therapies: misdiagnosis, failure to treat, failure of informed consent, fraud and misrepresentation (discussed under "Liability Risk Management"), abandonment, vicarious liability, and breach of privacy and confidentiality (Schouten and Cohen 2004). Some of these theories and their application to the provision of integrative mental health care are discussed below.

Misdiagnosis

Misdiagnosis refers to a caregiver's failure to diagnose a condition accurately or at all; it is malpractice when the failure occurred by virtue of providing care below generally accepted professional standards, pursuant to which the patient was injured. Misdiagnosis could occur if, for example, a mental health care practitioner recommends breathing (relaxation) techniques and fails to recognize the presence of a major medical condition, such as a major depressive disorder compounded by attention-deficit/hyperactivity disorder and, as a result of such failure, the patient injures himself or herself or another person.

Failure to Treat

Failure to treat through conventional care can lead to malpractice liability if the patient is injured through such failure. To take an obvious example, if a mental health care practitioner offers to treat severe depression through a CAM therapy such as St. John's wort, where the evidence to date fails to suggest effectiveness of the therapy, and the severely depressed patient continues to deteriorate (and/ or injures himself or herself or others), the practitioner could conceivably be liable for failure to properly treat the patient.

In general, if the medical evidence supports the safety and efficacy of a CAM therapy, liability is unlikely, and the practitioner can and should recommend the treatment; if the medical evidence indicates either serious risk to or inefficacy of a CAM therapy, liability is probable, and the practitioner should avoid and actively discourage the patient from using the treatment; if the medical evidence supports the safety of the CAM treatment but evidence regarding its efficacy is inconclusive, or the evidence supports the treatment's efficacy but evidence regarding safety is inconclusive, then the mental health care practitioner should caution the patient and, while accepting the patient's choice to try the CAM therapy, continue to monitor the therapy's efficacy and safety and stand ready to intervene with conventional treatment when medically necessary (Cohen and Eisenberg 2002). If a condition can be readily cured by conventional care, there is a strong imperative to provide such care. Delay in doing so does not by itself constitute negligence, but delay that aggravates the patient's condition or leads to irreversible progression of the disease might be considered negligent (Cohen and Eisenberg 2002). This example goes back to the earlier definition of malpractice as providing substandard care and, in so doing, causing patient injury.

Many dietary supplements, such as vitamins, minerals, amino acids, and herbs, have uncertain safety as well as efficacy. In line with the above framework, the mental health care practitioner should recommend dietary supplements only when the evidence supports their safety and efficacy and should avoid and discourage use of dietary supplements for which the evidence suggests risk of harm or inefficacy. When the evidentiary record for a dietary treatment is mixed, caution is advised. The practitioner should bear in mind that the U.S. Food and Drug Administration regulates dietary supplements as foods, not drugs, and therefore allows supplements to be sold in interstate commerce without prior proof of safety or efficacy. Dietary supplements may be adulterated or mislabeled or may interact adversely with conventional medication. Quality assurance is difficult, as is consistency of products from batch to batch, and often research has not yet disclosed the active ingredient(s) responsible for the supplement's potency, if any.

Mental health care practitioners should be especially cautious about selling dietary supplements as a condition of treatment. The American Medical Association has opined that physician sale of dietary supplements for profit may present an impermissible conflict of interest between good patient care and profit and thus may be ethically objectionable. Several states have enacted laws limiting or prohibiting physician sales of dietary supplements (Dumoff 2000). State medical boards also could discipline physicians who recommend or sell supplements, based on statutory provisions that allow physician discipline for such acts; for example, Ohio regulations define such acts as the "failure to maintain minimal standards applicable to the selection or administration of drugs, or failure to employ acceptable scientific methods in the selection of drugs or other modalities for treatment of disease" (Ohio Rev. Code Ann. §4731.22).

Failure of Informed Consent

The legal obligation of *informed consent* is to provide patients with all the information material to their making a treatment decision—in other words, information that would make a difference in the patient's choice to undergo or forgo a given therapeutic protocol. This obligation applies across the board, whether CAM or conventional therapies are involved (Cohen 1998, pp. 61–62; Ernst and Cohen 2001). *Materiality* refers to information about risks and benefits that is reasonably significant to a patient's decision to undergo or forgo a particular therapy; about half of the states judge materiality by the "reasonable patient's" notion of what is significant, whereas the other half judge materiality by the "reasonable physician" standard (Ernst and Cohen 2001). Shared decision making takes informed consent a step further by requiring full and fair conversations in which patients feel empowered and participatory in medical decisions affecting their care.

These norms apply across the board, whether a therapy is labeled "conventional" or "CAM"; such evenhandedness was, in fact, a principal conclusion in the 2005 report "Complementary and Alternative Medicine" issued by the Institute of Medicine at the National Academy of Sciences (Committee on the Use of Complementary and Alternative Medicine 2005).

Updating the patient about changes in medical evidence is an important part of the informed consent obligation. If the discussion involves an herbal product, the practitioner should let the patient know that the fact that the product is marketed as "natural" does not necessarily mean the product is safe (Ernst 1999; Fugh-Berman 2000; Piscitelli et al. 2000). Informing the patient about the changing medical evidence also may shift (in one direction or another) the patient's willingness to accept the known risks and benefits of the CAM therapy or even to use the therapy. Shared decision making improves patients' perceptions of their physicians; it has been shown that a practitioner who is perceived by patients as being arrogant tends to have increased liability exposure (Gutheil and Appelbaum 2000). In one twist, as more medical evidence begins to support the safety and efficacy of CAM therapies and these therapies become more generally accepted within the medical community, mental health care practitioners who fail to recommend safe and effective CAM therapies could conceivably be liable for *inadequate* informed consent (Cohen 1998, pp. 59–62; *Moore v. Baker* 1993).

Abandonment

Abandonment refers to the unilateral and unjustified termination of a treatment relationship by a caregiver that results in patient injury (Adams et al. 2002). As the term "unjustified" indicates, there are situations in which it is reasonable and appropriate to unilaterally terminate the treatment relationship; these include situations involving threatening or violent patients, patients who repeatedly fail to keep appointments, and patients who are noncompliant to the point that the clinician can no longer justify seeing them (Fentiman et al. 2000). Even when termination of the relationship may seem to be justified, it is advisable for the clinician to consult with one or more colleagues to see how they assess the situation, make arrangements for emergency coverage until the patient can find another caregiver, and, whenever possible, help facilitate the identification of a new physician and transfer of patient care.

Vicarious Liability

Although there are few judicial opinions setting precedent regarding referrals to CAM therapists, the general rule in conventional care is that there is no liability merely for referring to a specialist. Because the law related to health care is the same whether the practitioner is offering conventional or CAM therapies, referral by a conventional caregiver to a CAM practitioner or a conventional practitioner who uses CAM therapies should not in itself confer general liability (Studdert et al. 1998). Notable exceptions in which practitioners may be considered liable include when their referral delays or defers necessary medical care, when they refer a patient to someone the practitioner knows or should know is incompetent, and in cases of joint treatment, in which clinicians (e.g., a psychiatrist and an acupuncturist) collaborate to develop a plan to treat and monitor the patient (Cohen 2000, pp. 47–58). To avoid liability in these cases, it is advisable for clinicians to continue monitoring patients through conventional means, stand ready to intervene with conventional therapy when medically necessary, and try to assess the competence of the practitioner receiving the referral (i.e., understand the practitioner's credentials and proposed treatment plan and determine whether the patient is likely to receive substandard treatment or be injured) (Cohen and Eisenberg 2002).

LIABILITY RISK MANAGEMENT

As suggested above, a principal strategy clinicians can follow to help reduce their liability risk involves their paying attention to the therapeutic relationship, as bad outcomes compounded by bad feelings can lead to litigation (Gutheil and Appelbaum 2000). Good communication with patients, which includes tailoring the communication content and style to the needs of the individual patient, has been shown to enhance a patient's perception of the physician's competence and to reduce the risk of malpractice (Adamson et al. 1989; Moore et al. 2000).

Other risk management strategies include monitoring patients for potential adverse reactions between conventional and CAM therapies (e.g., adverse herb-drug interactions), particularly where the patient is ingesting dietary supplements concurrently with medication or surgery (Cohen and Eisenberg 2002). A clinician who continues to monitor a patient through conventional means and intervenes with conventional therapy when medically necessary will meet the standard of care and minimize the possibility of patient injury. For example, the physician and patient may wish to try a CAM therapy for a predefined period of time in lieu of conventional care (e.g., a combination of herbal products and lifestyle changes) and then return to conventional care (e.g., a standard psychopharmacological therapy) when it becomes necessary. From a liability perspective, the more acute and severe the patient's condition (and the more curable it is using conventional therapies), the more important it is to monitor and intervene using conventional means.

Another risk reduction measure is the practice of obtaining consultation and documenting such consultative opinions in the patient's record. These measures serve to establish the standard of care in the community, can provide valuable input into clinical decision making, and show that the clinician is willing to take extra steps for the benefit of the patient (Gutheil and Appelbaum 2000). In general, it is advisable to keep complete and accurate medical records that document the patient's medical history concerning the use of CAM therapies and conversations with the patient about the inclusion of such therapies. Such thorough documentation can help prove that informed consent requirements were satisfied and also may help protect against undue disciplinary action by state boards (Cohen and Eisenberg 2002). Physicians also should familiarize themselves with documentation standards suggested by the FSMB guidelines and determine whether these are applicable in their state or home institution (see below).

Finally, there is a legal doctrine known as *assumption of risk,* which provides that the practitioner may have a defense to malpractice when the treatment rendered was not substandard and the patient chose a particular therapeutic course despite the practitioner's efforts to dissuade him or her from doing so (Cohen 2000, pp. 26–31; *Schneider v. Revici* 1987). Not all states, however, adopt this approach; in addition, courts tend to disfavor forms by physicians and hospitals that ask patients to waive claims of liability for medical malpractice (*Tunkl v. Regents* 1963). Again, mental health care providers should engage patients in detailed conversations concerning CAM therapies and clearly document such discussions in the medical record as well as foster a positive relationship with patients that can help mitigate the prospect of litigation (see Appendix 2-A).

Health Care Fraud

Health care fraud refers to the legal concern for preventing intentional deception of patients. Overbroad claims sometimes can lead to charges of fraud, and its related legal theory, *misrepresentation* (Cohen 1998, pp. 68–70). If a clinician or institution submits a reimbursement claim for a treatment that was known or should have been known to be medically unnecessary, this also might be grounds for a finding of fraud and abuse under federal law (Cohen 1998, pp. 104–108).

Fraud and misrepresentation involve the knowing inducement of reliance on inaccurate or false information for the benefit of the person committing the fraud and to the detriment of the victim. The practitioner must know the information or representation is false or must recklessly fail to discover its falsity, and the victim must reasonably rely on the representation. For example, telling a patient that a particular yoga posture will cure a severe mental health condition might be considered fraudulent because there is no medical evidence to prove the claim.

Because it involves intentionality or recklessness as opposed to a lack of due care, fraud presents a higher level of culpability than negligence in most malpractice cases. As such, a fraud claim typically opens the defending physician to the possibility of punitive damages (Cohen 2000). At the same time, fraud is harder to substantiate because it requires proving a mental state (intention or recklessness) and not simply a negligent act. Nonetheless, fraud is a potent tool to curb misconduct relevant to provision of CAM therapies (Cohen 2004).

FEDERATION OF STATE MEDICAL BOARDS GUIDELINES

As noted, the FSMB has passed model guidelines for "(1) physicians who use CAM in their practices, and/or (2) those who co-manage patients with licensed or otherwise state-regulated CAM practitioners" (Federation of State Medical Boards 2002). The FSMB guidelines are suggestive but not binding in any given state, unless adopted by that state's medical board. They offer a framework for individual state medical boards to regulate physicians integrating CAM therapies. They should be read in conjunction with existing medical board guidelines in the state in which the physician practices, as the FSMB guidelines provide ways for medical boards to think about integrative practices.

In general, the FSMB guidelines "allow a wide degree of latitude in physicians' exercise of their professional judgment and do not preclude the use of any methods that are reasonably likely to benefit patients without undue risk." They also recognize that "patients have a right to seek any kind of care for their health problems" and that "a full and frank discussion of the risks and benefits of all medical practices is in the patient's best interest." To this extent, the FSMB guidelines implicitly recognize both shared decision making and patients' interest in integrative care.

At the same time, in trying to assess whether an integrative care practice is violative and should trigger physician discipline, the FSMB guidelines ask whether the therapy fits into any of the following categories:

- *Is it effective and safe?* Is there adequate scientific evidence of its efficacy and/ or safety or to substantiate its greater safety compared with other established treatment models for the same condition?
- *Is it effective, but with some real or potential danger?* Is there evidence of its efficacy but also of adverse side effects?
- *Has it been inadequately studied but is safe?* Is there insufficient evidence of its clinical efficacy but reasonable evidence to suggest its relative safety?
- *Is it ineffective and dangerous?* Has it been proven to be ineffective or unsafe through controlled trials or documented evidence or as measured by a risk–benefit assessment?

Some of these standards may be difficult to establish. For example, the first category includes any CAM therapy for which there is evidence showing it has greater safety and/or efficacy than the applicable conventional treatment; however, there may or may not be available evidence to this effect. Moreover, the FSMB guidelines list these four categories but do not offer suggestions for how to use them in clinical decision making.

In addition to the above standards, the FSMB guidelines provide an extensive checklist of items to which the physician must attend when offering CAM therapies. Psychiatrists practicing integrative care should review these items with their legal counsel and determine which are advisable and practical. For example, these items include documentation regarding the following:

- What medical options have been discussed, offered, or tried and to what effect, or a statement indicating whether the patient or patient's guardian refused certain options

- Whether proper referral has been offered for appropriate treatment and the risks and benefits of using the recommended treatment, to the extent known, have been appropriately discussed with the patient or patient's guardian
- Whether the physician has determined the extent to which the treatment could interfere with any other recommended or ongoing treatment

The FSMB guidelines also provide that the CAM treatment should

- Have a favorable risk–benefit ratio compared with other treatments for the same condition.
- Be used based on a reasonable expectation that it will result in a favorable patient outcome, including preventive practices.
- Be used based on the expectation that a greater benefit will be achieved than that which can be expected with no treatment.

ETHICAL ANALYSIS

Adams et al. (2002) offered seven factors to consider in assessing the ethics of whether or not to offer a patient a CAM therapy:

1. Severity and acuteness of illness
2. Curability with conventional treatment
3. Invasiveness, toxicities, and side effects of conventional treatment
4. Quality of evidence of safety and efficacy of the CAM treatment
5. Degree of understanding within the health care community of the risks and benefits of conventional and CAM treatments
6. Knowledge and voluntary acceptance of any known risks by the patient
7. Persistence of patient's intention to use CAM treatment

The above factors dovetail with the liability approach described earlier. Thus, if the illness is not severe or acute, is not easily curable with conventional treatment, or the conventional treatment is invasive and carries toxicities or side effects that are unacceptable to the patient, then, assuming the CAM therapy has not been proven to be unsafe or ineffective, it may be ethically compelling to try the CAM approach for a limited period while monitoring the patient through conventional means. The ethical posture is even further improved if the patient understands the risks and benefits of the CAM therapy, is willing to assume the risk of trying such an approach, and insists on taking this route. In this case, a monitoring "wait-and-see" approach respects the patient's autonomy interest while satisfying the clinician's obligation to do no harm.

One example of implementing this approach could be the use of hypnosis to reduce a patient's need for painkillers and anesthesia and reduce his or her anxiety (O'Connell 2002). Such a therapeutic technique, in conjunction with conventional care, if likely safe and potentially effective, would be ethically compelling, assuming the clinician held a full and fair conversation with the patient about the potential benefits and risks of such an approach. On the whole, integrative care suggests the need for such conversations. Even though the legal obligation of informed consent mandates a caregiver disclose risks and benefits to a patient, the premise of integrative care suggests the importance of fully engaging patients in shared decision making.

CONCLUSION

The integration of CAM therapies into mental health care requires a balance between caution and conversation, a balance that ultimately can become "clinically responsible, ethically appropriate, and legally defensible" (Cohen 2005). In accordance with such a balance, the National Center for Complementary and Alternative Medicine at the National Institutes of Health currently defines *integrative medicine* as health care that "combines mainstream medical therapies and CAM therapies for which there is some high-quality scientific evidence of safety and effectiveness" (National Center for Complementary and Alternative Medicine 2004). Such a definition implicitly recognizes the potential value of combining conventional and CAM therapies, provided that such therapies have "some high-quality" evidentiary base, but does not set an evidentiary threshold, leaving the clinician to make delicate judgments of good clinical and legal sense. Nonetheless, the integration of evidence-informed CAM therapies into psychiatry and mental health counseling can present clinicians with legal and ethical dilemmas when their preferences and perspectives clash with those of their patients. Individual clinicians as well as hospitals and medical and other professional organizations may wish to consider the suggestions in this chapter as input for continued reflection.

REFERENCES

Adams KE, Cohen MH, Jonsen AR, et al: Ethical considerations of complementary and alternative medical therapies in conventional medical settings. Ann Intern Med 137:660–664, 2002

Adamson TE, Tschann JM, Gullion DS, et al: Physician communication skills and malpractice claims: a complex relationship. West J Med 150:356–360, 1989

American Medical Association: Liability insurance requirements. Available at: www.ama-assn.org/ama/pub/category/print/4544.html. Accessed March 9, 2004.

Cohen MH: Complementary and Alternative Medicine: Legal Boundaries and Regulatory Perspectives. Baltimore, MD, Johns Hopkins University Press, 1998

Cohen MH: Beyond Complementary Medicine: Legal and Ethical Perspectives on Health Care and Human Evolution. Ann Arbor, University of Michigan Press, 2000

Cohen MH: Healing at the borderland of medicine and religion: regulating potential abuse of authority by spiritual healers. J Law Relig 18:373–426, 2004

Cohen MH: Legal Issues in Integrative Medicine. Washington, DC, NAF Publications, 2005

Cohen MH, Eisenberg DM: Potential physician malpractice liability associated with complementary/integrative medical therapies. Ann Intern Med 136:596–603, 2002

Cohen MH, Ruggie M: Integrating complementary and alternative medical therapies in conventional medical settings: legal quandaries and potential policy models. Cincinnati Law Review 72:671–729, 2004

Committee on the Use of Complementary and Alternative Medicine by the American Public: Complementary and Alternative Medicine in the United States. Board on Health Promotion and Disease Prevention, Institute of Medicine. Washington, DC, National Academies Press, 2005

Dumoff A: Medical board prohibitions against physician supplements sales. Alternative/Complementary Therapies 6:226–236, 2000

Eisenberg DM, Cohen MH, Hrbek A, et al: Credentialing complementary and alternative medical practitioners. Ann Intern Med 137:965–973, 2002

Ernst E: Second thoughts about safety of St John's wort. Lancet 354:2014–2016, 1999

Ernst EE, Cohen MH: Informed consent in complementary and alternative medicine. Arch Intern Med 161:2288–2292, 2001

Federation of State Medical Boards: Model Guidelines for Physician Use of Complementary and Alternative Therapies in Medical Practice. April 2002. Available at: www.fsmb.org/pdf/2002_grpol_Complementary_Alternative_Therapies.pdf. Accessed February 5, 2004.

Fentiman LC, Kaufman G, Merton V, et al: Current issues in the psychiatrist-patient relationship: outpatient civil commitment, psychiatric abandonment and the duty to continue treatment of potentially dangerous patients: balancing duties to patients and the public. Pace Law Review 20:231–262, 2000

Fugh-Berman A: Herb–drug interactions. Lancet 355:134–138, 2000

Gutheil TG, Appelbaum PS: Malpractice and other forms of liability, in Clinical Handbook of Psychiatry and the Law, 3rd Edition. Philadelphia, PA, Lippincott Williams & Wilkins, 2000, pp 135–214

Moore v Baker, 98 F.2d 1129 (11th Cir. 1993)

Moore PJ, Adler NE, Robertson PA: Medical malpractice: the effect of doctor-patient relations on medical patient perceptions and malpractice intentions. West J Med 173:244–250, 2000

National Center for Complementary and Alternative Medicine. Available at: www.nccam.nih.gov. Accessed February 4, 2004.

O'Connell S: It won't hurt you one bit. The Times (London), June 24, 2002

Piscitelli SC, Burstein AH, Chaitt D, et al: Indinavir concentrations and St John's wort. Lancet 355:547–548, 2000

Schneider v Revici, 817 F.2d 987 (2d Cir. 1987)

Schouten R, Cohen MH: Legal issues in integration of complementary therapies into cardiology, in Complementary and Integrative Therapies for Cardiovascular Disease. Edited by Frishman WH, Weintraub MI, Micozzi MS. New York, Elsevier, 2004, pp 20–55

Studdert DM, Eisenberg DM, Miller FH, et al: Medical malpractice implications of alternative medicine. JAMA 280:1610–1615, 1998

Tunkl v Regents of the University of California, 383 Pacific Reporter 2d 441 (Cal. 1963)

APPENDIX 2-A

Model Standard Consent Form for Use of Complementary and Alternative Medicine Therapies

APPENDIX 2-A. Model Standard Consent Form for Use of Complementary and Alternative Medicine Therapies

Documentation of Informed Consent

By signing this form, I, _____ *[name of patient],* agree that _____ *[name of clinician]* has disclosed to me sufficient information, including the risks and benefits, to enable me to decide to undergo or forgo _____ *[name of therapy or course of treatment]* for _____ *[name of patient's condition].*

Our discussion has included: 1) the nature of my condition and procedures to be performed; 2) the nature and probability of material risks involved; 3) benefits to be reasonably expected of the procedure; 4) the inability of the practitioner to predict results; 5) the irreversibility of the procedure, if that is the case; 6) the likely result of no treatment or procedure; and 7) the available alternatives, including their risks and benefits. _____ *[name of clinician]* has informed me that he or she has recorded an accurate, written description of the above in my medical record.

I have [refused the following recommended diagnostic and therapeutic interventions, and] elected to use the following [CAM] therapies: _____ *[list therapies].* [I understand that *[treatment X]* is not approved by the U.S. Food and Drug Administration.]

My consent to this course of treatment is given voluntarily, without coercion, and may be withdrawn, and I am competent and able to understand the nature and consequences of the proposed treatment or procedure.

Assumption of Risk and Release of Liability

The specific risks in making this choice of treatment are: _____ *[list of risks provided by clinician].* I knowingly, voluntarily, and intelligently assume these risks and agree to release, indemnify, and defend _____ *[name of clinician]* and his or her agents from and against any and all claims which I (or my representatives) may have for any loss, damage, or injury arising out of or in connection with my treatment.

I have carefully read this form and acknowledge that I understand it. No representations, statements, or inducements, oral or written, apart from the foregoing written statement, have been made. This form shall be governed by the laws of the state of _____ *[name of state],* which shall be the forum for any lawsuits filed under or incident to this form. If any portion of this form is held invalid, the rest of the document shall continue in full force and effect.

_____ *[patient signature]*   _____ *[date]*

_____ *[clinician signature]*   _____ *[date]*

Note. This form is a model that must be adapted by an attorney licensed to practice law within the client's state. It includes elements of informed consent and assumption of risk. It should be noted that in some states, physicians are not allowed to include an assumption-of-risk clause, and inclusion of such a clause could potentially invalidate the entire agreement.

Source. Reprinted from Cohen MH: *Legal Issues in Alternative Medicine.* Berne, NC, Trafford Publishing, 2004. Copyright 2004, Michael H. Cohen. Used with permission.

3

Patient Safety

Brian J. Ellinoy, Pharm.D.
James Lake, M.D.
Christopher Hobbs, L.Ac.

This chapter introduces a practical framework for weighing the relative risks and benefits of integrating alternative and conventional treatments in mental health care. It addresses challenges posed by the absence of definitive safety information on the range of complementary and alternative medicine (CAM) treatment approaches used in mental health care. High-quality "safety pearls" extracted from the peer-reviewed medical literature are presented, with the goal of providing clinically relevant information to psychiatrists and other mental health professionals. Safety data on herbals and other nonconventional biological therapies are presented in tables for easy reference and include comments on tolerability, contraindications, important adverse effects, and frequently encountered interactions. This chapter is intended as a general overview of safety issues that the clinician must keep in mind when any CAM modality is being considered. The reader is referred to Part II of this book, "Review of the Evidence and Clinical Guidelines," for more detailed discussions of specific safety concerns associated with the various biological, somatic, and mind–body treatments. Resources for identifying quality natural products and locating competent local practitioners of the alternative modalities discussed in this book are provided in Appendix C.

SAFETY ISSUES RELATED TO NONCONVENTIONAL APPROACHES IN MENTAL HEALTH CARE

Unresolved Safety Issues With Conventional Pharmacological Treatments

The focus of this chapter is safety issues associated with herbals, other natural products, and mind-body treatments. However, it is important to view these concerns in the broader context of documented safety problems associated with the use of conventional pharmacological treatments. One widely recognized safety issue is the risk of patients' developing the metabolic syndrome with chronic use of most atypical antipsychotics and other conventional drugs, resulting in weight gain and increased risk of type 2 diabetes. Infrequent serious risks associated with conventional pharmacological treatments include the risk of tardive dyskinesia and neuroleptic malignant syndrome in patients taking first-generation antipsychotics and serotonin syndrome in patients taking selective serotonin reuptake inhibitors (SSRIs) or combinations of SSRIs (or other antidepressants that affect brain serotonin levels) and monoamine oxidase inhibitors (MAOIs). Less serious but common safety issues include well-documented adverse effects or drug–drug interactions associated with SSRIs, antipsychotics, mood stabilizers, benzodiazepines, and other widely used synthetic psychotropic medications, such as loss of libido or erectile dysfunction, gastrointestinal distress, excessive perspiration, rash, fatigue, agitation or insomnia, weight gain, hair loss, dependence and tolerance (i.e., with prolonged benzodiazepine use), elevations in liver enzymes that deleteriously affect serum levels of other medications, heart rhythm disturbances, and movement disorders (Coupland et al. 1996; Leo 1999). Considerable public attention has recently been directed at concerns over adverse effects that commonly take place when antidepressants and other conventional psychotropic medications are abruptly discontinued after prolonged use (Schatzberg et al. 1997). Patients sometimes choose to continue taking antidepressants even in the absence of serious mood symptoms for prolonged periods because they are afraid of "withdrawing" from these medications. Examples of symptoms that occur after discontinuation of some antidepressants include excessive perspiration, agitation or jitteriness, panic attacks, insomnia, and feelings of disorientation or dread. Pharmaceutical companies acknowledge that unpleasant adverse effects take place after the discontinuation of many conventional drugs, but to date there are no effective treatments for these side effects.

In response to growing concerns about drug safety in general, the U.S. Food and Drug Administration (FDA) has directed the Institute of Medicine to review current procedures used by pharmaceutical manufacturers to monitor drug safety, especially in the postmarketing phase (Mechcatie 2005). Out of similar concerns, in 2002, the American Psychiatric Association Board of Trustees established a Committee on Patient Safety (Herzog et al. 2002). The broad goals of the committee include developing workshops on safety issues at annual American Psychiatric Association meetings, developing a series of publications on safety for psychiatrists, and establishing a national Listserve for the discussion and exchange of information pertaining to safety. One of the chief priorities of the Committee on Patient Safety is the promotion of effective strategies to prevent adverse medication effects.

Safety Considerations When Consulting on Hospitalized Patients

Mental health professionals often think about safety issues pertaining to alternative medicine only in the context of high-functioning outpatients. It is certainly true that a patient's level of acuity and ability to commit to regularly attending appointments in the therapist's office or the local community mental health clinic should be part of any discussion of the appropriateness of alternative therapies. However, many psychiatrically or medically hospitalized patients are treated (or self-treat) with herbals or other natural products before hospitalization. It is therefore important to keep in mind a range of safety issues associated with alternative therapies when caring for hospitalized patients.

Psychiatric inpatients are often reluctant to admit to using alternative treatments: "Why talk about it? Doctors won't believe in that anyway!" Many psychiatrically hospitalized patients lack the capacity to disclose their prehospitalization use of herbals or other natural products, and the admitting team seldom inquires about the use of such products or other alternative treatments. Medically hospitalized patients seen in consultation by a psychiatrist often use herbal medicines or other natural products concurrently with several prescribed drugs, including antibiotics, antihypertensives, immunosuppressives, and other synthetics that could pose a significant interaction potential. Debilitated medically hospitalized patients often have a diminished physiological capacity to remove foreign substances from the body because of impaired liver or renal function, resulting in toxic blood levels of certain substances from the ingestion of natural products (or synthetic drugs) at doses that are therapeutic in healthy adults (Crone and Wise 1998). This becomes problematic when interactions or adverse effects interfere with these patients' conventional medical treatment or result in a worsening of their medical or psychiatric problems.

Evaluating the Safety of Complementary and Alternative Therapies

Evaluating the general safety of CAM therapies used in mental health care, including herbs, other nutritional supplements, and mind-body modalities, can be challenging. Many patients who use nonconventional therapies believe these approaches are completely safe because they are "natural." Many approaches are apparently safe on the basis of their established use in traditional systems of medicine over centuries or longer; however, there is limited reliable information on potential risks associated with most nonconventional treatments (Ernst and Barnes 1998), and most have associated direct or indirect risks, including adverse effects. Furthermore, the issue of identifying a competent alternative medical practitioner sometimes poses risks, especially when there are few or no requirements for minimum standards of professional training or credentialing (Ernst et al. 1997). Growing numbers of patients use alternative remedies in the absence of professional consultation after reading popular self-help books or viewing television talk shows (Ernst and Armstrong 1988). Most information on the safety of these remedies comes from case reports that may be poorly documented and is therefore unreliable. More ambiguity is added to the search for clear answers when individual reviewers emphasize different data or cite different references when supporting claims of adverse effects (Barrett et al. 1999). Case reports of adverse effects or herb–drug interactions are often based on assumptions that unsafe outcomes are likely when a specified herb and a specified drug are combined on the basis of a known physiological effect profile or presumed incompatibility between the respective mechanisms of action. However, most case reports are not clearly substantiated by a high degree of evidence. Because of the popularity of St. John's wort to treat or self-treat depression, the greatest number of case reports of adverse effects or herb–drug interactions is associated with this herb. By mid-2003, nine case reports were published of possible serotonin syndrome when St. John's wort was combined with a conventional antidepressant (Fugh-Berman and Ernst 2003). However, very few of the claims in those reports were able to be substantiated as "likely interactions" on the basis of compelling evidence of a cause-effect relationship between concurrent use of St. John's wort and an antidepressant.

Manufacturing Standards for and Regulation of Herbal Medicines and Other Natural Product Treatments

A large telephone survey showed that 86% of Americans believe that all products labeled "natural" are safe (National Consumers League 2002). However, the medicinal use of many herbals and other natural products poses significant safety issues, especially in the United States. In contrast to Western Europe, where herbals and other natural products are regulated, sold, and prescribed as medicines, in the United States natural products are marketed and regulated as food supplements under the provisions of the Dietary Supplement Health and Education Act of 1994.

The FDA recently announced several new initiatives to further improve standards of quality, safety, and evidence for natural products marketed in the United States (U.S. Food and Drug Administration 2004). The FDA's National Center for Toxicological Research is collaborating with the National Institutes of Health's Office of Dietary Supplements, the National Center for Complementary and Alternative Medicine, the National Toxicology Program in the U.S. Department of Health and Human Services, and the National Center for Natural Products Research at the University of Mississippi to improve the quality of medical evidence used to determine acceptable standards of quality and safety of natural products. In public hearings held in November 2004, the FDA sought comments from the public about the type and quality of evidence that natural product manufacturers should be required to disclose about their products. These comments are currently under review and will affect future policy decisions. In addition, extensive documentation pertaining to good manufacturing practice requirements is under review, including more stringent requirements for evidence supporting therapeutic claims for natural products. The goal of this work is to apply the stringent quality assurance standards used for synthetic drugs to determine acceptable standards of quality, efficacy, and safety of biologically active natural products.

Although the FDA has established quality standards for natural products, they are not stringently enforced because of inadequate funding and other more pressing safety concerns, such as monitoring serious potential adverse effects and toxicities of conventional drugs. However, the importation of many natural products and the absence of standardized manufacturing practices have resulted in complex safety issues, including adulteration of natural products with synthetic drugs, pesticides, heavy metals, or other potentially toxic substances and the failure of some supplement companies to meet stated minimum contents of bioactive constituents (Gurely et al. 2000; Huggett 2001). Some imported Chinese herbal medicines are adulterated with steroids, phenobarbital, acetaminophen, and other drugs (Huang et al. 1997). However, Chinese medical practitioners who prescribe herbals in the United States and other Western countries typically use traditional Chinese herbal formulas produced under rigorous quality control standards, including batch testing for herbicides, pesticides, and heavy metals. Batches that fail to meet minimum U.S. federal safety standards are rejected and never go to market.

The magnitude of potential safety issues associated with the use of herbals and other natural products is evident from examining the growing U.S. demand for all natural products. Between 1991 and 1999, sales of all herbal products and other dietary supplements doubled every 2 years (Zeisel 1999). In 2001, total sales of dietary supplements reached $17 billion, and herbal medicines accounted for 25% of that amount (Natural Marketing Institute 2002). In view of the vast amount of herbals and other natural products taken in the United States, serious adverse effects or toxicities are relatively uncommon. Indeed, it is estimated that 20%–25% of all U.S. adults—approximately 20 million people—who use conventional drugs also use herbal medicines, yet very few actual case reports exist of serious adverse effects or toxicities from herb–drug interactions. This fact suggests that concern over the efficacy of natural substances used for medicinal purposes should be regarded as a more pressing issue than the safety of these substances. For example, some unethical suppliers of herbals or other natural substances promote products based on pseudoscience or very limited scientific evidence.

The careful selection of herbal and other natural products to be recommended to patients by mental health practitioners is critical to patient safety. The lack of FDA quality assurance regulations and uneven quality of manufacturing practices of medicinal herbs or other natural products can potentially interfere with a product's desirable therapeutic results or compromise patient safety. To ensure patients are directed to products that meet the highest standards for both safety and quality, mental health professionals should familiarize themselves with resources provided by U.S. Pharmacopoeia (USP), ConsumerLab.com, NSF International, or other third-party evaluators and provide patients with information about specific products that are approved by USP for the intended treatment application and highly rated by these third-party evaluators. These organizations provide independent safety and quality ratings for hundreds of natural products. In addition, the Web sites for these organizations (provided in Appendix C) include reports of product recalls or warnings. In collaboration with experts in botanical medicine, USP has published approximately 1,000 monographs on herbs, vitamins, and other natural products. The USP Web site lists hundreds of natural products that have been "USP verified" by rigorous quality assurance and safety tests. Safety documentation is available free of charge to consumers. ConsumerLab.com issues a free monthly electronic newsletter for consumers. (See also the Web sites listed in Appendix C related to safety information on natural products.)

Judicious Referrals to Alternative Practitioners

Just as important as careful product selection is the referral to competent practitioners of the various mind-body modalities. Many alternative practitioners are poorly trained or do not have the specialized skills necessary to work with serious psychiatric disorders, and there is often little or no oversight of their clinical work (Ernst et al. 1997). Alternative practitioners also sometimes recommend to patients that they discontinue or change medications without first consulting their prescribing physician. These issues may result in inappropriate alternative treatments or delays in more effective alternative or mainstream treatments. The referring physician should verify that the alternative therapy practitioner has the appropriate training, credentials, and licensure (if required) before making the referral. A practitioner's level of interpersonal skills is also a consideration in referring patients with a mental health disorder; for example, practitioners who treat depressed or anxious patients must have personal and intuitive skills that empower patients on their healing journeys. Qualified alternative practitioners are often found by word of mouth from patients or colleagues. They should be chosen with great care, as patients' overall progress often depends on positive interactions between alternative practitioners and patients. Licensure requirements for CAM practitioners and the names and contact information of profes-

sional alternative medical associations that can provide referrals to qualified practitioners in different geographic regions of the United States are provided in
Appendix C.

POTENTIAL ADVERSE EFFECTS
OF HERBAL SUPPLEMENTS

For the most part, herbal supplements seem to be well tolerated and have a relatively low incidence of adverse effects, especially when compared with prescription medications. However, the literature on their safety is incomplete, especially with regard to use in young children, pregnant and nursing women, and
patients with significant liver or kidney disease, where maximum safe doses
presently remain unknown.

All herbal medicines and other natural products contain biologically active
constituents that can potentially cause adverse effects or interact with synthetic
drugs, other natural products, or foods. Mental health clinicians should be aware
of possible adverse effects when recommending an herbal product and should
consider the potential for adverse effects on a case-by-case basis after a careful
review of a patient's medical history and concurrent use of conventional medication. The selection of a quality brand (see above) is also important, especially
in view of reports of contamination or questionable efficacy of some brands.

Another cause for concern is patients' lack of disclosure to their physician
about natural products they may be using to self-treat a psychiatric problem for
which they are contemporaneously taking a prescribed medication. Adverse effects or interactions can be frequently missed. Because of the widespread lack of
disclosure, the type, severity, and frequency of adverse effects and interactions
associated with most natural products have not been clearly established, and
most data on these events come from case reports.

Although herbs used to treat mental health problems can have adverse physiological effects, certain herbal products used in mental health treatment also have
psychiatric adverse effects. St. John's wort, for example, can induce mania or hypomania in susceptible individuals; ephedra-containing compounds (e.g.,
Mahuang) have been reported to cause psychosis (Jacobs and Hirsch 2000); excessive use of ginseng can result in restlessness, nervousness, insomnia, or agitation; and use of kava has been linked with extrapyramidal symptoms (Spollen et
al. 1999). U.S. sales of ephedra were banned in 2003 because of growing concerns about its safety (U.S. Department of Health and Human Services 2003). St.
John's wort can result in a photosensitive rash and should not be used by patients
who are likely to experience prolonged exposure to sunlight. Kava may cause loss
of uterine tone and should not be used by pregnant women. Nursing women
should also avoid kava use because the active constituents (kavapyrones) pass into
breast milk and may have sedating effects on a nursing infant. Kava may result in

excessive sedation and worsening of vegetative symptoms when used by severely depressed patients, and its use should be avoided in this population. Kava should not be used concurrently with sedative–hypnotics or alcohol, both of which may potentiate the sedative and muscle relaxant effects of kava.

Table 3–1 summarizes general safety concerns associated with the use of herbal supplements that are frequently recommended by alternative practitioners or are used by patients to self-treat mental health problems.

HERB–DRUG INTERACTIONS

In general, combining an herbal and conventional drug should be advised against when there is a reasonable basis for assuming that their combined use will result in a potentially unsafe interaction or in the absence of clear evidence that the substances can be safely combined. For example, phenothiazines or other drugs that potentially cause photosensitivity reactions should never be used in conjunction with herbals known to cause photosensitivity including kava or St. John's wort. Kava and valerian potentiate the sedating effects of benzodiazepines and therefore generally should not be used in combination with drugs in this class. Exceptions include the daytime use of kava in a patient who uses a benzodiazepine at bedtime to help induce sleep and the careful titration of kava to manage withdrawal effects or recurring anxiety in a patient whose benzodiazepine dosage is being gradually tapered. (General considerations of integrative treatment planning in mental health care are addressed in Chapter 4.)

It is prudent to avoid concurrent use of certain herbals or other natural products (e.g., tea, coffee, kola nut, soft drinks containing caffeine, ephedra [Mahuang], ginseng, guarana) in bipolar or schizophrenic patients taking conventional mood stabilizers or antipsychotics (Brown 1997). All of these herbals can cause insomnia, agitation, and worsening of psychosis or manic symptoms. Although the commercial sale of ephedra in the United States was banned in 2003, it is still relatively easy to obtain the substance at Chinese medical pharmacies or by mail order. Mental health professionals should continue to ask patients who are being treated by a Chinese medical practitioner about the specific herbal formulas that are being used or contact the prescribing Chinese medical practitioner when the patient cannot provide detailed information. Ginseng can also potentiate MAOIs, possibly resulting in a hypertensive crisis. Several case reports of interactions between ginseng and phenelzine have been reported. Although most case reports are anecdotal and poorly substantiated, they warrant caution when ginseng or other stimulant herbals are being considered in a patient who is already taking an antidepressant. Guarana, kola nut, and yerba maté are stimulants that should be avoided by bipolar or schizophrenic patients taking conventional synthetic medications because of numerous case reports of agitation, mania, and insomnia occurring with their use in this population. Valerian

TABLE 3–1. General safety concerns associated with herbal supplements widely used to treat mental health problems

Herb	Adverse effects	Comment
Ginkgo (*Ginkgo biloba*)	Very few adverse effects documented; most common are gastrointestinal discomfort (21 cases), skin allergy, dizziness, headache	Substantiated in pooled clinical trials of almost 10,000 people
	Very rare reports of subdural hematoma and hyphema	Case reports
		Ginkgo has anticoagulant action (decreases blood viscosity, antiplatelet activity); bleeding risk may be increased if it is used before surgery or labor/delivery
	Recurrent seizures in epilepsy patients with prior symptom control	Case reports
		Possible electroencephalographic changes
		Possible seed contamination of ginkgo leaf products
	Stevens–Johnson syndrome	Case report
	Cytotoxic and allergenic alkylphenols (e.g., ginkgolic acids) may be present in some extracts	Toxins removed from approved German products
	Anti–vitamin B_6 neurotoxin (ginkgotoxin) in seeds	Possible product contamination problem
		Ginkgo seeds are rarely sold to the public, and the leaves of *G. biloba* are used in most products

TABLE 3–1. General safety concerns associated with herbal supplements widely used to treat mental health problems *(continued)*

Herb	Adverse effects	Comment
Kava (*Piper methysticum*)	Generally well tolerated	Widespread, long-term recreational use in South Pacific seemingly without major problems
	Most common adverse effects are gastrointestinal discomfort (generally mild), allergic skin rashes, mild headache	1.5%–2.3% incidence of untoward reactions reported in two studies involving a total of 7,000 patients using dosages up to 800 mg/day of 30% kavalactone extract; both incidence and severity were dosage dependent
	Severe hepatotoxicity (necrotizing hepatitis), liver failure	Case reports
		Idiosyncratic reactions?
		Germany, Switzerland, and U.K. no longer permit public sales of kava products; American and Canadian governments are considering stopping sales of kava products
		Hepatotoxicity may be related to contamination from materials in the stem; most kava products are prepared from root or rhizome extracts and have no demonstrable hepatotoxicity (Nerurkar et al. 2004)
		Caution is required in patients with hepatic risk factors; routine liver function tests are suggested for kava patients

TABLE 3–1. General safety concerns associated with herbal supplements widely used to treat mental health problems *(continued)*

Herb	Adverse effects	Comment
Kava (*Piper methysticum*) *(continued)*	Dystonic reactions	Case reports
	Increased symptoms in Parkinson disease patient	Case report
	Dry, scaly rash	Due to use of high dosages (400 mg/day kavalactones) over long term; rash disappeared when kava was discontinued
St. John's wort (*Hypericum perforatum*)	Low incidence of adverse effects; most common are mild stomach discomfort, allergic skin rashes, tiredness, restlessness	2.4% of 3,250 patients in a study reported side effects; occurrence rates for all effects were 0.6% or less
	Manic episodes	Case reports
	Psychotic episode	Case report involving elderly patient with Alzheimer's disease
	Serotonin syndrome–like symptoms	Case report
	Photosensitivity; hypericin known to cause photosensitivity reactions, especially in animals	Case reports, two involving topical use of herb, one in which individual received intensive ultraviolet B therapy after oral use of herb
		Evidence of possible increased risk of cataract occurrence due to hypericin photoactivation in lens of eye

TABLE 3–1. General safety concerns associated with herbal supplements widely used to treat mental health problems *(continued)*

Herb	Adverse effects	Comment
Valerian (*Valeriana officinalis*)	Generally well tolerated	Unpleasant odor may be unacceptable to some
	Morning grogginess; headache	Clinical study Reported in 2 of 61 patients
	Impaired vigilance for a few hours after ingestion (no residual morning sedation when used at night)	Use of automobile or other hazardous machinery not recommended immediately after ingestion
	Withdrawal syndrome (sinus tachycardia, delirium after no herb postoperatively)	Case report involving patient using high doses over long term

may potentiate the effects of alcohol and conventional sedative-hypnotics, including benzodiazepines. Other caveats the clinician should be aware of include the following (Miller 1998):

- Avoid concurrent use of any herbal tincture (which can contain up to 75% alcohol) and alcohol, conventional anxiolytics, or hypnotics.
- Avoid red ginseng or processed Panax ginseng in patients with chronic insomnia, "nervousness," or hysterical symptoms or in schizophrenic patients with predominantly positive symptoms (excessive doses can cause insomnia or agitation). However, formulas containing *Panax quinquefolius* (American ginseng) or *Eleutherococcus senticosus* (eleutherococcus or Siberian ginseng) is not contraindicated in this population.
- Avoid concurrent use of a herbal diuretic, such as uva ursi, green tea, or dandelion leaf extract (often contained in over-the-counter weight loss or premenstrual syndrome remedies), and lithium carbonate; herbal diuretics can cause decreased renal lithium clearance and increased risk of lithium toxicity.
- Evening primrose oil or borage may unmask previously undiagnosed temporal lobe epilepsy due to high levels of γ-linoleic acid. Schizophrenic and other patients taking phenothiazines are at especially high risk for this complication.
- Avoid the use of hops (*Humulus lupulus*) in depressed patients, as hops can further depress central nervous system activity. Avoid concurrent use of herbal sedatives and conventional hypnotics or anxiolytics.
- Avoid concurrent use of MAOIs and herbals with sympathomimetic activity (e.g., ephedra, coffee, black tea, guarana, kola nut, yerba maté, caffeinated soft drinks, *Atropa belladonna, Datura,* and hyoscyamine. *Atropa belladonna, Datura,* and hyoscyamine are available only by prescription. Avoid concurrent use of phenothiazines and herbs with antimuscarinic activity, as this can result in decreased plasma phenothiazine levels.
- Avoid concurrent use of St. John's wort and an MAOI, as this combination can lead to a hypertensive crisis. Avoid ginseng-containing products in patients taking MAOIs; ginseng can potentiate MAOIs, possibly leading to a hypertensive crisis.
- Recommend that patients taking caffeine, other stimulants (e.g., guarana), or hormonal therapies not take ginseng. Avoid guarana-containing products in schizophrenic or other patients taking hypnotics or anxiolytics.
- Special safety considerations must be addressed when a patient is considering combining Chinese herbal medicines with conventional drugs, including psychotropics. In view of limited available safety information, it is reasonable to consider combining Chinese herbals and Western synthetic drugs only in cases where a licensed traditional Chinese medical practitioner is working collaboratively with a conventionally trained physician (Chen 1998/1999; Huang et al. 1997; Lake 2004).

Table 3–2 lists clinically important interactions that have been documented to occur when herbs commonly used in mental health treatment are combined with prescription drugs or other natural products. (Because documentation evidence is limited, some hypothetical interactions have been included to increase the practitioner's awareness of potentially serious scenarios.) One comprehensive literature review of herb–drug interactions concluded that warfarin was the most frequently reported drug and St. John's wort the most frequently reported herb in documented incidents of herb–drug interactions from case reports or controlled clinical trials (Brazier 2003). Although many cases of interactions between St. John's wort and warfarin (or other coumarin anticoagulants) have been reported, most of these probably resulted from additive anticoagulant effects and thus were not true herb–drug interactions. Interpreting reports of herb–warfarin interactions can be problematic, because most cases are from animal studies or individual case data. Further research is needed to determine the clinical significance of these reports (Heck et al. 2000). It is important to note that *Ginkgo biloba* potentially prolongs bleeding time at the platelet level, specifically by interfering with platelet aggregation factor, and has been associated with bleeding even in the absence of warfarin.

POTENTIAL ADVERSE EFFECTS OF NONHERBAL SUPPLEMENTS

Many natural supplements other than herbals are used to treat or self-treat a range of psychiatric problems. These include docosahexanoic acid and other essential fatty acids, phosphatidyl serine, amino acids and their precursors, vitamins, and minerals. Based on an evaluation of the current peer-reviewed medical literature, these substances are generally well tolerated and have few serious adverse effects, especially when compared with prescription medications. However, the literature is incomplete with regard to the safety of most supplements in young children, pregnant and nursing women, and patients with significant liver or kidney disease. In all of these cases, maximum safe doses have not been clearly established; clinicians should therefore use conservative dosing strategies as well as closely monitor patients for treatment-emergent adverse effects. Table 3–3 summarizes general safety concerns associated with nonherbal supplements in current widespread use to treat or self-treat mental health problems.

NONBIOLOGICAL ALTERNATIVE THERAPIES

Acupuncture, yoga, qigong, and other energetic or mind–body modalities are extensively used to treat psychiatric disorders in North America and western Europe. In general, alternative energetic or mind–body modalities have good safety profiles and relatively few contraindications or complications, especially when they are administered by a qualified practitioner. Table 3–4 summarizes safety issues pertaining to alternative nonbiological modalities used in mental health care.

TABLE 3–2. Herb–drug and herb–supplement interactions

Herb	Drug/Supplement	Interaction	Comment/Reference
Chinese red sage (*Salvia miltiorrhiza*)	Warfarin	Increased bleeding tendency	Chan 2001
Dong quai (*Angelica sinensis*)	Warfarin	Increased bleeding tendency	Lo et al. 1995
Ginkgo (*Ginkgo biloba*)	Aspirin	Hyphema	Case report
			Ginkgo is a potent inhibitor of platelet-activating factor
	Warfarin	Increased bleeding tendency	Concomitant use of warfarin and ginkgo is **CONTRAINDICATED**
			Preliminary data, based on ginkgo's effects on platelet function
	Other drugs affecting hemostasis (anticoagulants, antiplatelet agents)	Increased bleeding tendency	Hypothetical, based on ginkgo's antiplatelet activity
	Anticonvulsant agents	Diminished anticonvulsant effectiveness	Preliminary data, based on possible contamination of ginkgo products with the neurotoxin 4′-O-methylpyridoxine
	Garlic, phosphatidylserine, policosanol, vitamin E (at high dosages), ginger	Increased tendency for bleeding	Hypothetical, based on the combined anticoagulant effects of these natural products and ginkgo

TABLE 3–2. Herb–drug and herb–supplement interactions (continued)

Herb	Drug/Supplement	Interaction	Comment/Reference
Kava (Piper methysticum)	Barbiturates	Potentiation of barbiturate sedative effects	Preliminary data
	Benzodiazepines	Central nervous system depression (lethargy, disorientation)	Case report with alprazolam Concomitant use not recommended
	Antipsychotics (e.g., phenothiazines, haloperidol)	Increased risk of dystonic reactions	Preliminary data Case reports indicate that kava may have central dopamine-blocking activity
	Anti-parkinsonian medications (e.g., carbidopa/levodopa)	Decreased control of Parkinson's disease	Hypothetical, based on postulated kava dopamine blockade
	Metoclopramide, other dopamine blockers	Increased risk of dystonic reactions	Hypothetical
	Hops, passion flower, valerian (sedative herbs)	Increased risk of excessive sedation	Hypothetical
St. John's wort (Hypericum perforatum)	Cyclosporine	Transplant rejection (subtherapeutic cyclosporine levels)	Case reports Enzyme induction of CYP3A4 and intestinal p-glyco-protein by St. John's wort, causing increased drug metabolism and decreased drug absorption

TABLE 3–2. Herb–drug and herb–supplement interactions (*continued*)

Herb	Drug/Supplement	Interaction	Comment/Reference
St. John's wort (*Hypericum perforatum*) (*continued*)	Digoxin	Decreased digoxin serum levels	Clinical study Decreased digoxin intestinal absorption
	Indinavir (other HIV protease inhibitors?)	Decreased indinavir serum levels (increased risk of treatment failure or antiretroviral resistance in HIV patients)	Small clinical study involving healthy volunteers Increased indinavir metabolism
	Nevirapine (other nonnucleoside reverse transcriptase inhibitors?)	Decreased serum levels of nevirapine	
	Oral contraceptives	Decreased oral contraceptive effectiveness, unwanted pregnancies	Case reports Increased metabolism of ethinylestradiol
	Serotonergic drugs	Serotonin syndrome	Case reports
	"Statin" drugs (except pravastatin)	Possible decreased statin effectiveness	Increased metabolism of statins
	Theophylline	Increased theophylline serum levels after stopping St. John's wort	Case report Increased metabolism of theophylline

TABLE 3–2. Herb–drug and herb–supplement interactions (*continued*)

Herb	Drug/Supplement	Interaction	Comment/Reference
St. John's wort (*Hypericum perforatum*) (*continued*)	Tricyclic antidepressants (TCAs)	Possible decreased TCA effectiveness	Increased TCA metabolism
	Photosensitizing agents and proton pump inhibitors	Increased risk of photosensitivity reactions	Hypothetical
	Warfarin	Reduced anticoagulation	Case reports
Valerian (*Valeriana officinalis*)	Barbiturates and benzodiazepines	Potentiation of sedative effects	Preliminary studies
	Hops, kava, passion flower (sedative herbs)	Increased risk of excessive sedation	Hypothetical

TABLE 3–3. General safety concerns of nonherbal nutritional supplements

Supplement	Adverse effects	Comment
5-Hydroxytryptophan	Absence of significant side effects in clinical trials At usual dosages (50–100 mg po tid), mild nausea, dry mouth, stomach irritation, drowsiness can occur	Serotonin precursor Contaminant "peak X" (previously associated with eosinophilic myalgia with L-tryptophan) found in one product batch in 1998; rare case reports; causality weak; no U.S. Food and Drug Administration action; some recommend obtaining 6-month eosinophil levels; others consider this supplement unsafe
Huperzine A	Absence of significant side effects in clinical studies in China; however, inhibition of acetylcholinesterase might cause dry mouth, fatigue, nausea, diarrhea Safely used in short-term clinical trials (1–3 months)	Appears to have fewer side effects than synthetic acetylcholinesterase inhibitor congeners (e.g., donepezil, physostigmine, tacrine)

TABLE 3–3. General safety concerns of nonherbal nutritional supplements *(continued)*

Supplement	Adverse effects	Comment
L–Tryptophan	Crosses the blood–brain barrier and is synthesized into serotonin; uncommon adverse effects include drowsiness, dry mouth, blurred vision	1,500 cases of eosinophilia-myalgia syndrome (EMS) were attributed to one contaminated batch of L-tryptophan in the late 1980s; L–Tryptophan has remained in widespread use, and no subsequent cases of EMS have been reported No cases of serotonin syndrome or other serious adverse effects have been reported when L-tryptophan was combined with fluoxetine or other conventional antidepressants
Omega–3 fatty acids (from flaxseed or fish oil)	Generally considered safe; usually well tolerated at low doses taken orally; nausea and loose stools at higher doses; fishy-smelling "burps" common; gastrointestinal side effects may be minimized by taking oil with meals Mild blood-thinning activity but no bleeding problems caused when used alone or with aspirin Transiently elevates low-density lipoprotein Eicosapentaenoic acid component might suppress natural killer cell activity (preliminary findings)	Cod liver oil (as a fish oil source) contains high levels of vitamins A and D; increased risk of vitamin toxicity associated with long-term use or high dosages Pharmaceutical grade of product purity required to avoid contamination from heavy metals, polychlorinated biphenyls, organochlorines Single case report implies that use in patient with history of major depressive disorder may have caused hypomanic episode

TABLE 3–3. General safety concerns of nonherbal nutritional supplements *(continued)*

Supplement	Adverse effects	Comment
Phosphatidylcholine	Generally considered safe Oral dosages up to 30 g/day for 6 weeks were well tolerated (one reference) Gastrointestinal upset (e.g., abdominal discomfort, diarrhea, nausea) and reduced appetite may occur at dosages exceeding 10 g/day	Component of lecithin
Phosphatidylserine	Generally considered safe Side effects rare; higher dosages (300–600 mg/day) can result in gastrointestinal upset, insomnia	Now derived from soy or cabbage; most research based on bovine cortex products, which are no longer available due to concerns over mad cow disease
SAMe (S-adenosylmethionine)	Generally considered safe Well tolerated orally; mild digestive distress is most common side effect At high doses, more intense gastrointestinal symptoms (e.g., nausea, vomiting, diarrhea) and central nervous system symptoms (e.g., mild insomnia, nervousness) have been reported Anxiety reported in depressed patients; manic episodes reported in bipolar patients	Butanedisulfonate salt more bioavailable and more stable than tosylate salt, making product selection extremely important

TABLE 3–3. General safety concerns of nonherbal nutritional supplements *(continued)*

Supplement	Adverse effects	Comment
Theanine	Generally well tolerated; crosses blood–brain barrier, where it is synthesized into γ-aminobutyric acid, resulting in general calming effect without sedation	No reports of adverse effects or interactions
Vinpocetine	Generally well tolerated	Clinical studies
	Reversible agranulocytosis	Case report
Vitamin E	Few adverse effects at therapeutic doses	Safe upper intake limit for adults is 1,500 IU/day α-tocopherol ("natural" vitamin E)
	Mild antiplatelet activity at high doses	Clinical study (50 IU/day)
		Caution required when considering use in patients having surgery or giving birth or who have a bleeding disorder
	Inhibition of chemotherapy versus protection against chemotherapy side effects without interference?	Medical controversy

TABLE 3–4. General safety profiles of nonbiological alternative modalities used in mental health care

Modality	Overall safety	Comments
Acupuncture	Generally considered safe when performed by a trained practitioner Side effects may include transient pain, tiredness, bruising, fainting, vomiting, aggravation of symptoms Serious complications are rare (e.g., pneumothorax, nerve damage) Infection from needles is very unlikely in the United States, where only sterile, disposable needles are used	Studies have revealed a slightly higher probability of significant adverse events when acupuncture is delivered by practitioners with limited training (100–200 hours) compared with Chinese medical practitioners who have completed a conventional 4-year program Pregnant patients should not have certain acupuncture points stimulated
Biofeedback	Few safety risks reported	Caution should be used in patients who have heart conditions or implantable electrical devices; some biofeedback equipment emits a weak electrical current
Chiropractic	Generally considered safe Minor side effects include transient local discomfort after therapy, headache, and fatigue Serious complications caused by manipulation of neck are rare (e.g., stroke, vertebral fracture)	Complication rate estimated at 1 per million sessions Not recommended in patients with osteoporosis, recent fractures, bone tumors, bone or joint infections, spinal cord disease, bone marrow disease, ligament damage, fused spine
Guided imagery	Generally considered safe	Mindfulness techniques such as guided imagery, autogenic training, meditation, and relaxation response have no known safety risks

TABLE 3–4. General safety profiles of nonbiological alternative modalities used in mental health care *(continued)*

Modality	Overall safety	Comments
Homeopathy	Homeopathic remedies very safe; no toxic reactions reported in 200 years U.S. Food and Drug Administration is responsible for quality control of homeopathic remedies	Patients may experience a "healing crisis" or "healing aggravation," a mild worsening of symptoms usually lasting only a few days
Massage	Generally considered safe Can transiently exacerbate pain; bone fractures and other internal injuries are possible if treatment is too forceful To be avoided on abdomen, legs, and feet during the first 3 months of pregnancy	Not recommended in patients with recent fractures, areas of bleeding, unhealed wounds, rash, phlebitis, skin infections, or varicose veins; to be avoided near tumors, recent surgical incisions
Qigong	Generally considered safe	Cases of transient psychosis or agitation during qigong practice have been reported by patients diagnosed with personality disorders or schizophrenia
Tai chi	Considered to be as safe as other exercise or mind–body practices	Special accommodations are required for patients with reduced mobility, impaired balance, or inability to stand
Yoga	Considered to be as safe as other exercise or mind–body practices	Advanced postures may result in injury to inexperienced practitioners

REFERENCES

Barrett B, Kiefer D, Rabago D: Assessing the risks and benefits of herbal medicine: an overview of scientific evidence. Altern Ther Health Med 5:40–49, 1999

Brazier NC, Levine MA: Drug-herb interaction among commonly used conventional medicines: a compendium for health care professionals. Am J Ther 10:163–169, 2003

Brown R: Potential interactions of herbal medicines with antipsychotics, antidepressants and hypnotics. European Journal of Herbal Medicine 3:25–28, 1997

Chan TY: Interaction between warfarin and danshen (*Salvia miltiorrhiza*). Ann Pharmacother 35:501–504, 2001

Chen J: Recognition and prevention of herb-drug interactions. Medical Acupuncture 10:9–13, 1998/1999

Coupland N, Bell C, Potokar JP: Serotonin reuptake inhibitor withdrawal. J Clin Psychopharmacol 16:356–362, 1996

Crone C, Wise T: Use of herbal medicines among consultation-liaison populations: a review of current information regarding risks, interactions, and efficacy. Psychosomatics 39:3–13, 1998

Ernst E, Armstrong N: Lay books on complementary/alternative medicine: a risk factor for good health? International Journal of Risk and Safety in Medicine 11:209–215, 1988

Ernst E, Barnes J: Methodological approaches to investigating the safety of complementary medicine. Complement Ther Med 6:115–121, 1998

Ernst E, Siev-Ner I, Gamus D: Complementary medicine: a critical review. Isr J Med Sci 33:808–815, 1997

Fugh-Berman A, Ernst E: Herb-drug interactions: review and assessment of report reliability. Br J Clin Pharmacol 52:587–595, 2003

Gurely B, Gardner S, Hubbard M: Content versus label claims in ephedra-containing dietary supplements. Am J Health Syst Pharm 57:1–7, 2000

Heck AM, DeWitt BA, Lukes AL: Potential interactions between alternative therapies and warfarin. Am J Health Syst Pharm 57:1221–1227, 2000

Herzog A, Shore M, Beale R, et al: Patient safety and psychiatry: recommendations to the board of trustees of the American Psychiatric Association. The American Psychiatric Association Task Force on Patient Safety. November 24, 2002. Available at: www.psych.org/edu/other_res/lib_archives/archives/tfr/tfr200301.pdf

Huang W, Wen K, Hsiao M: Adulteration by synthetic therapeutic substances of traditional Chinese medicines in Taiwan. J Clin Pharmacol 37:334–350, 1997

Huggett D: Organochlorine pesticides and metals in select botanical dietary supplements. Bull Environ Contam Toxicol 66:150–155, 2001

Jacobs K, Hirsch K: Case reports: psychiatric complications of Ma-Huang. Psychosomatics 41:58–62, 2000

Lake J: The integration of Chinese medicine and Western medicine: focus on mental illness. Integr Med 3:20–28, 2004

Leo R: Movement disorders associated with the serotonin selective reuptake inhibitors. J Clin Psychiatry 57:449–454, 1999

Lo AC, Chan K, Yeung JH, et al: Danggui (*Angelica sinensis*) affects the pharmacodynamics but not the pharmacokinetics of warfarin in rabbits. Eur J Drug Metab Pharmacokinet 20:55–60, 1995

Mechcatie E: FDA plans to strengthen drug safety program. Clinical Psychiatry News, January 2005, p 8

Miller L: Herbal medicinals: selected clinical considerations focusing on known or potential drug-herb interactions. Arch Intern Med 158:2200–2211, 1998

National Consumers League: "Natural" or "plant-derived" labelling can mislead. January 17, 2002. Available at: nclnet.org/news/2002/natural_labeling.htm

Natural Marketing Institute: The Dietary Supplement Trends Report. Philadelphia, PA, Natural Marketing Institute, April 1, 2002. Available at: www.marketresearch.com

Nerurkar PV, Dragull K, Tang CS: In vitro toxicity of kava alkaloid, pipermethystine, in HepG2 cells compared to kavalactones. Toxicol Sci 79:106–111, 2004

Schatzberg A, Haddad P, Kaplan E, et al: Serotonin reuptake inhibitor discontinuation syndrome: a hypothetical definition. Discontinuation Consensus Panel. J Clin Psychiatry 58 (suppl 7):5–10, 1997

Spollen J, Spollen S, Markowitz J: Psychiatric side effects of herbal medicinals. Journal of Pharmacy Practice 12:196–209, 1999

U.S. Department of Health and Human Services: FDA announces plans to prohibit sales of dietary supplements containing ephedra. December 30, 2003. Available at: www.hhs.gov/news/press/2003pres/20031230.html

U.S. Food and Drug Administration: FDA Announces Major Initiatives for Dietary Supplements. November 4, 2004. Available at: www.fda.gov/bbs/topics/news/2004/NEW01130.html

Zeisel S: Regulation of "neutraceuticals." Science 285:1853–1855, 1999

4

Integrative Approaches

James Lake, M.D.

This chapter reviews the conceptual foundations and methods of integrative medicine, especially as they pertain to mental health care. (A more in-depth treatment of this topic is available in Lake [2006].)

APPROACH OF CURRENT MEDICAL SYSTEMS

The primary role of psychiatrists and family practice physicians is increasingly becoming to treat illness through medication prescription and management; other nonconventional approaches to treatment are frequently excluded as being unscientific, even before the available evidence is appraised. Alternative medical practitioners are guilty of a similar myopic perspective when they encourage patients to accept only the treatments they recommend and dismiss conventional Western medicine as too conservative, rigid, or parochial. In mental health care, the situation is further complicated by the fact that conventionally trained psychotherapists provide psychotherapy only and refer patients to psychiatrists for medication management consultations (but not adjunctive psychotherapy) only when psychological symptoms persist or become severe after a prolonged trial on a particular psychotherapeutic "regimen." These three perspectives reflect the disparate professional trainings, personal values, and financial interests of Western physicians, psychotherapists, and alternative medical practitioners. Each perspective contains inherent biases rooted in different ideologies and approaches to professional clinical training. The lack of common ground among these conflicting perspectives potentially results in treatment delays, inappropriate or inadequate patient care, and poor outcomes.

Patients themselves are more frequently seeking care for mental health problems from several practitioners, each trained in disparate conventional and nonconventional approaches, and receiving many conventional or nonconventional treatments for the same complaint. When patients experience a lack of response to a particular conventional pharmacological, psychotherapeutic, or nonconventional treatment, they eventually pursue other treatment choices. This process often takes place with limited reliable information about the comparative efficacy or safety of different treatment choices. For patients being treated by several practitioners, there is typically little or no dialogue among the conventionally trained physicians, alternative medical practitioners, and psychotherapists who work with the same patient, sometimes resulting in patients receiving contradictory advice from these practitioners. The practical consequences of this lack of dialogue include misdiagnoses or missed diagnoses, treatment delays, or treatment combinations that are not synergistic, are incompatible, or are potentially unsafe. Integrative medicine can help to resolve these problems by providing methods for identifying treatment combinations that address the patient's unique symptoms, history, needs, preferences, and circumstances.

UNDERSTANDING INTEGRATIVE MEDICINE
Philosophy

Integrative health care is difficult to characterize because of the highly divergent perspectives of patients and medical practitioners and the complex degrees of integration possible when biomedical and nonconventional treatments are used together. It is anchored on two premises: 1) that combining approaches from disparate traditions of medicine can be beneficial and 2) that the most effective or relevant treatment regimen should always be determined on a case-by-case basis with the active involvement of the patient.

First, integrative medicine takes the perspective that combining biomedical, complementary, and alternative treatments on a case-by-case basis offers significant advantages over any specific treatment or single system of medicine. Thus, the methods of integrative medicine are broader and more encompassing than those of a particular treatment approach or healing tradition. The practical methods of integrative medicine aimed at ensuring safety and efficacy are still under development.

Second, the effectiveness of a particular conventional, alternative, or integrative treatment regimen will probably vary considerably in relation to the unique symptoms and circumstances of every patient. Treatment planning methods in integrative medicine address these issues by considering the patient's unique symptoms in the context of realistic constraints on treatment cost and the availability of qualified conventional or nonconventional practitioners. The peer-reviewed literature on integrative medicine suggests that the key aspects of this patient-oriented medicine are a collaborative partnership between patient and practitioner, the interdisciplinary blending of conventional and nonconventional treatments, and an emphasis on enhanced cost-effectiveness of treatment through combining disparate therapies (Boon et al. 2004). Integrative health care neither rejects conventional biomedical treatments nor uncritically accepts alternative and complementary medicine (CAM) approaches (Gaudet 1998).

Role of Clinician and Patient in Integrative Medicine

In conventional biomedicine, the clinician's primary goals are to diagnose and treat pathological conditions. Patients assume that the end point of treatment will be a return to good health. In contrast, the central goals in integrative health care include the exploration of ways to achieve a greater "balance" in their lives, a spiritual harmony, or healthy lifestyle changes that promote self-healing, including improved nutrition and exercise and possibly also enhanced self-awareness through a regular mind–body practice. The clinician's responsibilities to the patient depend on the kind of conventional or nonconventional treatment provided. The patient's responsibilities to the treatment process include compliance with agreed-on nutritional or lifestyle changes, mind–body practices, or conventional medications.

When developing an individualized integrative treatment plan, the clinician and patient work together to clarify target symptoms and agree on outcomes. As in conventional biomedicine, in integrative health care, the clinician and patient must agree on the meaning of treatment as well as specific treatment goals and a time frame in which beneficial effects can reasonably be expected to be achieved. Integrative treatment planning should be flexible and responsive to changing symptoms, circumstances, or patient preferences.

EVOLUTION OF TRADITIONAL MEDICINE TOWARD AN INTEGRATIVE MEDICAL SYSTEM

Recognition of Philosophical Differences

Attempts to understand how to combine research methods and treatments from disparate systems of medicine lead to important philosophical problems. Disparate assumptions about the nature of phenomenal reality are implicit in different systems of medicine and are the basis of efficacy claims pertaining to the range of theories and practices in each system. Thus, from the perspective of biomedicine and other established systems of medicine, there is seldom a motivation to develop objective methods (i.e., methods that are outside of any particular paradigm) for substantiating beliefs about the causes or conditions of illness and health because such beliefs are implicit in the philosophical structure of each system. A frequently described example is the belief in Chinese medicine that a universal energetic process (*qi*) exists independently of conventional models of space and time or biological functioning and determines the essential energetic balance that is manifested as health or illness. Ayurveda, perhaps the oldest system of medicine, bases an analogous energetic model of illness and health on a postulated vital energy called *prana*. In these systems, energy states that correspond to particular symptoms are subjectively knowable and can be clearly described by the patient and unambiguously interpreted by a trained clinician. The basic tenets of biomedicine no longer rely on vitalist interpretations of natural phenomena such as the causes or conditions of illness and health. On the other hand, contemporary biomedicine incorporates the broad philosophical assumptions of Western science, declaring that fundamental realities, including the brain and other complex biological systems, are ultimately material in nature (although this distinction admittedly does not hold in contemporary Western science at the level of subatomic particles, which are formalized in terms of energy, probability distributions, and fields) and that health or illness phenomena are reducible to certain basic physical, chemical, and biological processes.

Different assumptions about primary categories of existence embedded in disparate systems of medicine correspond to different methodological approaches for validating claims of treatment mechanisms or verifying that claimed outcomes actually take place. Just as practitioners of Western biomedicine do not see a need to substantiate the ideas and methods of that paradigm in terms of traditional Chinese medicine, Ayurveda, or other world systems of medicine, practitioners of these so-called nonconventional systems of medicine do not see a need to reconcile their theories and techniques with Western biomedicine. Thus, claims of energetic and material processes that underlie health or illness are asserted as factual statements that are implicit assumptions in Chinese medicine and Western biomedicine, respectively. It follows that there is no need (from either perspective) to argue toward energetic or material phenomena in illness and health from first principles.

Because of the above-noted fundamental conceptual gaps between major world systems of medicine, efforts to achieve a common philosophy of integrative medicine are bound to fail. However, the problem of developing integrative assessment and treatment approaches can be addressed at the practical levels of compatibility and outcomes.

Growth of Integrative Health Care Around the World

Integrative approaches are in wide use despite the absence of compelling scientific evidence for most specific treatment combinations. Approximately half of the adult populations of all industrialized countries use nonconventional (i.e., nonbiomedical) treatments on a regular basis (Bodeker 2001). In many countries, multiple approaches to healing are used contemporaneously with little or no guidance from health professionals, regulatory oversight bodies, or government policies regarding safe or effective integration of these approaches. The results of a large survey conducted in 2002 showed that over half of the U.S. adult population used nonconventional treatments in an integrative fashion (Barnes et al. 2004). Most individuals who use any nonconventional approach do so out of the belief that combining nonconventional treatments with conventional biomedical treatments will have beneficial results.

Different countries have addressed this problem in two general ways: making disparate treatments available as separate medical services that patients may choose to combine with other treatments and formally integrating disparate treatments at the levels of medical education and clinical services. The national health services of the United Kingdom, other European Union countries, India, and South Korea have adopted the former model, whereas Taiwan and China follow the latter approach (Steering Committee 1997). In contrast to the United Kingdom's successful efforts to integrate nonconventional approaches into mainstream medicine, government-backed efforts to "modernize" Chinese medicine through the integration of Western drugs and other biomedical approaches have not succeeded in Taiwan and China. In both countries, traditional (Chinese) medicine and Western biomedical services coexist in parallel and are provided by qualified clinicians, but patients are seldom treated in a truly integrative manner (Chi 1994). In Taiwan, it is estimated that roughly two-thirds of all adults use Western drugs in combination with Chinese herbs or acupuncture treatments for a variety of medical and psychiatric problems. The Chinese approach to integration through modernization has been criticized in recent decades because the government has prioritized biomedical treatments and Western style research over traditional Chinese healing approaches. For example, traditional medical education in China requires students to master fewer acupuncture points than was required before the mid-1960s and the Cultural Revolution. The same trend is taking place in the United States, where conventionally trained physicians are regarded as qualified to perform acupuncture after becoming familiar with only a few acupuncture points and basic protocols during brief, intensive "medical acupuncture" training programs. There is a concern that if this trend continues, efforts to simplify and "extract" techniques from highly evolved systems of medicine and adapt them to biomedicine may eliminate the therapeutic benefits of many nonconventional modalities (Gaudet 1998).

Integrative Health Care as the De Facto Standard in the United States

Growing numbers of conventionally trained U.S. physicians believe that nonconventional medical treatments are effective and routinely refer patients to alternative medical practitioners while continuing to manage the patients' conventional medical care (Astin et al. 1998; Ernst et al. 1995). For example, when all medical and psychiatric indications are considered, 43% of conventionally trained physicians refer patients to acupuncturists, 40% refer to chiropractors, and 21% refer to massage therapists (Astin et al. 1998). In the United States, 26% of doctors believe that homeopathy is a legitimate form of therapy and refer patients to homeopaths or prescribe homeopathic remedies themselves. Many medical doctors are trained in at least one nonconventional medical approach and actively incorporate it in their medical practice (Astin et al. 1998). These trends clearly demonstrate that because of changing beliefs and shifting practice patterns of conventionally trained physicians and a growing public interest in nonconventional medicine, the broad base of orthodox medicine in the United States and other industrialized countries is rapidly evolving into a de facto system of integrative health care. However, many integrative regimens are frequently used in the absence of compelling evidence for their efficacy or safety. For example, in mental health care, although certain natural products have synergistic effects when combined with antidepressants, at present little evidence supports the combined use of most natural products and conventional drugs. (Combinations of folic acid or certain omega-3 fatty acids with a conventional antidepressant are examples of integrative regimens for which there is emerging evidence.)

Factors to Consider in Regard to Increasing the Integration of Medical Systems

The future of integrative health care as an important social trend and an emerging paradigm in Western medicine remains unclear, with many basic questions about the efficacy and safety of integrative approaches not yet having been answered. In addition, many complex factors favor or interfere with the movement of Western biomedicine toward integration with nonconventional approaches.

The coexistence of disparate systems of medicine in the same country raises complex ethical, medicolegal, and regulatory issues. For example, although some societal frameworks favor the coexistence of disparate systems of medicine and their respective ideological foundations (i.e., medical pluralism), others favor novel combined uses of disparate healing approaches and the creation of truly integrative regimens. The dynamic balance of factors favoring medical pluralism versus integration ultimately depends on the social, cultural, and economic background in which diverse healing methods are practiced in a particular country or world region. For these reasons, the "shape" of medical culture is substantially different within countries and over time in any given country (Steering Committee 1997).

Factors Against Increasing Integration

It has been argued that most CAM modalities are unproven and have unknown risks. On this basis, an accurate risk-benefit analysis of nonconventional medical approaches is not possible at this time, and the integration of nonconventional approaches into mainstream medical treatments based on unsubstantiated claims would be irresponsible. Furthermore, in many countries, there are no minimum standards of competence for nonconventional medical practitioners, thus making it difficult for patients and referring providers to identify qualified practitioners. Finally, prematurely combining nonconventional therapies and biomedical treatments before rigorous studies have verified their safety and effectiveness almost always results in disappointment (Ernst 1997).

Bias among practitioners also presents seemingly insurmountable hurdles to integration. Nonconventional medical practitioners seldom refer patients to physicians and other conventionally trained medical practitioners because they regard them as being focused on only one narrow dimension of health and illness (i.e., biological functioning). In a similar vein, conventional medical practitioners seldom refer patients to nonconventional practitioners because their methods are viewed as unscientific. The situation is complicated by the fact that most insurance providers do not cover the cost of nonconventional therapies. In addition, physicians and other conventionally trained medical practitioners who administer treatments that are not acknowledged to be within the scope of their medical specialty are liable to malpractice. Physicians also assume liability when referring patients to nonconventional medical practitioners and may face disciplinary action from their state medical board, resulting in probation, suspension, or possibly revocation of their medical license (Green 1996). (See Chapter 2 for a review of important medicolegal issues pertaining to referral of patients to CAM practitioners.)

Factors in Favor of Increasing Integration

The above criticisms of CAM treatments should apply equally to all traditions of medicine. Many patients seek a nonconventional practitioner after expensive conventional treatments have failed and their physician is unable to advise them about appropriate nonconventional treatment choices. The holistic perspective of nonconventional practitioners emphasizes inexpensive treatments using natural products and healthy lifestyle changes and helps patients feel they have greater control over their illness (Rees 2001). In developing countries, traditional medical practitioners continue to fulfill most health care needs, and the World Health Organization actively encourages the integration of traditional healing approaches and biomedical treatments. Herbal medicines and other treatments derived from natural products that have demonstrated efficacy are widely used to treat a range of medical and mental health problems (Zhang 2000).

OBTAINING RELIABLE INFORMATION ABOUT NONCONVENTIONAL APPROACHES

It is often difficult to obtain reliable research or clinical practice information about nonconventional approaches. Textbooks are probably the most useful resources for general background information on theories and methods. Searching online databases is the most efficient approach to obtaining information about specific clinical or research questions (Guyatt and Rennie 2002). A useful resource for planning Internet searches on CAM treatments is *Complementary Therapies on the Internet* (Beckner and Berman 2003). The National Center for Complementary and Alternative Medicine and several programs in integrative medicine affiliated with medical centers have established excellent Web sites on CAM therapies, providing links to quality online resources that will be helpful for obtaining general information about a particular modality (Wilson et al. 2002a). Searching the *Cochrane Collaboration* databases is the most efficient method for obtaining reliable critically reviewed information on nonconventional treatments. There are several Cochrane databases. For modalities that have been extensively researched, the best starting place is the *Cochrane Systematic Reviews*. These reviews are probably more useful than other narrative reviews because inclusion and exclusion criteria are clearly stated and excluded studies are identified (Ezzo et al. 2002). The reader is thus aware of the specific studies examined or excluded and detailed reasons for these decisions. The *Cochrane Clinical Controlled Trials Registry* is probably the most useful database when searching for information about nonconventional approaches for which systematic reviews have not yet been done. The National Library of Medicine's *PubMed* (www.pubmed.gov) and other mainstream medical databases should be considered a second-tier resource, because they contain fewer than half of all published clinical trials on CAM therapies and few non–English articles and will therefore provide limited relevant information (Gray 2004).

Searching online resources is no longer a challenging task. There are four basic steps to searching for medical information on the Internet: 1) clearly formulating the question, 2) using appropriate search tools and methods, 3) conducting and refining searches, and 4) interpreting search findings and determining whether they apply to a particular patient (Beckner and Berman 2003; Wilson et al. 2002a). Formulating an unambiguous question is the most important step in searching for information on any subject. A clearly stated query containing specific key words is more likely to result in useful clinical information than a vaguely worded query containing ambiguous terms. Different search engines are available for conducting the online searches. Yahoo and Google are very inclusive search tools, whereas other search engines will probably result in fewer "hits" or relevant findings pertaining to CAM (Beckner and Berman 2003). The number and quality of results will depend in part on the search engine that is used. Following the same logic used when searching the Internet, four basic steps have been suggested for appraising evidence obtained from searches: 1) determining whether the study question was clearly formulated, 2) determining whether the study design adequately addressed the question, 3) appraising the quality of findings, and 4) determining whether the findings can be validly applied to a particular patient (Wilson et al. 2002b).

When there is little or no peer-reviewed literature on a particular nonconventional modality, expert consensus is a reasonable starting place for evaluating that modality. Most nonconventional medical practitioners are affiliated with a professional association that provides clinical practice guidelines based on expert consensus. The National Guideline Clearinghouse (www.guideline.gov) and the *Concise Guide to Evidence-Based Psychiatry* (Gray 2004; see especially page 30) are useful resources for obtaining high-quality practice guidelines. It is important to note that many guidelines are based on expert consensus and do not meet strict standards of evidence-based medicine. In the absence of published peer-reviewed articles and clinical practice guidelines, it is sometimes necessary to manually search conference proceedings or specialty journals on a particular nonconventional modality. Relevant journals can usually be identified by contacting CAM associations (see Appendix C).

TOWARD METHODS FOR PLANNING INTEGRATIVE HEALTH CARE

Qualitative Versus Quantitative Evidence for Integration of Modalities

The perceived utility of quantitative versus qualitative information on medical treatments is based on different epistemological assumptions. Quantitative information can be regarded as an index of rigor, whereas qualitative findings can be viewed as an index of a particular treatment's relevance to the needs of a particular patient (Richardson 2002). Both kinds of information are useful when assessing the safety, effectiveness, and cost-effectiveness of any integrative treatment plan. Quantitative evidence assumes that general conclusions about clinical treatment decisions can be validly inferred from specific findings and assessed on the basis of the statistical significance of findings; quantitative methods are the mainstay of biomedical research. In contrast, qualitative evidence is based on subjective, patient-centered criteria for determining satisfaction with treatment outcomes, including beneficial changes in social or occupational functioning (Liverani 2000). Qualitative methods are useful for assessing the impact of a treatment on quality of life.

Consistent, statistically significant positive outcomes from multiple randomized, double-blind, controlled trials are the gold standards of evidence for all biomedical treatment, and qualitative evidence is often overlooked. However, the value of randomized, controlled trials is limited because they only show effects that are statistically significant according to predefined criteria; they do not address why an intervention is effective, meaningful, or beneficial for a particular patient. In contrast, many nonconventional modalities are assessed (by practitioners and patients) only on the basis of qualitative evidence that is accepted as valid in the absence of corroborating research studies. Furthermore, many nonconventional modalities (including mind–body techniques, "energy" medicine, and others) are not susceptible to quantitative research methods because interventions are frequently complex and lack standardization, treatment goals and outcomes are often difficult or impossible to quantify, and identifying an appropriate placebo is usually difficult or impossible (Verhoef et al. 2002). When combining conventional and nonconventional modalities, it is appropriate and necessary to use both quantitative and qualitative criteria to adequately capture all pertinent evidence for rigor and relevance of an integrative approach with respect to a specified medical or psychiatric problem (Vuckovic 2002).

Much reliable information is available on some herbal medicines and other treatments derived from natural products. However, the use of other nonconventional approaches is based largely on open studies, case reports, or anecdotal information. Research programs sponsored by the National Center for Complementary and Alternative Medicine are in the early stages of identifying safe and efficacious integrative treatment strategies for addressing numerous medical and psychiatric illnesses (Riley and Heger 1999). At present, a paucity of clinically useful information is available for the purpose of planning integrative treatments addressing specific medical or psychiatric problems. Nevertheless, conventional biomedical treatments continue to be frequently used in combination with nonconventional modalities. The debate continues over what constitutes "sufficient" evidence for combining disparate modalities (Walach 2001).

Consideration of Patient Safety When Using Integrated Treatments

Safety issues are obviously important when considering whether to use two or more treatments together. At present, limited research findings from randomized, controlled studies support the clinical use of particular combinations of biomedical and nonconventional treatment when addressing specific medical or psychiatric problems.

Because there is limited reliable information on most nonconventional treatments, safety risks associated with combinations of certain nonconventional therapies and synthetic drugs are poorly understood. Practical, safe approaches to planning integrative health care must take into account the limitations of available information. In this context, only conservative strategies for integrating disparate treatments should be considered until further research can provide more answers on the safety and efficacy of combined treatments. Presented below are a few provisional guidelines presented as "levels of evidence" supporting clinical decisions when integration is being considered. These guidelines will be useful for physicians and alternative medical practitioners interested in finding safe and effective ways to combine different treatment approaches in integrative health care:

• It is reasonable to consider combining two (or more) disparate biomedical or nonconventional treatments when consistent findings from randomized controlled trials support the efficacy and safety of the specified combination for a designated medical or psychiatric problem.

- In the absence of strong research evidence, it is reasonable to consider combining two (or more) disparate treatments when consistent case reports suggest that the specified combination is both safe and effective when treating a specified problem.
- In cases where research evidence or consistent findings from case reports do not support the use of a particular treatment combination, it may be reasonable to consider the specified integrative approach if it is in widespread use among professional conventional or nonconventional medical practitioners and there is informal consensus over its use for a specified problem.
- Two (or more) disparate biomedical or nonconventional treatments should never be used in combination when findings from controlled trials show that the specified combination is unsafe, lacks efficacy for a specified problem, or both.
- Two (or more) disparate treatments should not be combined when consistent findings from case reports suggest that the specified integrative approach is unsafe, lacks efficacy for a specified problem, or both.
- Combinations of two (or more) disparate treatments for which there is limited or no research evidence or case reports should be avoided if conventional or nonconventional medical practitioners who are knowledgeable about the treatments in question believe that the specified approach is unsafe or lacks efficacy.

In practice, numerous CAM therapies are widely used in combination with synthetic drugs or other conventional biomedical therapies, and few serious safety issues have been reported. Combining synthetic drugs with nonconventional therapies that are not based on potent biological mechanisms of action and affect the body in general ways is probably safe in most cases. This is true because the general beneficial effects of improved nutrition, exercise, mindfulness training, and mind–body practices and possibly also energy therapies do not potentially interfere with the highly specific pharmacodynamic and pharmacokinetic actions of synthetic drugs, thus eliminating the danger of serious biologically mediated toxicities or adverse interactions.

Treating physicians should also be aware that almost two-thirds of patients who use nonconventional therapies do not disclose this fact to their physicians (Eisenberg et al. 1998). In 1997 (the last year for which accurate data are available), approximately 15 million U.S. adults used prescription medications concurrently with herbal remedies or high-dose vitamins, resulting in unknown risks of toxicities or interactions (Eisenberg et al. 1998). The number of users of multiple therapies and the potential magnitude of risk associated with this practice have probably continued to increase since that time.

INTEGRATIVE ASSESSMENT AND TREATMENT PLANNING IN MENTAL HEALTH CARE

This section provides a brief overview of methods for deriving safe, effective, and appropriate integrative approaches in mental health care. A more detailed treatment, including a comprehensive review of the evidence for specific non-conventional modalities, is available in Lake (2006). The primary goal of integrative mental health care is to develop a suitable treatment strategy that adequately addresses the patient's complaint and is both acceptable to the patient and realistic. This approach is based on a series of methods for constructing practical solutions to clinical problems. Integrative health care begins with taking a patient's history, progresses to treatment planning, and continues with outcome assessment. This process is intrinsically iterative in that emerging findings suggest new treatment approaches that may in turn lead to different outcomes calling for novel kinds of assessment and so forth.

Integrative assessment and treatment cannot be used as a substitute for psychotherapy in addressing primary psychological issues or life problems that cannot be resolved using biological, somatic, mind–body, or energetic therapies. Appropriate psychotherapy should be combined with thoughtful integrative mental health care when the patient has the capacity for insight and is motivated to do psychological work that will help him or her achieve insight or resolve conflicts. As is true of biomedicine and all nonconventional paradigms in medicine, the conceptual framework in which a medical or psychiatric problem is framed will determine the explanation that is regarded as sufficient and judgments about the most appropriate treatment, which in turn will define and limit potential outcomes. The same is true when approaching dynamic issues using psychotherapy. In this context, in contrast to conventional models of supportive therapy or cognitive-behavioral therapy, existential and transpersonal psychotherapies are based on a synthesis of Eastern and Western psychologies and thus permit insights into a broader range of psychodynamic issues and normal versus abnormal states of consciousness than does either tradition alone (Walsh 1996). These more "synthetic" approaches to psychotherapy are analogous to integrative mental health care in that they provide the patient with a broader range of interventions than are generally available through conventional forms of psychotherapy, thus enhancing opportunities for beneficial insights or beneficial psychological or spiritual growth.

Integrative Assessment

Like treatment planning, integrative assessment is a multidimensional process that takes into account a range of factors that may be causally related to the symptom pattern that is being addressed. The integration of conventional and nonconventional assessment approaches should be considered in cases where conventional approaches fail to provide specific accurate information about the causes of a mental health problem. Integrative assessment in mental health care will

- Be useful when the medical–psychiatric differential diagnosis is complicated or vague, requiring additional clarification.
- Use emerging approaches that are presently outside of mainstream medicine, including quantitative electroencephalography, serological studies of immunological or endocrine factors, and other approaches that may clarify underlying causes of psychiatric symptoms or provide specific markers for disorders.
- Clarify the etiologies of complex presentations related to psychological, biological, energetic, or other factors by combining assessment approaches from conventional biomedicine and nonconventional medical traditions.

Integrative Treatment Planning

A well-planned integrative assessment will result in a range of quantitative and qualitative findings that will permit patient-specific, effective, and cost-effective integrative treatment planning. The treatment plan will combine biomedical and nonconventional treatments to target disparate psychological, biological, somatic, mind–body, and possibly energetic or spiritual factors underlying psychiatric symptom patterns. Integrative treatment planning in mental health care

- Begins with a thorough review of history and previous treatments.
- Uses rigorous methods to identify appropriate, safe, and effective conventional and nonconventional treatment options.
- Endorses rigorous standards of evidence and treatment planning algorithms for developing individualized integrative treatment strategies.
- Requires a high degree of collaboration and communication between Western-trained physicians and nonconventional medical practitioners.
- Will take into account new findings on reviewing outcomes (or lack thereof), resulting in appropriate changes in an integrative treatment regimen that is realistic and acceptable to the patient.

Selection of a Core Treatment

The goal of integrative treatment planning is to identify the most substantiated, realistic, and patient-compatible regimen that is effective against the target symptom pattern. The first step in this process involves identifying the conventional or nonconventional treatment with the strongest evidence base that has not yet been tried for the target symptom pattern. If the patient reports that all validated treatments for his or her symptom pattern have already been tried but without benefit, the clinician should carefully review the patient's history to ensure that the dosing or duration of those treatments was adequate. In cases where a substantiated conventional or nonconventional approach was used appropriately and remained ineffective, the clinician should consider combination therapies. When considering which treatments, the clinician should recommend a core treatment around which an integrative treatment regimen can be constructed. A *core treatment* is a modality that is substantiated as effective and safe for the target symptom pattern being addressed. Biological, somatic, mind–body, or other approaches may qualify as core treatments depending on the available evidence supporting their use with respect to the target symptom pattern. When two or more core treatments are supported by evidence of equal weight (i.e., they are substantiated treatments that have not yet been tried by the patient or have been tried but within a subtherapeutic regimen), the practitioner and patient should identify the most appropriate core treatment on the basis of patient preferences while taking into account realistic constraints imposed by cost or availability. Examples of core biologically active treatments for depressed mood are the selective serotonin reuptake inhibitors or S-adenosylmethionine (SAMe). An example of a core somatic treatment for depressed mood is regular physical exercise.

Development of a Realistic Integrative Treatment Plan

After a core treatment has been selected, the practitioner and patient should work together to design a realistic integrative treatment plan that includes approaches that are compatible or synergistic with the core treatment and acceptable to the patient. Suggesting an integrative treatment plan that the patient cannot afford or is unmotivated to pursue will result in disappointment; thus, the patient's input is essential for successful integrative planning. One advantage of integrative treatments is that patients often feel more proactive in obtaining them and therefore more involved in their care.

If the selected core treatment is a biologically active substance (e.g., a synthetic drug, herb, other natural product), other biologically active treatments should be added only when there is strong evidence that the treatments are compatible and each treatment is efficacious against the target symptom. It is best to start with treatments that are synergistic—that is, when combined, they improve the outcome compared with either treatment alone. Examples of synergistic biologically active treatments of depressed mood include SAMe taken together with vitamin B_{12} and folate and selective serotonin reuptake inhibitors taken together with omega-3 fatty acids.

A biologically active core treatment can also be combined with nonbiological treatments, including somatic treatments, mind–body practices, treatments based on forms of energy that are validated by Western science, and treatments based on postulated subtle energies that are not validated by Western science. When considering which nonbiological treatment to use in conjunction with a core biological treatment, those treatments that have the strongest evidence base with respect to the target symptom pattern should be considered first. If two or more nonbiological treatments are supported by an equal weight of evidence, the patient and practitioner should identify the approach that is most affordable and available and that the patient is motivated to pursue. For example, although yoga practice is an effective core treatment for generalized anxiety, recommending daily yoga exercises to a busy corporate executive who expresses disdain for mind–body practices will almost certainly end in disappointment and treatment failure.

If the core treatment is a nonbiological approach (e.g., a somatic approach, a mind–body method, a treatment based on a form of energy that is validated by Western science) and the patient, after using the approach as prescribed or under appropriate supervision, has not improved within a reasonably expected time or the target symptoms have worsened, it is reasonable to consider changing the core treatment or adding another treatment. As noted above, treatments that are most substantiated with respect to the target symptom pattern should be considered first. The practitioner and patient should work together to identify an integrative treatment plan that combines compatible modalities that are affordable, locally available, and of interest to the patient. Table 4–1 lists integrative treatment strategies for many common psychiatric disorders.

Modifying the Treatment Plan

The process of integrative treatment planning is highly iterative; that is, new combinations are tried until an effective regimen is identified that is realistic for the patient receiving treatment. In cases where all substantiated treatments or treatment combinations have been tried for a particular symptom pattern without benefit, it is reasonable to consider integrative approaches that include less substantiated treatments. At this stage of treatment planning, it is reasonable to consider combining a provisional treatment that has not yet been tried with a substantiated treatment that the patient wishes to continue and that may be more effective when used in combination with the provisional treatment. As in conventional mental health care, the frequency of follow-up appointments will depend on symptom severity and the need to evaluate the patient's response to treatment. During follow-up appointments, the integrative treatment plan can be modified on the basis of emerging history, new assessment findings, and treatment response.

It is important for the practitioner to note that treatments that are considered to be substantiated with respect to a particular symptom pattern will change over time as new research findings emerge. For example, certain conventional or nonconventional treatments that are currently regarded as substantiated for the treatment of depressed mood will be viewed as provisional or ineffective treatments in the future. For this reason, it is important for the clinician to stay current with the research evidence for the range of conventional and nonconventional treatments.

TABLE 4–1. Integrative treatment strategies for common psychiatric disorders

Disorder	Validated integrative treatments	Comments
Major depressive disorder	Antidepressant efficacy is enhanced when SAMe is used with folate and vitamin B_{12} (Crellin et al. 1993).	Folate and B_{12} are essential cofactors for SAMe
	Combining an omega-3 fatty acid (the ethyl ester of eicosapentaenoic acid) 1–2 g/day with a conventional antidepressant may improve antidepressant response (Nemets et al. 2002).	Provisional finding; studies ongoing
	The mood-elevating benefits of exercise are enhanced by exposure to bright light (Partonen et al. 1998).	Greater antidepressant effect of combined approach compared with exercise or bright-light exposure alone
Bipolar disorder	EMPowerPlus, a nutrient formula, is a beneficial adjunctive treatment of both phases of bipolar illness (Kaplan et al. 2001).	*Caution:* Toxic interactions are possible when EMPowerPlus is combined with a conventional drug.
	Combining omega-3 fatty acids 1–2 g/day with a conventional mood stabilizer may reduce the severity and frequency of manic episodes (Stoll et al. 1999).	Provisional finding; studies ongoing
Schizophrenia	Combining an omega-3 fatty acid (the ethyl ester of eicosapentaenoic acid) 1–4 g/day with a conventional antipsychotic may improve outcomes (Peet et al. 2002).	Inconsistent findings; studies ongoing; large doses of omega-3 fatty acids may cause adverse gastrointestinal effects
	Combining estrogen with a conventional antipsychotic may improve response (Kulkarni et al. 2001).	*Caution:* Estrogen potentially increases the risk of breast cancer in susceptible women.

TABLE 4–1. Integrative treatment strategies for common psychiatric disorders *(continued)*

Anxiety disorders	Regular electromyogram, galvanic skin response, and electroencephalogram, and biofeedback may permit dosage reductions of conventional antianxiety drugs in patients with generalized anxiety disorder (Sarkar et al. 1999).	The benefits of biofeedback may not be sustained after treatment ends.
	Microcurrent electrical stimulation may permit dose reductions of conventional antianxiety drugs in phobic patients (Smith and Shiromoto 1992).	The residual benefits of this approach may continue for prolonged periods.
Dementia	Acetyl-L-carnitine (1.5–3 g/day) combined with omega-3 fatty acids or α–lipoic acid may slow progression in Alzheimer's disease and age–related memory loss (Hager et al. 2001; Lolic et al. 1997).	Acetyl-L-carnitine is well tolerated, with few adverse effects being reported.
	Regular physical exercise (Abbott et al. 2004), moderate wine consumption, and reduced dietary saturated fat reduce the risk of all categories of dementia (Grant 1997).	Medically ill or physically impaired individuals should consult their physicians before starting an exercise program or modifying their diets.
Alcohol abuse	Supplementation with certain amino acids may have beneficial effects in alcoholic individuals. SAMe (Lieber 2000) may reduce alcohol intake. Taurine may reduce alcohol withdrawal (Ikeda 1977). Acetyl-L-carnitine may enhance cognitive performance in abstinent alcoholic individuals (Tempesta et al. 1990); L-tryptophan may reduce alcohol cravings (Westrick et al. 1988).	A deficit in brain serotonin may be present in individuals with chronic alcoholism; supplementation with amino acids that increase central nervous system serotonin may have beneficial effects.

CONCLUSION

Physicians are increasingly referring patients to clinicians who practice outside the domain of orthodox Western medicine. On the basis of conventional medical research and critical examination of concepts from alternative systems of medicine, including the putative links among mental illness, stress, and endocrine and immunological dysfunction, novel integrative approaches to assessment and treatment will gradually emerge in the coming decades. This evolutionary process will result in novel models of disease and healing that will take into account the complex, dynamic interaction among social, biological, psychological, and possibly also spiritual and energetic factors, resulting in integrative assessment and treatment approaches that address the range of medical and psychiatric disorders. The continuing evolution of biomedicine and other major world systems of medicine toward a truly integrative paradigm will permit a deeper, more complete understanding of fundamental biological, informational, and energetic processes associated with disease and healing. In future decades, a truly integrative medicine will address mental and emotional symptoms on the basis of methods that combine effective, cost-effective, and relevant biomedical, mind–body, somatic, and possibly also spiritual and energetic approaches on a case-by-case basis.

REFERENCES

Abbott R, White L, Ross W, et al: Walking and dementia in physically capable elderly men. JAMA 292:1447–1453, 2004

Astin J, Marie A, Pelletier K, et al: A review of the incorporation of complementary and alternative medicine by mainstream physicians. Arch Intern Med 158:2303–2310, 1998

Barnes P, Powell-Griner E, McFann K, et al: Complementary and alternative medicine use among adults: United States, 2002. Seminars in Integrative Medicine 2:54–71, 2004

Beckner W, Berman B: Complementary Therapies on the Internet. St. Louis, MO, Churchill Livingstone, 2003

Bodeker G: Lessons on integration from the developing world's experience. BMJ 322:164–167, 2001

Boon H, Verhoef M, O'Hara D, et al: Integrative health care: arriving at a working definition. Altern Ther Health Med 10:48–56, 2004

Chi C: Integrating traditional medicine into modern health care systems: examining the role of Chinese medicine in Taiwan. Soc Sci Med 39:307–321, 1994

Crellin R, Bottiglieri T, Reynolds E: Folates and psychiatric disorders: clinical potential. Drugs 45:623–636, 1993

Eisenberg D, Davis R, Ettner S, et al: Trends in alternative medicine use in the United States, 1990–1997: results of a follow-up national survey. JAMA 280:1569–1575, 1998

Ernst E: Integrating complementary medicine? J R Soc Health 117:285–286, 1997

Ernst E, Resch K, White A: Complementary medicine: what physicians think of it: a meta-analysis. Arch Intern Med 155:2405–2408, 1995

Ezzo J, Wright K, Hadhazy V, et al: Use of the Cochrane electronic library in complementary and alternative medicine courses in medical schools: is the giant lost in cyberspace? J Altern Complement Med 8:681–686, 2002

Gaudet TW: Integrative medicine: the evolution of a new approach to medicine and to medical education. Integrative Medicine 1:67–73, 1998

Grant WB: Dietary links to Alzheimer's disease. Alzheimer's Disease Review 2:42–55, 1997

Gray G: Concise Guide to Evidence-Based Psychiatry. Washington, DC, American Psychiatric Publishing, 2004

Green J: Integrating conventional medicine and alternative therapies. Altern Ther Health Med 2:77–81, 1996

Guyatt G, Rennie D (eds): Users' Guide to the Medical Literature: Essentials of Evidence-Based Clinical Practice. Chicago, IL, American Medical Association Press, 2002

Hager K, Marahrens A, Kenklies M, et al: Alpha-lipoic acid as a new treatment option for Alzheimer type dementia. Arch Gerontol Geriatr 32:275–282, 2001

Ikeda H: Effects of taurine on alcohol withdrawal (letter). Lancet 2(8036):509, 1977

Kaplan BJ, Simpson JSA, Ferre RC, et al: Effective mood stabilization with a chelated mineral supplement: an open-label trial in bipolar disorder. J Clin Psychiatry 62:936–944, 2001

Kulkarni J, Riedel A, de Castella A, et al: Estrogen: a potential treatment for schizophrenia. Schizophr Res 48:137–144, 2001

Lake J: Textbook of Integrative Mental Health Care: Foundations and Clinical Methods. New York, Thieme Medical Publishers, 2006

Lieber CS: Alcoholic liver disease: new insights in pathogenesis lead to new treatments. J Hepatol 32 (suppl 1):113–128, 2000

Liverani A: Subjective scales for the evaluation of therapeutic effects and their use in complementary medicine. J Altern Complement Med 6:257–264, 2000

Lolic MM, Fiskum G, Rosenthal RE: Neuroprotective effects of acetyl-L-carnitine after stroke in rats. Ann Emerg Med 29:758–765, 1997

Nemets B, Stahl Z, Belmaker RH: Addition of omega-3 fatty acid to maintenance medication treatment for recurrent unipolar depressive disorder. Am J Psychiatry 159:477–479, 2002

Partonen T, Leppamaki S, Hurme J, et al: Randomized trial of physical exercise alone or combined with bright light on mood and health-related quality of life. Psychol Med 28:1359–1364, 1998

Peet M, Horrobin DF, E-E Multicentre Study Group: A dose-ranging exploratory study of the effects of ethyl-eicosapentaenoate in patients with persistent schizophrenic symptoms. J Psychiatr Res 36:7–18, 2002

Rees L: Integrated medicine imbues orthodox medicine with the values of complementary medicine. BMJ 322:119–120, 2001

Richardson J: Evidence-based complementary medicine: rigor, relevance and the swampy lowlands. J Altern Complement Med 8:221–223, 2002

Riley D, Heger M: Integrative medicine data collection network (IMDCN), in Proceedings of the Fourth Annual Alternative Therapies Symposium and Exposition. New York, NY, March 25–28, 1999

Sarkar P, Rathee SP, Neera N: Comparative efficacy of pharmacotherapy and biofeedback among cases of generalised anxiety disorder. Journal of Projective Psychology and Mental Health 6:69–77, 1999

Smith R, Shiromoto F: The use of cranial electrotherapy stimulation to block fear perception in phobic patients. Journal of Current Therapeutic Research 51:249–253, 1992

Steering Committee for the Prince of Wales's Initiative on Integrated Medicine: Integrated health care: a way forward for the next five years? a discussion document. London, The Prince of Wales's Foundation for Integrated Health, 1997

Stoll AL, Severus WE, Freeman MP, et al: Omega 3 fatty acids in bipolar disorder. Arch Gen Psychiatry 56:407–412, 1999

Tempesta E, Troncon R, Janiri L, et al: Role of acetyl-L-carnitine in the treatment of cognitive deficit in chronic alcoholism. Int J Clin Pharmacol Res 10:101–107, 1990

Verhoef MJ, Casebeer AL, Hilsden RJ: Assessing efficacy of complementary medicine: adding qualitative research methods to the "gold standard." J Altern Complement Med 8:275–281, 2002

Vuckovic N: Integrating qualitative methods in RCTs: the experience of the Oregon Center for CAM. J Altern Complement Med 8:225–227, 2002

Walach H: The efficacy paradox in randomized controlled trials of CAM and elsewhere: beware of the placebo trap. J Altern Complement Med 7:213–218, 2001

Walsh R: Toward a synthesis of Eastern and Western psychologies, in Healing East and West: Ancient Wisdom and Modern Psychology. Edited by Sheikh AA, Sheikh KS. Hoboken, NJ, Wiley, 1996, pp 542–555

Westrick ER, Shapiro AP, Nathan PE, et al: Dietary tryptophan reverses alcohol-induced impairment of facial recognition but not verbal recall. Alcohol Clin Exp Res 12:531–533, 1988

Wilson K, McGowan J, Guyatt G, et al: Teaching evidence-based complementary and alternative medicine, 3: asking the questions and identifying the information. J Altern Complement Med 8:499–506, 2002a

Wilson K, Mills EJ, Ross C, et al: Teaching evidence-based complementary and alternative medicine, 4: appraising the evidence for papers on therapy. J Altern Complement Med 8:673–679, 2002b

Zhang X: Integration of traditional and complementary medicine into national health care systems. J Manipulative Physiol Ther 23:139–140, 2000

Part II

Review of the Evidence and Clinical Guidelines

Nonconventional Biological Treatments

5

Western Herbal Medicines

Roberta Lee, M.D.
Pamela S. Yee, M.D.
Grace Naing, M.D.

Pharmacological treatments for medical conditions were initially produced from herbs. Until about 1930, herbal products represented a large portion of the U.S. pharmacopoeia. Today, many commonly used medicines are still derived from plants, such as colchicine, digoxin, ephedrine, vincristine, and others. Regulation of the medicinal uses of botanicals varies from country to country. In the Dietary Supplement and Health Education Act of 1994 passed by the U.S. Congress, botanical medicines were classified as food supplements. In other countries (e.g., Germany), botanical medicines are evaluated by a special committee of experts in the fields of botany, ethnobotany, pharmacology, and medicine. It is beyond the scope of this chapter to discuss these distinctions in detail; for more information, the reader may consult botanical reference texts such as *The ABC Clinical Guide to Herbs,* published by the American Botanical Council (Blumenthal 2003).

Herbal remedies are widely used in the United States. In the 1990s, sales of herbal products increased, reaching their highest retail sales volume in 1998 and subsequently leveling off in 2001 (Blumenthal 2003). The decline in consumer use has been ascribed to a variety of factors, including the release of negative media articles on botanicals, reports of poor-quality herbal products, and unreasonable consumer expectations. Complaints of fatigue, headache, insomnia, depression, and anxiety are the most frequent reasons patients seek alternative therapies (Unutzer et al. 2000). Furthermore, many patients are reluctant to accept a diagnosis of a psychiatric disorder, making the use of botanical alternatives a frequent choice.

There are important safety issues to be considered with regard to the use of botanicals. Although there have been fewer per capita reports of adverse events associated with herbal remedies in the United States than with prescription medications (Blumenthal 2003), a growing body of evidence suggests that significant pharmacological interactions are possible with some botanical plants. To further exacerbate the potential for drug–herb interactions, it has been reported that up to 70% of patients who use alternative therapies fail to disclose this fact to their physicians (Eisenberg et al. 1998). Thus, whether or not practitioners agree with integrating botanicals into their medical practice, it is an important part of clinical training for them to understand their efficacy and potential interactions with conventional drugs. This chapter discusses three botanicals commonly used to treat psychiatric disorders: kava (*Piper methysticum*), St. John's wort (*Hypericum perforatum*), and ginkgo root (*Ginkgo biloba*).

KAVA (*PIPER METHYSTICUM*)

Historical and Current Uses

Piper methysticum, commonly known as kava, kava-kava, ava–ava, *kawa,* or *awa,* is a plant of great cultural significance to Pacific Islanders that has been used for centuries (Lebot et al. 1998). Even today, the Melanesian, Polynesian, and Micronesian peoples grind fresh or dried roots of this plant to prepare a traditional beverage that serves as a ceremonial centerpiece for occasions of great social and political significance, including honoring a respected elder, buying a piece of land, and settling disputes. The botanist J. G. Forster (1777), who sailed with the eighteenth-century British explorer Captain James Cook on his second voyage, is credited with the first valid botanical description of this Pacific plant. However, the first scientific observations of its presence in the Pacific remain in question. The Dutch navigators Le Maire and Schoeten observed its use in the island of Futuna as early as 1616 (Lebot and Levesque 1989). Cook is commonly cited as the earliest person to record its presence in the Pacific islands. In his captain's log, he noted that those in his crew who sampled large amounts of this beverage seemed to be sedated as if they were taking opium (Steinmetz 1960). Cook's characterization of kava's pharmacological hallucinogenic properties ultimately was proven to be incorrect. Kava is now recognized as a mild narcotic and hypnotic (Lewin 1924; Schultes and Hofmann 1979). There have been many traditional medical uses of kava, including its use as a treatment for inflammation of the urogenital system, gonorrhea, menstrual problems, migraine headaches, chills, vaginal prolapse, rheumatism, dermatological conditions, and nervousness (Lebot et al. 1998). In the last 150 years, numerous scientific publications on the chemical and pharmacological properties of kava have given Western medicine greater insight into the potential value of this plant.

During the past 20 years, kava has gained popularity as an herbal treatment for anxiety, nervousness, insomnia, stress, management of benzodiazepine withdrawal, and anxiety related to menopause. In 1998, kava ranked fifth in the

North American botanical sales market (Mirasol 1998). However, its use and sales rapidly plummeted beginning in the fall of 2001 after many cases of hepatotoxicity were reported. By the end of 2001, public health authorities in Germany initiated a new evaluation of the risk–benefit ratio of kava. This soon led to the withdrawal of authorization for continued sales of kava products in Germany. Other public health authorities in Europe (including Switzerland) and countries around the world soon followed Germany's example (Blumenthal 2002). Today, strict warnings exist in countries where sales of kava are permitted, dampening the public and professional use of this botanical product.

Description and Standardization

P. methysticum is a slow-growing perennial belonging to the *Piperaceae* family. When cultivated, the plant is harvested when it reaches age 2–3 years or a height of 2–2.5 meters. The leaves are heart-shaped and approximately 8–25 cm long. Kava is cultivated for its rootstock or stump. The stump is a thick tuberous and knotty mass with a fringe of lateral roots. The rootstock color varies from white to dark yellow, depending on the concentration of kavalactones, which are the bioactive constituents responsible for the psychoactive characteristics of kava. The kavalactones are concentrated in the lateral roots. The spread of kava plants has occurred primarily through human cultivation, as most *P. methysticum* is propagated asexually by planting stem cuttings of the harvested plants. The roots are dried or freshly pounded to make a ceremonial beverage or dried and pulverized to make standardized liquid or solid extracts, alcohol-based tinctures, teas, and salves. Preparations vary in kavalactone content depending on the source of kava. There are 118 cultivar morphotypes or botanical variants labeled *P. methysticum* in different areas, and each morphotype has subtle variations in the proportion of kavalactones in the rootstock. The method of kavalactone extraction influences kavalactone content in medicinal preparations, as these constituents are lipophilic. Lesser quality products have included the stem peelings as well as the rootstock, thus diluting the concentration of active constituents and possibly contributing unwanted toxic compounds (Dragull et al. 2003). Standardized preparations are generally extracted to not less than 30% kavalactones in powdered dried extracts or not less than 50% kavalactones in semisolid (paste) extracts (Blumenthal 2003).

Pharmacology

Kava's psychoactive activity is attributed to a group of compounds known as *kavalactones* (or *kavapyrones*). These compounds consist of 13 carbon atoms, 6 of which form a benzene ring attached by a double bond to an unsaturated lactone. There are 15 kavalactones identified in the rhizome, but 7 major kavalactones are credited for most of the pharmacological activity: methysticin, dihydromethysticin, kavain, 7,8-dihydrokavain, 5,6-dehydrokavain, 5,6-dehydromethysticin, and yangonin. The concentration of these constituents is high in the roots (15%) and decreases to 5% in the stems. Although kavalactones such as kavain and methysticin can be synthesized, early studies evaluating the psychoactive effects of these singular compounds reveal that they are less active physiologically than the natural raw extracts. These findings support the hypothesis that the kavalactones as a group have synergistic pharmacological activity (Steinmetz 1960). Other constituents identified in the rhizome include flavokavains A, B, and C, which are phytosterols; the minerals potassium, calcium, magnesium, sodium, aluminum, and iron; and amino acids (Blumenthal 2003; Lebot et al. 1998).

The reported neuropharmacological effects of kava include analgesia, anesthesia, sedation, and hyporeflexia (Singh 1992). In animal experiments, kava has been shown to have anticonvulsive, antispasmodic, and central muscular relaxant effects. Antimycotic properties have also been reported (Hansel et al. 1966). More recent in vitro studies have identified antithrombotic activity as well (Gleitz et al. 1997).

Kava acts on several areas in the central nervous system (CNS), but its mechanism of action is not entirely clear. Differing results have been reported from in vitro and in vivo studies, and it is uncertain whether kava binds to γ-aminobutyric acid (GABA) receptors (Boonen and Halberlein 1998; Boonen et al. 2000; Davies et al. 1992; Jussofie 1993; Jussofie et al. 1994; all cited in Blumenthal 2003). A possible noradrenaline uptake effect has been reported in three kavalactones (Seitz et al. 1997). In an animal trial (Baum et al. 1998), it was reported that kava activates the mesolimbic dopaminergic neuron, resulting in the subject's becoming more relaxed and slightly euphoric. Other CNS interactions of kava have been reported with the glutamate receptors (Gleitz et al. 1996).

The modulation of sodium channel receptor sites is a potential mechanism for kava's anticonvulsant activity ("Piper methysticum" 1998); kava has been demonstrated to suppress seizures induced by strychnine (Klohs et al. 1959). In some studies, kava has relaxed skeletal muscle through direct action on the muscle fiber without inducing CNS depression (Singh 1983). Kavain, whether applied topically or injected subcutaneously, was found to induce local anesthesia, but higher doses caused paralysis of the peripheral nerves (Baldi 1980).

Kava at therapeutic doses does not appear to have sedative effects, a significant advantage of this botanical. However, no large trials have confirmed this aspect of kava. Many early trials were small and have been criticized as being methodologically flawed. In small comparative studies evaluating kava's effects on behavior and the CNS, event-related potentials during a memory task were significantly decreased in both speed and quality of response in the benzodiazepine arm versus the kava arm (Heinze et al. 1994; Herberg 1996; Munte et al. 1993).

Pharmacodynamics and Pharmacokinetics

When kava is orally administered, kavain and dihydrokavain are rapidly absorbed from the gut (10 minutes). In contrast, methysticin and its dihydro derivatives are more slowly absorbed (45 minutes) (Shulgin 1973). When 40 mg/kg of dihydrokavain was given orally, half of it was found in the urine within 48 hours in the form of hydroxylated derivatives (Duffield and Lidgard 1986). In one study, quantitative uptake of four kavalactones in mice brain indicated that kavain and dihydrokavain attain maximal brain concentrations within 5 minutes, whereas demethoxy-yangonin and yangonin entered the brain more slowly (Keledjian et al. 1988). It is generally agreed that kavain and dihydrokavain are the two kavalactones that most readily cross the blood-brain barrier. Peak levels for kavain occur at 1.8 hours, with an elimination half-life of approximately 9 hours and a distribution half-life of 50 minutes (Saletu et al. 1989). In test animals, the LD_{50} (lethal dose for 50% of subjects) of kavalactones is estimated to be 300–400 mg/kg (Meyer 1962).

Review of Clinical Evidence

Anxiety

Kava has been evaluated in 14 randomized clinical trials for anxiety in studies of 4–25 weeks' duration. A meta-analysis of randomized trials initially published in 2000 (Pittler and Ernst 2000) and updated in 2002 (Pittler and Ernst 2002) and 2003 (Pittler and Ernst 2003) concluded that kava had moderate efficacy in the treatment of anxiety. In the meta-analysis, 14 clinical trials were identified, but 7 were excluded from the analysis due to methodological flaws such as duplicate reporting, concurrent benzodiazepine use, or use of an isolated kavalactone. The remaining 7 clinical trials were evaluated for methodology, and 3 were selected for analysis, involving 198 patients. Pooled data from the 3 studies that used a common outcome measure, the Hamilton Anxiety Scale (Ham-A), found a significant reduction in the mean anxiety score of the kava group compared with that of the placebo group, with a mean difference of 9.69 points (95% confidence interval [CI] = 3.54–15.83 points) (Pittler and Ernst 2000). In the 2003 update of the meta-analysis, 11 trials involving 645 participants were eligible for inclusion in the analysis (Pittler and Ernst 2003). The 6 studies using the Ham-A as a common outcome measure showed that kava was effective for the treatment of anxiety and was "relatively safe for short-term treatment (1–24 weeks)" (Pittler and Ernst 2003).

Menopausal/Perimenopausal Anxiety

Three randomized, placebo-controlled clinical trials have evaluated kava 100 mg/day with hormone replacement therapy (De Leo et al. 2000, 2001) or kava 100–200 mg/day plus calcium (Cagnacci et al. 2003) as a treatment for perimenopausal and menopausal anxiety. All three trials used the Ham-A or State-Trait Anxiety Inventory as an outcome instrument to assess changes in anxiety. In each trial, the reduction in anxiety was more pronounced in the kava treatment versus the placebo arm.

Equivalence Trials

Several clinical trials (Boerner et al. 2003; Lindenberg and Pitule-Schodel 1990; Woelk et al. 1993) comparing kava with benzodiazepines have been conducted. In each of the trials, no significant difference was found on anxiety measures. However, the trials lacked placebo arms, and the sample sizes of the earlier trials were possibly too small to measure equivalence. In the largest randomized, controlled, multicenter trial, 129 patients were given 400 mg of LI 150 (kava), 10 mg of buspirone, or 100 mg of opipramol daily for 8 weeks. Subjects were evaluated for anxiety using the Ham-A scale, sleep quality, quality of life, and measures of general well-being. Approximately 70% were classified as responding to the treatment with a 50% reduction in Ham-A scores, and 60% achieved full remission (Boerner et al. 2003). In a small ($n=40$) randomized placebo-controlled trial, patients who were taking benzodiazepines for anxiety were given increasing amounts of kava (WS 1490), up to 300 mg/day, as their benzodiazepine dosage was tapered. The dosage adjustments were followed by 3 weeks of monotherapy with kava versus placebo. Patients were monitored for benzodiazepine withdrawal, subjective well-being, and anxiety. The results confirmed the anxiolytic efficacy of kava (Malsch and Kieser 2001).

Unresolved Safety Issues

In recommended doses over short periods of time, kava has been regarded as safe. However, the potential hepatotoxicity of kava has become a concern, with more than 30 cases of liver damage associated with its use being reported in Europe as of 2001. In several cases, liver transplants were required because of the extent of hepatic damage. An independent assessment of the adverse effects in these cases was undertaken by a noted expert in the field of hepatotoxicology, Donald Waller from the University of Illinois at Chicago. He concluded that there were only a few cases in which kava might be directly associated with liver damage and that those cases were likely due to hypersensitivity or idiosyncratic responses to kava (Waller 2002). At the time of this writing, the U.S. Food and Drug Administration has issued a warning to consumers concerning the use of kava, and many countries have removed kava from public access (Blumenthal 2002). The mechanism of action and doses and durations of kava use associated with hepatic damage currently remain unclear. Possible causes include the method of extraction of kava, resulting in an increased proportion of one or more kavalactone constituents that predispose some individuals to liver damage, and the contamination of kava preparations by toxic alkaloids. Serious adverse events associated with kava use are extremely rate. One published report estimated that approximately 250 million daily doses of ethanolic kava extract were administered in the 1990s, with only two causally related cases of hepatotoxicity (Schmidt and Nahrstedt 2002). In both cases of hepatotoxicity, kava was used at doses far beyond the recommended levels. Based on these two isolated cases, the rate of adverse event reports for kava was 0.008 report per 1 million daily doses. By contrast, benzodiazepines have a much higher rate of adverse event reports per 1 million daily doses: 0.90 for bromazepam, 1.23 for oxazepam, and 2.12 for diazepam. The authors concluded that transitioning patients who are using kava to a benzodiazepine could potentially increase the risk of adverse effects (Schmidt and Nahrstedt 2002).

Guidelines for Use in Psychiatric Disorders

Uses

Kava should be used primarily for anxiety and may be considered in some cases of sleep disorder, stress, and restlessness.

Safety

In December 2001, the American Botanical Council recommended that kava not be taken for more than 1 month without professional supervision (Blumenthal 2003). Botanical preparations should be avoided in patients who have known liver disease, a history of chronic alcohol abuse, or Parkinson's disease and in patients who are chronic users of benzodiazepines or other sedative-hypnotic medications.

Dosing

Typical dosing for adults using a standardized preparation of 30% kavalactones is a daily dosage equivalent of 60–120 mg of kavalactones or a total dose of 70–210 mg of kava. Most controlled clinical trials are based on three 100-mg doses of a dried extract standardized to 70 mg of kavalactones or 210 mg of kavalactones/day. The onset of response is generally within 2–4 weeks, comparable with that for prescriptive anxiolytic medications (Blumenthal 2003). Reputable brands used in clinical trials include Kavatrol, Laitan, and WS 1490.

Toxicology

There is considerable concern over cases of hepatotoxicity, as discussed above. Chronic heavy use of kava has been associated with renal dysfunction, hematological abnormalities, pulmonary hypertension, dermopathy, and choreoathetosis. These conditions have been cited in case reports; however, a causal relation linked to kava use remains unclear due to multiple confounding variables and/or incomplete reporting.

Adverse Effects

- *Dermatological:* A dermatological condition known as "kava dermopathy" can appear during prolonged and heavy use. This condition reverses after kava use is discontinued (Norton and Ruze 1994).
- *Neurological:* Several cases of extrapyramidal side effects (Meseguer et al. 2002) and the exacerbation of parkinsonian symptoms (Schelosky et al. 2002) have been reported after 1–4 days of use. Anecdotal cases of sedation have been reported, although small trials in humans suggest that kava does not cause neurological or psychological impairment.
- *Psychiatric:* Apathy has been noted with long-term use (Blumenthal 2003).
- *Pulmonary:* Pulmonary hypertension was proposed as the mechanism responsible for the shortness of breath observed in one study, in which chronic kava users frequently complained of having difficulty breathing (69%) and nonusers seldom reported this problem (25%) (Blumenthal 2003).
- *Hematological:* Antiplatelet activity was reported with kavain, a single kavalactone. Blood dyscrasias have been reported in Aborigine people who are heavy kava users (Blumenthal 2003).
- *Gastrointestinal:* Hepatotoxicity has been an ongoing concern and was discussed earlier in the chapter. Gastrointestinal upset has been reported infrequently as an adverse effect in some studies (Blumenthal 2003).

Drug Interactions

- *Alcohol:* Animal studies have reported increases in kava's sedative effects when it is coadministered with alcohol.
- *Sedative drugs/CNS depressants:* Kava has been found to potentiate some CNS depressants.
- *Dopamine, dopamine antagonists, dopamine agonists:* Kava has been reported to antagonize the effect of dopamine and elicit extrapyramidal effects.
- *Monoamine oxidase inhibitors:* Constituents of kava have been shown to have weak monoamine oxidase (MAO) inhibitory activity in vitro.
- *Anesthetics:* Kava has been shown in case reports to prolong the sedative action of anesthesia.
- *Antiplatelet agents:* Kavain, an isolated kavalactone, has been reported to have antiplatelet activity.
- *Hepatotoxic drugs:* More than 30 case reports of hepatotoxicity have been noted since 2001 (as discussed above).
- *Cytochrome P450 substrates:* Preliminary studies have indicated that kava may inhibit multiple cytochrome P450 substrates (e.g., 1A2, 2C9, 2C19, 2D69, 3A4) (Mathews et al. 2002).

Pregnancy and Lactation

Pregnant or nursing women should avoid using products that contain kava.

ST. JOHN'S WORT (*HYPERICUM PERFORATUM*)

Historical and Current Uses

Hypericum perforatum, commonly known as St. John's wort, is a perennial plant common in the United States, Europe, and Asia. Its traditional uses date back to the fifth century B.C.E., when Hippocrates first documented the medicinal qualities of St. John's wort in healing wounds. The herb has also been traditionally used to treat afflictions of the nervous system (e.g., hysteria, neurosis) and a wide of range of disorders (e.g., spinal injuries, rheumatism); has been used as a neuralgesic, diuretic, and astringent; and has been given for dysentery and parasites (Mills and Bone 1999).

St. John's wort has recently gained popularity as an herbal treatment, mostly for depression but also for mood disorders associated with premenstrual syndrome, seasonal affective disorder, perimenopausal symptoms, obsessive-compulsive disorder, and anxiety. In 1998, St. John's wort was the second highest-selling dietary supplement in the United States, but it fell to fifth place in 2000 because of negative publicity surrounding its potential for adverse interactions with many conventional drugs (Blumenthal et al. 2000).

Description and Standardization

St. John's wort is made using the dried tops, leaves, and stems procured during flowering season, which are prepared as standardized extracts, teas, alcohol-based tinctures, capsules and tablets, and topical oil infusions. These preparations may vary in constituents, depending on growing conditions and on climate, harvesting, and extraction methods, yielding products that vary significantly in content from manufacturer to manufacturer and batch to batch. St. John's wort is often standardized to 0.3% hypericin extract or 2%–4.5% hyperforin (Bruneton 1999). In earlier studies, hypericin was thought to be the primary constituent possessing antidepressant efficacy, but recent studies have indicated that hyperforin probably plays a more significant role. To date it is not known whether the antidepressant efficacy of St. John's wort comes from one or a combination of constituents present in the whole herb. A practical consequence of this uncertainty is that standardization is not a critical factor in determining the probable clinical effectiveness of different preparations (Linde and Mulrow 2002).

Pharmacology

The biologically active constituents that may contribute to the antidepressant effects of St. John's wort include the compounds naphthodianthrones (hypericin and pseudohypericin), phloroglucinols (hyperforin and adhyperforin), fla-vonoids, xanthones, oligomeric procyanidins, and amino acids (Nahrstedt and Butterweck 1997). As noted above, it is not yet clear which constituents have beneficial effects on mood; however, the research focus has recently shifted to hyperforin as the principal antidepressant constituent. St. John's wort exerts its effects on several neurotransmitters, specifically by inhibiting reuptake of sero-tonin (5-hydroxytryptamine [5-HT]), norepinephrine, dopamine, GABA, and L-glutamate in vitro. Animal models have demonstrated serotonin receptor (5-HT_1 and 5-HT_2) upregulation and downregulation of β_1-adrenergic receptors when St. John's wort is used for a long period (De Smet 2002; Di Carlo et al. 2001). In vitro binding to $GABA_A$, $GABA_B$, benzodiazepines, inositol, and MAO A and B receptors has also been confirmed (Cott 1997). There is a report of dose-dependent potentiation of animal behaviors affected by CNS serotonin levels, with the greatest effect being with a 38.8% hyperforin extract, in contrast to a more dopaminergic-mediated behavior with an extract of 4.5% hyperforin (Bhattacharya et al. 1998). A small study of healthy volunteers demonstrated in-creased cortisol levels after oral administration of 600 mg of WS 5570 (an extract of St. John's wort), suggesting central norepinephrine or serotonin activity (Schule et al. 2001).

Pharmacodynamics and Pharmacokinetics

In humans, the mean plasma concentration (150 ng/mL) of hyperforin is reached approximately 3.5 hours after oral administration of 5% hyperforin ex-tract. The elimination half-life is 9 hours (Biber et al. 1998). Clinical studies have demonstrated the induction of cytochrome P450 (CYP) enzymes by St. John's wort, resulting in increased metabolism and reduced plasma concentra-tions of many drugs. More recently, it has been suggested that the drug trans-porter P-glycoprotein, found in the gastrointestinal tract and the CNS, may also alter the bioavailability of many drugs (Zhou et al. 2004). Hyperforin, but not hypericin, has been found to induce CYP 3A4 expression in human hepatocytes (Moore et al. 2000; Wentworth et al. 2000). CYP 3A4 is the most clinically im-portant member of the CYP family of hepatic enzymes and is involved in the metabolism of many common pharmaceuticals. Induction of intestinal P-glyco-protein/multidrug resistance 1 (Pgp/MDR1) transport by St. John's wort and hepatic CYP 3A4 decreases intestinal absorption and increases first-pass clear-ance of many drugs (Dressler et al. 2003).

Review of Clinical Evidence

Depression

Many randomized controlled trials have been conducted using St. John's wort; at the time of this writing, six systematic reviews and meta-analyses have found the herb to be superior to placebo and as effective as conventional antidepressants for the short-term treatment of mild-to-moderate depression (Gaster and Holroyd 2000; Kim et al. 1999; Linde and Mulrow 2002; Linde et al. 1996; Whiskey et al. 2001; Williams et al. 2000). However, negative results were found in two recent studies evaluating the effectiveness of St. John's wort in severely depressed individuals, with Hamilton Rating Scale for Depression (Ham-D) scores higher than 20. Shelton et al. (2001) conducted a multicenter randomized, double-blind, placebo-controlled trial in 200 subjects over 4 weeks using LI 160, a preparation standardized to 0.3% hypericin, and concluded the herb had no effect on severe depressed mood. The study was criticized for the unusually low remission rates in both groups and the lack of a conventional antidepressant arm to ensure sensitivity. More recently, the Hypericum Depression Trial Study Group compared St. John's wort with sertraline and placebo for major depression. In that trial, 340 subjects were randomized to receive LI 160 (900–1,500 mg), sertraline (50–100 mg), or placebo over 8 weeks; outcomes were based on the Ham-D and Clinical Global Impression (CGI) scores (Hypericum Depression Trial Study Group 2002). Improvement was seen in all three groups, with no significant differences among the groups. In both studies, the significance of the findings was limited by the short study duration and the lack of adequate statistical power on which to base strong conclusions. In view of the above findings, the evidence supporting the use of St. John's wort for the treatment of severe depressed mood remains inconclusive; however, there is compelling evidence of the herb's beneficial effects in mild-to-moderate depression.

Anxiety Disorders

Case reports suggest that St. John's wort is an effective treatment for some anxiety disorders (Davidson and Connor 2001). However, here is insufficient evidence to recommend the use of St. John's wort for particular anxiety disorders.

Obsessive-Compulsive Disorder

Early studies suggested that St. John's wort may ameliorate symptoms of obsessive-compulsive disorder. The findings of one small 3-month study using a preparation standardized to 0.3% hypericin twice daily for 3 months showed clinical improvement based on CGI scores and the Yale-Brown Obsessive Compulsive Scale. However, the small sample size and the fact that the study was not controlled limited the significance of these findings (Taylor and Kobak 2000).

Mood Disorders Associated With Perimenopause

To date, no controlled studies have examined the effectiveness of St. John's wort as a treatment for dysphoria or other psychiatric symptoms associated with perimenopause. Small uncontrolled studies have been conducted, but the findings are inconclusive (Grube et al. 1999).

Premenstrual Syndrome

There is preliminary evidence that St. John's wort alleviates some symptoms of premenstrual syndrome. One small study ($n=19$) used a preparation standardized to 0.3% hypericin. Outcome measures using standardized rating scales showed a 50% decrease in symptom severity in two-thirds of the patients (Stevinson and Ernst 2000). Positive findings of this uncontrolled observational study suggest the need for further studies to clarify the possible clinical benefits of St. John's wort as a treatment of premenstrual syndrome.

Seasonal Affective Disorder

Preliminary findings suggest that St. John's wort improves symptoms of seasonal affective disorder (SAD). One small study examined St. John's wort 900 mg/day alone or in combination with light therapy for 1 month. There was significant improvement in mood with St. John's wort, but no incremental benefit when light exposure therapy was added (Kasper 1997). A larger nonrandomized 8-week trial found no differences between St. John's wort 300 mg tid alone and St. John's wort combined with bright-light therapy for mild-to-moderate symptoms of SAD; those researchers concluded that St. John's wort alone was an effective treatment of SAD (Wheatley 1999). The limitations of these findings do not provide sufficient evidence for recommending St. John's wort for SAD; further studies are warranted.

Depression in Children and Adolescents

Herbal therapies, perceived as safer alternatives to conventional psychotropic medications, have not undergone any rigorous placebo-controlled trials in children or adolescents to date. The findings of some studies indicate that St. John's wort has good short-term (4-week) tolerability in children and adolescents under age 16 years. An observational trial evaluated St. John's wort at dosages of 300–1,800 mg/day in 84 children ages 1–12 years who had depression or other mood symptoms (Hubner and Kirste 2001). Compliance and efficacy were assessed every 2 weeks. The results of the study suggested that St. John's wort is potentially safe in children. However, these findings were limited by missing data at each assessment point and the fact that only 76% of the initial sample remained at the end of the trial. A recent pilot study examined the effectiveness, safety, tolerability, and pharmacodynamics of St. John's wort in 33 children and adolescents ages 6–16 years (Findling et al. 2003). The patients were started on a standardized preparation of St. John's wort 150 mg tid. At 4 weeks, the dosage was increased to 900 mg/day in subjects who did not meet predefined treatment response criteria. At 8 weeks, 25 subjects showed significant clinical improvement, and St. John's wort was well tolerated (Findling et al. 2003).

Guidelines for Use in Psychiatric Disorders

Uses

St. John's wort is effective for mild-to-moderate depression. Because it is unknown whether a particular constituent or a combination of constituents is responsible for the herb's beneficial effects on mood, it is recommended that the same brands tested in clinical trials be used (e.g., Kira [LI 160] and Remotiv [ZE 117]). Other reasonable choices include reputable brands that are highly rated by third-party evaluators (e.g., see www.consumerlab.com).

Safety

Clinical trials confirm that St. John's wort is safe when used at recommended doses for less than 3 months and by individuals who are not concurrently taking conventional medications. The safety profile of St. John's wort beyond this period of time and for larger doses remains unclear.

Dosing

Typical adult dosing of standardized St. John's wort preparations of 0.3% hypericin or 3% hyperforin for the treatment of depression is 300 mg po tid. The onset of response is generally within 2–4 weeks, comparable with that of standard antidepressants (Agency for Health Care Policy and Research 1999). A maintenance dose has not been determined, and there are limited data supporting the use of St. John's wort in children. Anecdotal evidence suggests that St. John's wort 900 mg bid can be effective (Davidson and Connor 2001).

Toxicology

Animal data suggest chronic use of high levels of St. John's wort can lead to nonspecific symptoms of weight loss. These data also indicate that patients who have overdosed on St. John's wort should avoid sunlight for at least 1 week to avoid photodermatitis (Hammerly et al. 2004).

Adverse Effects

Gastrointestinal complaints, dizziness, fatigue, sedation, headache, and dry mouth are the most commonly reported adverse effects with St. John's wort.

- *Allergic:* Allergic skin reactions, including rash and pruritis, have been reported in clinical trials. Meta-analyses (Kim et al. 1999; Linde et al. 1996) have shown that adverse effects are comparable with placebo and occur less often than with conventional antidepressants. Anecdotal reports suggest that St. John's wort may affect blood pressure and heart rate during surgery (Voelker 1999).

- *Dermatological:* A photosensitive rash has been reported after exposure to ultraviolet light. This adverse effect is more common in individuals infected with HIV or hepatitis C. Hypericin is thought to be the causative bioactive constituent for this reaction. Patients should be advised to use caution when combining St. John's wort with medications that cause photosensitivity such as tetracycline or fluoroquinolones.
- *Psychiatric:* Cases of anxiety, mania, psychosis, and serotonin syndrome have been reported with St. John's wort. Two possible cases of symptomatic worsening in schizophrenic patients taking St. John's wort have been reported. However, in both cases, the individuals who became worse had stopped their antipsychotic medications prior to taking St. John's wort. There has been one case report of possible withdrawal symptoms when St. John's wort was discontinued after chronic use (Hammerly et al. 2004).
- *Cardiovascular:* Case reports of hypertensive episodes unrelated to serotonin syndrome have been reported with St. John's wort. There was one report of a hypertensive crisis in a patient taking no other medications or supplements who reportedly consumed tyramine-containing foods the night of the hospital admission. As noted above, in vitro studies have shown that St. John's wort has weak MAO inhibitory activity (Hammerly et al. 2004).
- *Genitourinary:* In one series, anorgasmia was reported in 25% of patients compared with 32% receiving sertraline and 16% receiving placebo. Increased urinary frequency was also reported in the same study.

Drug Interactions

Many studies have examined the pharmacokinetic and pharmacodynamic properties of St. John's wort because of its widespread use and potential interactions with many conventional drugs metabolized by the same liver enzymes. Both synergistic effects and antagonistic interactions with certain conventional drugs may result in toxicities or decreased efficacy. CYP 3A4 is the enzyme most commonly induced by St. John's wort. Because 50% of all conventional medications are metabolized through this pathway, potential safety issues resulting from interactions with St. John's wort must be taken into account. CYP 2D6 is not altered by St. John's wort (Markowitz et al. 2003).

The following is a partial list of potential interactions between St. John's wort and widely used conventional drugs:

- *Anticoagulants:* When combined with St. John's wort, the effectiveness of warfarin is decreased. This effect is reversed when St. John's wort is stopped or the dose of warfarin is increased. Strokes have not been reported when St. John's wort is combined with warfarin.
- *Anticonvulsants:* Carbamazepine showed no changes in serum levels when combined with St. John's wort in healthy subjects. However, close monitor-

ing is necessary when carbamazepine and St. John's wort are used together because of the potential for interaction between the two substances. The same risk applies to phenytoin, although cases of possible interactions have not been reported.

- *Antidepressants:* There are case reports of serotonin syndrome when tricyclic antidepressants are combined with St. John's wort. Tricyclic antidepressant serum levels are reduced in patients concurrently taking St. John's wort. There have been reports of serotonin syndrome when St. John's wort is combined with selective serotonin reuptake inhibitors (SSRIs) and at least one case report of possible mania. There is a theoretical risk of potentiation of MAO inhibitors, resulting in serotonin syndrome, although there have been no documented cases of this adverse effect. Two cases of serotonin syndrome were reported when St. John's wort was combined with venlafaxine or nefazodone; these combinations should be avoided (Hammerly et al. 2004).
- *Antiretrovirals:* St. John's wort significantly decreases serum levels of indinavir and nevirapine. The risk of this effect should be extrapolated to all protease inhibitors because of the serious implications of treatment resistance and failure in HIV-related illness (Zhou et al. 2004).
- *Cardiovascular drugs:* Cases of decreased digoxin serum levels have been reported when that drug is taken together with St. John's wort. This effect is increased with prolonged use of St. John's wort. Concentrations of the 3-hydroxy-3-methylglutaryl coenzyme A reductase inhibitor simvastatin are reduced when the drug is taken with St. John's wort. This effect was not seen with a related drug, pravastatin, possibly because simvastatin, unlike pravastatin, is a substrate of the P-glycoprotein (Zhou et al. 2004). Reductions in serum levels of nifedipine, a widely used antihypertensive agent, have also been reported (Hammerly et al. 2004).
- *Immunosuppressants:* Interactions between St. John's wort and cyclosporine are well documented. Because of the narrow therapeutic index and widespread use of cyclosporine in transplant patients, concomitant use of St. John's wort is contraindicated. Case reports cite decreases in cyclosporine serum levels and two cases of acute transplant rejection. Serum levels of the immunosuppressant tacrolimus have also been reduced when St. John's wort is taken concurrently. However, this effect has not been reported with mycophenolic acid. The reason is probably related to the fact that cyclosporine and tacrolimus both use the CYP 3A4 pathway, whereas mycophenolic acid is principally metabolized by other hepatic enzymes including the uridine diphosphate glycosyltransferases 1A8, 1A9, and 1A10 (Zhou et al. 2004).
- *Anticancer drugs:* Reports of decreased concentrations of irinotecan and imatinib through induction of CYP 3A4 by St. John's wort have been documented; the combined use of St. John's wort with these drugs should be avoided.

- *Oral contraceptives:* Oral contraceptives are metabolized by CYP 3A4, and cases of breakthrough bleeding and unwanted pregnancy have been reported by patients who use St. John's wort concurrently with these contraceptives.

Pregnancy and Lactation

Toxic effects of St. John's wort on fetuses have not been shown in animal and in vitro studies. The in vitro studies have shown uterine stimulant activity associated with St. John's wort; however, there have also been case reports of women taking St. John's wort during pregnancy without adverse effects. It is recommended that St. John's wort be avoided during pregnancy because of possible uterine contractions. Traces of hyperforin have been found in breast milk. No adverse effects on nursing infants have been reported; however, because of the absence of strong safety data, we cannot recommend the use of St. John's wort in women who breast-feed (Hammerly et al. 2004).

GINKGO (GINKGO BILOBA)

Historical and Current Uses

Ginkgo biloba is thought to be the oldest living tree species, having originated in China 200 million years ago. A ginkgo tree can live up to 1,000 years and is tolerant of harsh environmental conditions, including extreme cold and pollution, which has led to its abundance in many urban areas. Ginkgo is also resistant to insects, bacteria, fungi, and plant viruses. The wild tree is virtually extinct now, but cultivars are widely distributed in many world regions for medicinal purposes.

The ginkgo nut has historically been used for at least 5,000 years in Chinese remedies for various conditions, including respiratory ailments, circulatory problems, and urinary disturbances (Mills and Bone 2000). Ginkgo was introduced to Germany in the 1960s, and standardized extracts of the leaf are now widely prescribed in Europe and are among the best-selling herbs in the United States. Ginkgo is used in the treatment of many psychiatric and medical problems, including dementia (both Alzheimer's type and multi-infarct dementia), cognitive impairment related to stroke or cerebral insufficiency, pain associated with intermittent claudication, erectile dysfunction, altitude sickness, premenstrual syndrome, retinopathy, and macular degeneration, as well as being used as a memory-enhancing agent in healthy individuals.

Most research on *G. biloba* was conducted during the past 30 years using standardized extracts of the ginkgo leaf. Over 400 studies have been conducted to date, mostly in Germany (Blumenthal et al. 2000). The value of many early studies was limited by faulty research designs, including poor randomization, inadequate exclusion criteria, small sample sizes, and ambiguous rating scales or outcome parameters. Recent studies conducted in the United States show promising results; however, improved methodology and larger sample sizes are still needed. An ongoing study of 3,000 elderly subjects by the National Center for Complementary and Alternative Medicine is investigating ginkgo's putative preventive role in dementia (National Institutes of Health 2006).

The German Commission E, which is one of the foremost authorities on evidence-based recommendations for herbal preparations, approved the use of ginkgo for dementia, intermittent claudication, and vertigo and tinnitus caused by vascular disease (Blumenthal et al. 2000). The World Health Organization (WHO) subsequently approved ginkgo as a treatment for Raynaud's disease, acrocyanosis, and postphlebitis syndrome (Mills and Bone 2000).

Standardization

The active components of the ginkgo leaf are standardized according to the content of flavonoids (flavonol glycosides, including quercetin, kaempferol, and isorhamnetin) and terpenoids (ginkgolides and bilobalide). The ginkgolides can be further broken down into ginkgolide A, B, C, and J (Mills and Bone 2000). EGb 761, made by Schwabe Pharmaceuticals, is the standardized extract most widely used in research trials. This product is standardized to 24% ginkgo flavone glycosides and 6% terpenoids and is found in many brands, including Tebonin, Tanakan, and Rökan. Another standardized ginkgo preparation LI 1370 (Kaveri), made by the German company Lichtwer Healthcare, is standardized to 25% ginkgo flavone glycosides and 6% terpenoids (Blumenthal et al. 2000).

Pharmacology

The pharmaceutical actions of *G. biloba* are believed to be associated with its neuroprotective, antioxidant, and anti-inflammatory properties as well as its vasodilatory and anti–platelet-activating factor (PAF) activity (Blumenthal et al. 2000). Its beneficial effects on cognitive performance are probably related to the flavonoid components, which have potent antioxidant activity, may stimulate release of catecholamines and other neurotransmitters, inhibit reuptake of serotonin, protect MAO activity, and promote activity of endothelial-derived relaxing factor mechanisms in the brain (Blumenthal et al. 2000). The ginkgolides and bilobalide provide their indirect neuroprotective effects by enhancing cerebral circulation, thus reducing or preventing hypoxic and ischemic brain damage. These fractions also improve microcirculation in the brain by inhibiting PAF activity (Mills and Bone 2000).

Pharmacodynamics and Pharmacokinetics

The bioavailability of the ginkgolides A and B and bilobalide from orally administered *G. biloba* has been estimated at 98%–100%. Absorption is primarily

through the small intestine. Peak plasma levels are reached 2–3 hours after ingestion, and the duration of action is approximately 7 hours.

Review of Clinical Evidence

Enhancing Cognitive Functioning

G. biloba has been studied most extensively for its putative cognitive-enhancing
effects, especially in Alzheimer's type or vascular dementia. Many trials have
been done on G. biloba as a symptomatic treatment of cerebral insufficiency, including impaired memory and cognition, fatigue, headaches, dizziness, tinnitus,
depressed mood, and anxiety. In elderly populations, these symptoms may be a
part of normal aging; however, in some cases, they may be early symptoms of
the onset of dementia. Meta-analyses have documented significant positive effects of ginkgo on symptoms of cerebral insufficiency when a standardized preparation is administered for at least 4–6 weeks (Hopfenmuller 1994; Kleijnen and
Knipschild 1992).

The use of ginkgo to enhance memory in healthy individuals is another area of
research interest; however, to date, the studies have been limited. One small double-
blind, placebo-controlled study of adults with normal cognitive functioning found
that a high dose of ginkgo (600 mg) improved short-term memory when taken 1
hour before subjects were tested (Subhan and Hindmarch 1984). Findings of other
studies have been inconsistent, and most of the reports of improved cognitive performance are in elderly subjects with mild-to-moderate memory impairment and
not in healthy young or elderly subjects with intact memory (Rai et al. 1991; Solomon et al. 2002). These findings suggest a dose-response relation when ginkgo is
used to enhance cognitive functioning in healthy individuals.

Major Depressive Disorder

Studies of G. biloba for depression are limited, but the research evidence suggests
that ginkgo is probably ineffective against major depressive disorder and SAD.
Another trial found no improvement in symptoms in SAD patients who used
ginkgo alone for 10 weeks (Lingaerde et al. 1999). Combining ginkgo with
trimipramine resulted in no incremental improvement in patients diagnosed
with major depressive disorder, but the patients' sleep was improved (Hemmeter
et al. 2001). One study of elderly depressed patients with comorbid cognitive
impairment showed moderate improvement in mood and cognitive functioning
with ginkgo (Schubert and Halama 1993).

Several studies have examined the use of G. biloba for the treatment of sexual
dysfunction caused by antidepressants. One study found a 64% response rate
with doses titrated up to 120 mg bid for 1 month (Cohen and Bartlik 1998).
However, this study was criticized for its poor methodology and design flaws.

Another study found no beneficial effects of ginkgo on SSRI-induced sexual dysfunction (Kang et al. 2002).

Schizophrenia and Other Psychotic Disorders

In one study, combining a standardized ginkgo preparation with haloperidol improved symptoms of schizophrenia and possibly reduced extrapyramidal symptoms associated with haloperidol (Zhang et al. 2001).

Alzheimer's Type and Other Forms of Dementia

A recent Cochrane Systematic Review (Birks et al. 2002) examined *G. biloba* for age-related cognitive impairment and dementia. Of the 33 studies published before June 2002 that satisfied inclusion criteria, all but 1 used a standardized preparation of ginkgo. Daily doses ranged from 80 to 600 mg and were generally lower than 200 mg. The duration of treatment was 3–52 weeks (average: 12 weeks). Meta-analyses of trials with dosages above or below 200 mg/day were performed separately. Analyses of all dosage and duration categories showed that *G. biloba* was beneficial compared with placebo, as measured with standardized rating scales and outcome measures, including the CGI and Activities of Daily Living scales. The authors of the meta-analysis noted that some earlier trials had flawed methodologies and some more recent trials had inconsistent results. On this basis, they concluded that the evidence of improvement in cognition and cognitive functioning associated with ginkgo is "promising" and recommended further clinical trials using standardized methods and larger sample sizes.

A separate review examining the use of ginkgo in all types of dementia (Ernst and Pittler 1999) reported similar conclusions. The authors remarked that standardized ginkgo preparations were effective in delaying the progress of dementia and improved many symptoms of dementia. However, the authors also noted the flawed research methodologies used and indicated that further studies were needed before definitive conclusions about the efficacy of ginkgo could be made.

In a systematic review and meta-analysis of the efficacy of ginkgo in Alzheimer's-type dementia (Oken et al. 1998), four randomized, placebo-controlled, double-blind studies met inclusion criteria (Hofferberth 1994; Kanowski et al. 1996; Le Bars et al. 1997; Wesnes et al. 1987). This meta-analysis included only studies using patients who had been diagnosed with Alzheimer's type dementia and in which the standardized ginkgo extract EGb 761 had been used. Based on these four studies, the authors calculated an overall effect size of 0.4, which represented significant clinical improvement in cognitive functioning according to the Alzheimer Disease Assessment Scale. This finding compared favorably with those achieved with donepezil (Rogers et al. 1998), which has dose-dependent effect sizes of 0.42 and 0.48 at 5 mg/day and 10 mg/day, respectively. The authors cited the need for more research before specific recommendations could be made.

Of particular interest is a study that evaluated the standardized extract EGb 761 as a long-term maintenance treatment for dementia (Le Bars et al. 1997). The findings of this study resulted in significant media attention and increased sales of ginkgo preparations in the United States. The 202 elderly male and female subjects with mild-to-moderate dementia completed the 1-year randomized double-blind, placebo-controlled multicenter study. Cognitive function was assessed using the Alzheimer Disease Assessment Scale, the Geriatric Evaluation by Relatives Rating Instrument, and the CGI. The findings were limited by a high dropout rate and the fact that control patients were switched to ginkgo if any signs of deterioration were observed during the study. Analysis was done on data obtained from patients who completed at least 6 months of the trial. This study concluded that EGb 761 stabilized and, in many cases, improved symptoms of mild-to-moderate dementia when treatment lasted for 6 months to 1 year.

Alcoholism and Substance Abuse

One small 10-week randomized, double-blind, placebo-controlled trial of *G. biloba* in cocaine dependence showed no differential effect of ginkgo on relapse prevention compared with piracetam or placebo (Kampman et al. 2003).

Unresolved Safety and Other Issues

When used in standardized doses, *G. biloba* leaf extract is generally safe, but rare side effects do occur, including mild gastrointestinal upset, headaches, muscle weakness, dizziness, and allergic skin reactions. The ginkgo fruit pulp has been associated with contact dermatitis, stomatitis, and proctitis. The ginkgo seed should be avoided due to its high concentration of ginkgo toxin (4′-O-methylpyridoxine), a neurotoxin that has reportedly caused seizures and coma, particularly in infants. Trace amounts of ginkgo toxin in the leaves are not enough to cause toxicity. However, there have been reports of seizures in patients with known seizure disorders. Ginkgo may lower the seizure threshold and should be used with caution in seizure-prone populations. Only standardized extracts of ginkgo leaves should be used, which contain no more than 5 ppm of ginkgolic acid, compared with crude extracts that contain potentially toxic concentrations.

The most serious safety issue associated with *G. biloba* is the increased risk of bleeding due to its anti-PAF activity. Several cases of bleeding complications have been linked to the use of standardized ginkgo preparations, including subarachnoid hemorrhage, subdural hematoma, intracerebral hemorrhage, vitreous hemorrhage, and postoperative bleeding. In some cases, ginkgo was not the only supplement or medication being used, so that a direct causal relationship could not be inferred. However, caution should be exercised when ginkgo is taken with conventional drugs or supplements that have antiplatelet or anticoagulant effects, including aspirin, warfarin, nonsteroidal anti-inflammatory drugs, ticlopidine (Ticlid), clopidogrel (Plavix), enoxaparin (Lovenox), and heparin.

Guidelines for Use in Psychiatric Conditions

Uses

Ginkgo can be used for a number of conditions, including dementia and cerebral insufficiency. There is little evidence for using ginkgo for treating depression or SAD.

Safety

Ginkgo is safe when recommended doses are taken orally. Ginkgo may increase bleeding and should be avoided in individuals with known clotting disorders. Ginkgo preparations should be discontinued 2 weeks before surgery.

Dosing

Only the standardized 50:1 ginkgo leaf extract containing 24%–25% ginkgo flavone glycosides and 6% terpenoids should be used. Optimum doses for cognitive-enhancing benefits have not been clearly established. Based on previous studies for dementia and cerebral insufficiency, a reasonable daily dosage regimen is 80–240 mg in two to three divided doses; 4–6 weeks of treatment may be required before symptomatic improvement is noticeable.

Toxicity

Ingestion of the seeds of ginkgo is potentially lethal. The seeds have been reported to cause tonic-clonic seizures.

Adverse Effects

Healthy adults generally tolerate standardized ginkgo preparations without adverse effects, but some effects have been noted.

- *Allergic:* Cases of severe allergic reactions or hypersensitivity have been reported. Cross-reactivity may be seen in individuals who are allergic to mango rind, sumac, poison ivy, poison oak, and cashews.
- *Genitourinary:* It is possible that high serum concentrations of ginkgo may reduce both male and female fertility.
- *Hematological:* Cases of bleeding associated with ginkgo have been reported, as discussed above.
- *Miscellaneous:* Infrequent cases of headache, dizziness, gastric discomfort, hypotension, and restlessness have been reported.

Drug Interactions

- *MAO inhibitors:* One in vitro animal study found MAO inhibition with ginkgo (Sloley et al. 2000); however, other human and animal studies failed to demonstrate this effect (Fowler et al. 2000; Porsolt et al. 2000). The current recommendation is to avoid concomitant use of ginkgo with MAO inhibitors.
- *SSRIs:* Caution is advised when ginkgo is used with SSRIs because ginkgo may have some serotonergic activity and combining it with an SSRI can potentially cause serotonin syndrome.
- *Thiazide diuretics and other antihypertensive medications:* There is evidence that ginkgo reduces blood pressure; however, there is one case report indicating that combining ginkgo with a thiazide diuretic increases blood pressure. The effects of combining ginkgo with thiazide diuretics and antihypertensives remain unclear (Shaw et al. 1997).
- *Drugs metabolized by CYP enzymes:* The ginkgo leaf extract affects some CYP enzymes, especially CYP 2C9 and CYP 3A4, and thus should be not be used in combination with drugs that are metabolized by these enzymes. These include warfarin, glyburide, glipizide, amitriptyline, phenytoin, lovastatin, ketoconazole, itraconazole, fexofenadine (Allegra), triazolam, trazodone, and others (National Medicines Comprehensive Database 2004).
- *Anticoagulants:* There have been no reports of increased bleeding risk when anticoagulants such as warfarin are combined with ginkgo.

Pregnancy and Lactation

The safety of ginkgo has not been clearly established in pregnant or nursing women. and its use should be avoided in these populations.

REFERENCES

Blumenthal M: The ABC Clinical Guide to Herbs. Edited by Goldberg A, Kunz T, Dinda K. Austin, TX, American Botanical Council, 2003

Eisenberg DM, Davis RB, Ettner SL, et al: Trends in alternative medicine use in the United States, 1990–1997: results of a follow-up national survey. JAMA 280:1569–1575, 1998

Unutzer J, Klap R, Sturm R, et al: Mental disorders and the use of alternative medicine: results from a national survey. Am J Psychiatry 157:1851–1857, 2000

Kava (*Piper methysticum*)

Baldi D: Sulle proprieta farmacologischedel *Piper methysticum*. Terapia Moderna 4:359–364, 1980

Baum SS, Hill R, Rommelspacher H: Effect of kava extract and individual kavapyrones on neurotransmitter levels in the nucleus accumbens of rats. Prog Neuropsychopharmacol Biol Psychiatry 22:1105–1120, 1998

Blumenthal M: Kava safety questioned due to case reports of liver toxicity. HerbalGram 55:26–32, 2002

Blumenthal M: Kava, in The ABC Clinical Guide to Herbs. Edited by Goldberg A, Kunz T, Dinda K. Austin, TX, American Botanical Council, 2003, pp 259–272

Boerner RJ, Sommer H, Berger W, et al: Kava-kava extract LI 150 is as effective as opipramol and buspirone in generalized anxiety disorder: an 8-week randomized, double-blind multicenter clinical trial in 129 outpatients. Phytomedicine 10 (suppl): 38–49, 2003

Boonen G, Haverlein H: Influence of genuine kavapyrone enantiomers on the GABA-A binding site. Planta Medica 64:504–506, 1998

Boonen G Pramanik A, Rigler R, et al: Evidence for specific interactions between kavain and human cortical neurons monitored by fluorescence correlation spectroscopy. Planta Medica 66:7–10, 2000

Cagnacci A, Arangino S, Renzi A, et al: Kava-kava administration reduces anxiety in perimenopausal women. Maturitas 44:103–109, 2003

Davies LP, Drew CA, Duffield P, et al: Kava pyrones and resin: studies on GABA-A, GABA-B, and benzodiazepine binding sites in rodent brain. Pharmacol Toxicol 71:120–126, 1992

De Leo V, La Marca A, Lanzetta D, et al: Assessment of the association of kava-kava extract and hormone replacement therapy in the treatment of postmenopausal anxiety. Minerva Ginecol 52:263–267, 2000

De Leo V, La Marca A, Morgante G, et al: Evaluation of combining kava extract with hormone replacement therapy in the treatment of postmenopausal anxiety. Maturitas 39:185–188, 2001

Dragull K, Yoshida WY, Tang CS: Piperidine alkaloids from *Piper methysticum*. Phytochemistry 6:193–198, 2003

Duffield A, Lidgard R: Analysis of kava resin by gas chromatography and electron impact and negative ion chemical ionization mass spectrometry: new trace constituents of kava resin. Biol Mass Spectrom 13:621–626, 1986

Gleitz J, Beile A, Peters T: Kavain inhibits the veratridine- and KCl-induced increase in intracellular $Ca2+$ and glutamate release of rat cerebrocortical synaptosomes. Neuropharmacology 35:179–186, 1996

Gleitz J, Beile A, Wilkens P, et al: Antithrombotic action of the kava pyrone (+)-kavain prepared from *Piper methysticum* on human platelets. Planta Med 63:27–30, 1997

Hansel R, Sauer H, Rimpler H: Fungistatic effect of kava. Archiv der Pharmazie 229:507–512, 1966

Heinze HJ, Munthe TF, Steitz J, et al: Pharmacopsychological effects of oxazepam and kava kava extract in a visual search paradigm assessed with event-related potentials. Pharmacopsychiatry 27:224–230, 1994

Herberg KW: Safety-related performance after intake of kava-extract, bromazepam and their combination. Z Allgemein Med 72:973–977, 1996

Jussofie A: Brain specific differences in the effects of neuroactive steroids on the GABA-A receptor complexes following acute treatment with anesthetically active steroids. Acta Endocrinol 129:480–485, 1993

Jussofie A, Schmiz A, Hiemke C: Kavapyrone enriched extract from *Piper methysticum* as modulator of the GABA binding site in different regions of rat brain. Psychopharmacology (Berl) 116:469–474, 1994

Keledjian J, Duffield P, Jamieson DD, et al: Uptake into mouse brain of four compounds present in the psychoactive beverage kava. J Pharm Sci 77:1003–1006, 1988

Klohs M, Keller F, Williams R, et al: A chemical and pharmacological investigation of *Piper methysticum* Forst. J Med Pharm Chem 1:95–103, 1959

Lebot V, Levesque J: The origin and distribution of kava (*Piper methysticum* Forst. f., *Piperaceae*): a phytochemical approach. Allertonia 5:223–281, 1989

Lebot V, Merlin M, Lindstrom L: Kava: The Pacific Drug. New Haven, CT, Yale University Press, 1998

Lewin L: Phantastica: Narcotic and Stimulating Drugs. London, Routledge, Kegan Paul, Trench, Trubner, 1924, pp 180–182

Lindenberg D, Pitule-Schodel H: D,L-Kavain in comparison with oxazepam in anxiety disorders: a double-blind study of clinical effectiveness. Fortschr Med 108:277–282, 1990

Malsch U, Kieser M: Efficacy of kava-kava in the treatment of not-psychotic anxiety, following pretreatment with benzodiazepines. Psychopharmacology (Berl) 157:277–283, 2001

Mathews JM, Etheridge AS, Black SR: Inhibition of human cytochrome P450 activities by kava extract and kavalactones. Drug Metab Dispos 30:1153–1157, 2002

Meseguer E, Taboada R, Sanchez V, et al: Life-threatening parkinsonism induced by kava-kava. Mov Disord 17:195–196, 2002

Meyer HG: Pharmacology of the active principles of kava root (*Piper methysticum* Forst) [in German]. Arch Int Pharmacodyn Ther 138:505–536, 1962

Mirasol F: Botanicals industry posts strong growth in U.S. Chemical Market Reporter 4:12–13, 1998

Munte TF, Heinze HJ, Matke M, et al: Effects of oxazepam and an extract of kava roots (*Piper methysticum*) on event related potentials in a word recognition task. Neuropsychobiology 27:46–73, 1993

Norton SA, Ruze P: Kava dermopathy. J Am Acad Dermatol 31:89–97, 1994

Piper methysticum (kava kava). Altern Med Rev 3:458–460, 1998

Pittler MH, Ernst E: Efficacy of kava extract for treating anxiety: systematic review and meta-analysis. J Clin Psychopharmacol 20:84–89, 2000

Pittler MH, Ernst E: Kava extract for treating anxiety. Cochrane Database Syst Rev (2): CD003383, 2002

Pittler MH, Ernst E: Kava extract for treating anxiety. Cochrane Database Syst Rev (1): CD003383, 2003

Saletu B, Grunberger J, Linzmayer L, et al: EEG brain mapping, psychometric and psychophysiological studies on central effects of kavain: a kava plant derivative. Hum Psychopharmacol 4:169–190, 1989

Schelosky L, Raffauf C, Jendroska K, et al: Kava and dopamine antagonism. J Neurol Neurosurg Psychiatry 58:639–640, 1995

Schmidt M, Nahrstedt A: Is kava hepatotoxic? Deutsche Apotheker-Zeitung 142:58–63, 2002

Seitz U, Schule A, Gleitz J: 3H Monoamine uptake inhibition properties of kava pyrones. Planta Med 63:548–549, 1997

Shulgin A: The narcotic pepper: the chemistry and pharmacology of *Piper methysticum* and related species. Bull Narc 25:59–74, 1973

Schultes RE, Hofmann A: Plants of the Gods. New York, McGraw-Hill, 1979, pp 13, 26

Singh YN: Effects of kava on neuromuscular transmission and muscle contractility. J Ethnopharmacol 7:267–276, 1983

Singh YN: Kava: an overview. J Ethnopharmacol 37:13–45, 1992

Steinmetz EF: Kava Kava (*Piper methysticum*): Famous Drug Plant of the South Sea Islands. San Francisco, CA, Level Press, 1960

Waller DP: Report on Kava and Liver Damage. Silver Spring, MD, American Herbal Products Association, 2002

Woelk H, Kapoula O, Lehri S, et al: Treatment of patients suffering from anxiety—a double-blind study: kava special extract versus benzodiazepines [in German]. Z Allgemein Med 69:271–277, 1993

St. John's Wort (*Hypericum perforatum*)

Agency for Health Care Policy and Research: Treatment of Depression: Newer Pharmacotherapies. Evidence Report/Technology Assessment No 7 (AHCPR Publ No 99-E014). Rockville, MD, U.S. Department of Health and Human Services, 1999

Bhattacharya SK, Chakrabarti A, Chatterjee SS: Activity profiles of two hyperforin containing hypericum extracts in behavioral models. Pharmacopsychiatry 31 (suppl 1): 22–29, 1998

Biber A, Fischer H, Romer A, et al: Oral bioavailability of hyperforin from hypericum extracts in rats and human volunteers. Pharmacopsychiatry 31 (suppl 1):36–43, 1998

Blumenthal M, Goldberg A, Brinckmann J (eds): Herbal Medicine: Expanded Commission E Monographs. Austin, TX, Integrative Medicine Communications, 2000

Bruneton J: Pharmacognosy, Phytochemistry, Medicinal Plants, 2nd Edition. Paris, Lavoisier, 1999

Cott JM: In vitro receptor binding and enzyme inhibition by *Hypericum perforatum* extract. Pharmacopsychiatry 30 (suppl):108–112, 1997

Davidson JR, Connor KM: St. John's wort in generalized anxiety disorder: three case reports. J Clin Psychopharmacol 21:635–636, 2001

De Smet PA: Drug therapy: herbal remedies. N Engl J Med 347:2046–2056, 2002

Di Carlo G, Borrelli F, Ernst E, et al: St. John's wort: Prozac from the plant kingdom. Trends Pharmacol Sci 22:292–297, 2001

Dressler GK, Schwarz UI, Wilkinson GR, et al: Coordinate induction of both cytochrome P450 3A and MDR1 by St. John's wort in healthy subjects. Clin Pharmacol Ther 73:41–50, 2003

Findling RL, McNamara NK, O'Riordan MA, et al: An open-labeled pilot study of St. John's wort in juvenile depression. J Am Acad Adolesc Psychiatry 42:908–914, 2003

Gaster B, Holroyd J: St. John's wort for depression: a systematic review. Arch Intern Med 160:152–156, 2000

Grube B, Walper A, Wheatley D: St. John's wort extract: efficacy for menopausal symptoms of psychological origin. Adv Ther 16:177–186, 1999

Hammerly M, Rouse J, Spoerke DG: St. John's wort: alternative medicine evaluation, in AltMedDex System. Edited by Klasko RK. Greenwood Village, CO, Thompson MICROMEDEX, 2004

Hubner WD, Kirste T: Experience with St. John's wort (*Hypericum perforatum*) in children under 12 years with symptoms of depression and psychovegetative disturbances. Phytother Res 15:367–370, 2001

Hypericum Depression Trial Study Group: Effect of *Hypericum perforatum* (St. John's wort) in major depressive disorder: a randomized controlled trial. JAMA 287:1807–1814, 2002

Kasper S: Treatment of seasonal affective disorder with hypericum extract. Pharmacopsychiatry 30 (suppl 2):89–93, 1997

Kim HL, Streltzer J, Goebert D: St. John's wort for depression: a meta-analysis of well-defined clinical trials. J Nerv Ment Dis 187:532–539, 1999

Linde K, Mulrow CD: St. John's wort for depression. Cochrane Database Syst Rev (2): CD000448, 2002

Linde K, Ramirez G, Mulrow CD, et al: St. John's wort for depression: an overview and meta-analysis of randomized clinical trials. BMJ 313:253–258, 1996

Markowitz JS, Donovan JL, DeVane CL, et al: Effect of St. John's wort on drug metabolism by induction of cytochrome P450 3A4 enzyme. JAMA 290:1500–1504, 2003

Mills S, Bone K: Principles and Practice of Phytotherapy: Modern Herbal Medicine. London, Churchill Livingstone, 1999

Moore LB, Goodwin B, Jones SA, et al: St. John's wort induces hepatic drug metabolism through activation of the pregnane X receptor. Proc Natl Acad Sci U S A 97:7500–7502, 2000

Nahrstedt A, Butterweck V: Biologically active and other chemical constituents of the herb *Hypericum perforatum*. Pharmacopsychiatry 30 (suppl 2):129–134, 1997

Schule C, Baghai T, Ferrera A, et al: Neuroendocrine effects of *Hypericum* extract WS 5570 in 12 healthy male volunteers. Pharmacopsychiatry 34 (suppl 1):S127–S133, 2001

Shelton RC, Keller MB, Gelenberg A, et al: Effectiveness of St. John's wort in major depression: a randomized controlled trial. JAMA 285:1978–1986, 2001

Stevinson C, Ernst E: A pilot study of *Hypericum perforatum* for the treatment of premenstrual syndrome. BJOG 107:870–876, 2000

Taylor LH, Kobak KA: An open-label trial of St. John's wort (*Hypericum perforatum*) in obsessive-compulsive disorder. J Clin Psychiatry 61:575–578, 2000

Voelker R: Herbs and anesthesia. JAMA 281:1882, 1999

Wentworth JM, Agostini M, Love J, et al: St. John's wort, a herbal antidepressant, activates the steroid X receptor. J Endocrinol 166:R11–R16, 2000

Wheatley D: Hypericum in seasonal affective disorder. Curr Med Res Opin 15:33–37, 1999

Whiskey E, Werneke U, Taylor D: A systematic review and meta-analysis of *Hypericum perforatum* in depression: a comprehensive clinical review. Int Clin Psychopharmacol 16:239–252, 2001

Williams JW Jr, Mulrow CD, Chiquette E, et al: A systematic review of newer pharmacotherapies for depression in adults: evidence report summary. Ann Intern Med 132:743–756, 2000

Zhou S, Chan, E, Pan SQ, et al: Pharmacokinetic interactions of drugs with St. John's wort. J Psychopharmacol 18:262–276, 2004

Ginkgo (*Ginkgo biloba*)

Birks J, Grimley EV, Van Dongen M: *Ginkgo biloba* for cognitive impairment and dementia. Cochrane Database Syst Rev (4):CD003120, 2002

Blumenthal M, Goldberg A, Brinckmann J (eds): Herbal Medicine: Expanded Commission E Monographs. Newton, MA, Integrative Medicine Communications, 2000, pp 160–169

Cohen AJ, Bartlik B: *Ginkgo biloba* for antidepressant-induced sexual dysfunction. J Sex Marital Ther 24:139–143, 1998

Ernst E, Pittler MH: Ginkgo biloba for dementia. A systematic review of double-blind, placebo-controlled trials. Clin Drug Invest 17:301–308, 1999

Fowler JS, Wang G-J, Volkow ND, et al: Evidence that *Ginkgo biloba* extract does not inhibit MAO A and B in living human brain. Life Sci 66:141–146, 2000

Hemmeter U, Annen B, Bischof R, et al: Polysomnographic effects of adjuvant *Ginkgo biloba* therapy in patients with major depression medicated with trimipramine. Pharmacopsychiatry 34:50–59, 2001

Hofferberth B: The efficacy of EGb 761 in patients with senile dementia of the Alzheimer type: a double-blind, placebo-controlled study on different levels of investigation. Hum Psychopharmacol 9:215–222, 1994

Hopfenmuller W: Evidence for a therapeutic effect of *Ginkgo biloba* special extract: meta-analysis of 11 clinical studies in patients with cerebrovascular insufficiency in old age. Arzneimittelforschung 44:1005–1013, 1994

Kampman K, Majewska MD, Tourian K, et al: A pilot trial of piracetam and *Ginkgo biloba* for the treatment of cocaine dependence. Addict Behav 28:437–448, 2003

Kang B, Lee S, Kim M, et al: A placebo-controlled, double-blind trial of *Ginkgo biloba* for antidepressant-induced sexual dysfunction. Hum Psychopharmacol 17:279–284, 2002

Kanowski S, Herrmann WM, Stephan K, et al: Proof of efficacy of the *Ginkgo biloba* special extract EGb 761 in outpatients suffering from mild to moderate primary degenerative dementia of the Alzheimer type or multi-infarct dementia. Pharmacopsychiatry 29:47–56, 1996

Kleijnen J, Knipschild P: *Ginkgo biloba* for cerebral insufficiency. Br J Clin Pharmacol 34:352–358, 1992

Le Bars PL, Katz MM, Berman N, et al: A placebo-controlled, double-blind, randomized trial of an extract of *Ginkgo biloba* for dementia. JAMA 278:1327–1332, 1997

Lingaerde O, Foreland AR, Magnusson A: Can winter depression be prevented by *Ginkgo biloba* extract? a placebo-controlled trial. Acta Psychiatr Scand 100:62–66, 1999

Mills S, Bone K: Principles and Practice of Phytotherapy: Modern Herbal Medicine. Toronto, Canada, Churchill Livingstone, 2000

National Institutes of Health: Ginkgo biloba prevention trial in older individuals (NCT00010803). Available at: http://clinicaltrials.gov/ct/show/NCT00010803. Accessed August 2006.

Natural Medicines Comprehensive Database: Ginkgo leaf (Ginkgo leaf extract), 2004. Available at: www.naturaldatabase.com. Accessed August 2004.

Oken BS, Storzbach DM, Kaye JA: The efficacy of *Ginkgo biloba* on cognitive function in Alzheimer disease. Arch Neurol 55:1409–1415, 1998

Porsolt RD, Roux S, Drieu K: Evaluation of a *Ginkgo biloba* extract (EGb 761) in functional tests for monoamine oxidase inhibition. Arzneimittelforschung 50:232–235, 2000

Rai GS, Shovlin C, Wesnes KA: A double-blind, placebo controlled study of *Ginkgo biloba* extract ("Tanakan") in elderly outpatients with mild to moderate memory impairment. Curr Med Res Opin 12:350–355, 1991

Rogers SL, Farlow MR, Doody RS, et al: A 24-week, double-blind, placebo-controlled trial of donepezil in patients with Alzheimer's disease. Neurology 50:136–145, 1998

Schubert H, Halama P: Depressive episode primarily unresponsive to therapy in elderly patients: efficacy of *Ginkgo biloba* (EGB 761) in combination with antidepressants. Geriatr Forschung 3:45–53, 1993

Shaw D, Leon C, Kolev S, et al: Traditional remedies and food supplements: a 5-year toxicological study (1991–1995). Drug Saf 17:342–356, 1997

Sloley BD, Urichik LJ, Morley P, et al: Identification of kaempferol as a monoamine oxidase inhibitor and potential neuroprotectant in extracts of *Ginkgo biloba* leaves. J Pharm Pharmacol 52:451–459, 2000

Solomon PR, Adams F, Silver A, et al: Ginkgo for memory enhancement: a randomized controlled trial. JAMA 288:835–840, 2002

Subhan Z, Hindmarch I: The psychopharmacological effects of *Ginkgo biloba* extract in normal healthy volunteers. Int J Clin Pharmacol Res 4:89–93, 1984

Wesnes K, Simmons D, Rook M, et al: A double-blind placebo-controlled trial of Tanakan in the treatment of idiopathic cognitive impairment in the elderly. Hum Psychopharmacol 2:159–169, 1987

Zhang X, Zhou D, Zhang P, et al: A double-blind, placebo-controlled trial of extract of *Ginkgo biloba* added to haloperidol in treatment-resistant patients with schizophrenia. J Clin Psychiatry 62:878–883, 2001

6

Nutritional Supplements

Janet E. Settle, M.D.

Psychological symptoms are often the first sign of micronutrient deficiency, making psychiatrists with their medical training uniquely qualified to identify and treat such deficiencies. In vitamin-deprivation studies, behavioral and mental performance changes are the first and often the only findings. The possibility that undetected micronutrient deficiencies cause or contribute to common psychiatric illnesses is receiving increased attention. Such deficiencies may result from dietary inadequacies at the individual or societal level. Alternatively, as may be the case with depression and folate, the genetic or biochemical features of a disorder may increase micronutrient requirements, rendering usual intake inadequate. Regardless of whether or not deficiencies contribute to common psychopathology, micronutrients are powerful agents in normal neuronal functioning, which independently justifies investigation into their potential as therapeutic molecules.

The study of micronutrient therapies is hindered by a long-standing bias against nutritional supplements in medicine. Goodwin and Tangum (1998) offered an entertaining and enlightening discussion of this bias. The bias against micronutrients is evidenced by unquestioning acceptance of toxic effects, reluctance to accept evidence of their beneficial effects, and the use of a dismissive, scornful tone, unusual in academic dialogue, when reviewing supplements in medical textbooks.

Medicine has traditionally been closed to innovation by outsiders. The original proponents of micronutrients were often nonphysicians who, rejected as partners and contributors by the medical community, took their message directly to the public. Goodwin and Tangum (1998) highlighted parallels between this situation and the case against Galileo, a mathematician who published his hypothesis that the universe revolves around the sun in Italian, the language of the masses. He was allegedly persecuted for this proposal, although it had been made previously by others, including Copernicus, without political repercussion. Galileo's true crimes were bypassing the intellectual elite, who communicated in Latin, and stepping outside the bounds of mathematics to trespass on the territory of philosophers, who outranked mathematicians. The attempts of the intellectual establishment to discredit Galileo were a response to his unorthodox methods more than his ideas.

Proponents of micronutrients have received much the same treatment from medicine. Linus Pauling, a chemist who offended the medical establishment by advocating the use of megavitamins, was initially received in print with ridicule and condemnation. The reputations of Galileo and Pauling were later resurrected from heretic to genius status. The question of whether Galileo, Pauling, or current innovators in holistic medicine are right or wrong is not the point. The social context within which we practice medicine powerfully influences our appraisal of new ideas about diseases and treatments. By obtaining insight into our biases, we have the opportunity to avoid errors of judgment created by contextually defined blind spots.

Of course, a bias in favor of micronutrients can be just as dangerous. As physicians, we have a responsibility to do our due diligence in comparing micronutrients with existing therapies in terms of efficacy, risk, and cost. In some cases, the benefits are similar to those of established therapeutic agents. In others, early uncontrolled data look promising, but controlled studies have not yet been reported. Given the absence of financial incentives to develop patentable natural products, the depth of evidence we have come to expect in Western science may never be available for these treatments.

Inundated by a sea of medical information, physicians have largely deferred to the U.S. Food and Drug Administration (FDA) and pharmaceutical companies to sanction a menu of appropriate treatment options. This arrangement, while effective in organizing the use of pharmaceuticals, places a heavier burden on the clinician to independently evaluate the evidence on nonpharmaceutical treatments. In the current medical climate, venturing outside the territory of FDA-approved options involves a calculated risk. Accurately determining the risk–benefit ratio of micronutrient supplementation requires considerable data.

Are there enough data to justify recommending micronutrient treatment strategies to patients? In the current landscape of imperfect pharmaceutical options and inadequate data on complementary approaches, this becomes a personal question, the answer to which varies on a case-by-case basis. Factors influencing each individual's decision about micronutrient supplementation include severity of illness, responsiveness to conventional treatment, the side-effect profiles of options being considered, the attitudes and preferences of the patient, and the comfort of the physician.

Within practical limits, this chapter provides the level of detail about available research data that is necessary to allow the reader to weigh the adequacy of clinical information on the use of the following natural product supplements in mental health care: S-adenosyl-L-methionine, folate, multivitamins, EMPowerPlus (a proprietary multivitamin–multimineral supplement), 5-hydroxytryptophan, inositol, chromium, and acetyl-L-carnitine. The discussion of each supplement begins with its general relevance to mental health treatment followed by a concise review of evidence for its use, guidelines for use, safety concerns, and discussion. Most data on the use of nutritional supplements in mental health care apply to the treatment of mood disorders, particularly depression. This chapter is therefore organized by supplement, not by disorder. Findings pertaining to natural product treatments of bipolar disorder can be found in the sections on chromium, inositol, and folate. The section on EMPowerPlus deals exclusively with the treatment of bipolar disorder. One study on the benefits of micronutrients in schizophrenia is presented in the section on folate. Data on treating anxiety disorders are presented in the sections on inositol and 5-hydroxytryptophan. One study on eating disorders is presented in the section on inositol. Data on the treatment of dysthymia are presented in the sections on chromium and acetyl-L-carnitine.

It is important to note that most supplements are not standardized. Patients should be advised to purchase supplements from reputable suppliers. ConsumerLab.com (www.consumerlab.com), an independent laboratory, analyzes individual brands of natural products to verify that preparations actually contain the compounds listed on the product label. Important safety data pertaining to the natural products reviewed in this chapter are summarized in Chapter 3, "Patient Safety."

S-ADENOSYL-L-METHIONINE

Interest in the role of methylation in the etiology of mental and physical illness is gaining momentum. In a cycle called *one-carbon metabolism* (or the one-carbon cycle), methylfolate, the biologically active form of folate, combines with homocysteine in a B_{12}-dependent reaction to form methionine. With the addition of adenosine 5′triphosphate (ATP), methionine becomes S-adenosyl-L-methionine (SAMe). SAMe serves as a methyl group donor in more than 35 reactions throughout the body and brain, facilitating synthesis of the monoamine neurotransmitters, membrane phospholipids, proteins, and nucleotides. By donating a methyl group, SAMe is converted back into homocysteine to feed the cycle again. The amount of SAMe in the body determines a person's methylation capacity, which may be impaired in depression and schizophrenia and can be excessive in mania. The similarity in the antidepressant efficacy of two methyl group donors, folate and SAMe, supports the hypothesis that methylation and one-carbon metabolism are important factors in mood regulation and the pathogenesis of mood disorders.

The specific methylation reactions responsible for the beneficial effects of SAMe are unknown but may involve improved membrane fluidity and enhanced neurotransmitter synthesis. SAMe donates a methyl group to phosphatidylethanolamine, yielding phosphatidylcholine, which increases cell membrane fluidity and may increase neurotransmission. Both SAMe and folate are methyl group donors that impact the rate-limiting step in the biosynthesis of dopamine, norepinephrine, and serotonin.

Studied in Europe since the 1970s and reportedly taken by more than 1 million Europeans for depression, fibromyalgia, liver disease, and arthritis, SAMe has been available in the United States only since 1999. Advocates argue that the beneficial effects of SAMe are equivalent to those of conventional antidepressants with quick onset of action and few adverse effects.

Decreased SAMe levels are found in depression, Alzheimer's and Parkinson's diseases, HIV neuropathies, and vitamin B_{12} and folate deficiency. SAMe supplementation results in increased cerebrospinal (CSF) fluid levels of SAMe and the monoamine neurotransmitters. Research findings also show that SAMe supplementation increases protein methylation, receptor numbers, receptor binding, serotonin and dopamine activity, and membrane fluidity.

Evidence for Use

Three decades of research make SAMe one of the most thoroughly studied dietary supplements. Between 1973 and 1995, 1,359 patients were studied in 39 published reports on the antidepressant efficacy of SAMe. Of the 25 controlled studies, 11 were placebo-controlled and 14 compared SAMe with tricyclic antidepressants (TCAs). The findings of two meta-analyses of controlled studies are discussed here. Early studies used parenteral (intravenous or intramuscular) delivery of SAMe, which was standard practice before difficulties with the stability of SAMe preparations were resolved. Subsequent research has confirmed good absorption and antidepressant efficacy with oral SAMe, but head-to-head trials comparing oral and parenteral delivery have not been done.

Bressa (1994) published conclusions based on two meta-analyses of studies of SAMe in the treatment of depression conducted between 1973 and 1992. In the first of these meta-analyses, which examined six double-blind studies involving a total of 198 subjects, SAMe was determined to be far superior to placebo in efficacy, outperforming placebo by a greater margin than did conventional antidepressants. In the second meta-analysis, which examined seven double-blind studies involving 201 subjects, SAMe and TCAs were found to have comparable antidepressant efficacy.

Pancheri et al. (1997) published a meta-analysis of controlled studies on SAMe in depression that used Hamilton Rating Scale for Depression (Ham-D) criteria for enrollment and response. An effect size was calculated for each study based on the percentage change in Ham-D scores. In four of six placebo-controlled studies (total of 216 subjects), SAMe was shown to have superior antidepressant efficacy compared with placebo. Significant differences in outcomes between studies using parenteral versus oral SAMe were not found. In six TCA-controlled studies of parenteral SAMe, two found that SAMe was superior to TCAs, one showed TCA to be superior, and three showed comparable efficacy. Two TCA-controlled studies of oral SAMe showed comparable efficacy.

The significance of many of the controlled studies included in these meta-analyses was limited by the fact that the studies were conducted in heterogeneous populations with relatively small numbers of subjects. Despite these problems, an analysis of cumulative research findings shows that the antidepressant efficacy of SAMe is equivalent to that of TCAs (as determined by Ham-D scores) and that SAMe has a rapid onset of action. Extensive additional data are available from larger well-designed studies. Bell et al. (1994) reported the results of a 4-week double-blind study comparing treatment with oral SAMe and desipramine in depressed patients. In the SAMe group, 62% of patients improved compared with 50% in the desipramine group. Responders in both groups had significantly increased serum SAMe levels, consistent with the hypothesis that increased methylation capacity is related to antidepressant response.

Three large randomized, double-blind multicenter trials have recently been published, with the results laying to rest charges of inconclusive data regarding SAMe. The large diagnostically homogeneous patient populations in the trials gave these studies sufficient power to detect clinically significant differences among the drugs under investigation. The control treatment used in these studies was imipramine, long considered a gold standard in the pharmacological treatment of depression. The findings of these well-designed multicenter trials confirmed three decades of research pointing to the antidepressant efficacy of SAMe.

Pancheri et al. (2002) reported on outcomes in 293 outpatients with nonpsychotic, moderately severe (Ham-D score ≥ 18) unipolar depression who were randomized to receive SAMe 400 mg/day intramuscularly versus imipramine 150 mg/day in a 4-week double-blind study. Both treatments were effective in reducing the severity of depression, and no significant differences in efficacy were found. Imipramine reduced Ham-D scores by 50.4%, compared with 51.8% for SAMe. SAMe was found to be better tolerated by patients. Intramuscular administration of SAMe ensured rapid onset of action and maximal bioavailability. The authors suggested that initial parenteral administration followed by a transition to oral administration could be a potential treatment strategy.

Delle Chiaie et al. (2002) published two double-blind, randomized multicenter studies of nonpsychotic outpatients (ages 18–70 years) with unipolar depression ($n = 576$). Subjects were diagnosed with major depressive disorder (DSM-IV; American Psychiatric Association 1994) of at least moderate severity (Ham-D score ≥ 18). The first study compared oral SAMe at 1,600 mg/day

($n=143$) with imipramine at 150 mg/day ($n=138$) for 6 weeks. In the second study, intramuscular SAMe at 400 mg/day ($n=147$) was compared with imipramine at 150 mg/day ($n=148$) for 4 weeks. In both studies, both SAMe and imipramine resulted in significant reductions in the severity of depression. Oral SAMe, intramuscular SAMe, and imipramine had equivalent antidepressant efficacy. Significantly fewer adverse events were reported in the SAMe groups. A significant clinical response was achieved with SAMe at oral doses of 1,200–1,600 mg/day, and SAMe at an intramuscular dose of 400 mg/day was effective, was well tolerated, and had higher bioavailability compared with the oral form.

Guidelines for Use

Research data support the efficacy of oral SAMe at 1,200–1,600 mg/day for the treatment of major depressive disorder. A reasonable starting dose is 400 mg/day, which is increased by 200–400 mg every other day to 800 mg/day, then incrementally up to 1,600 mg/day in divided doses as tolerated or until a therapeutic response is achieved. Anecdotal reports suggest that oral doses of SAMe as low as 400 mg/day are effective; however, studies evaluating the antidepressant efficacy of lower doses have not been performed. Enteric-coated tablets offer optimal stability, absorption, and tolerability. Oral SAMe should be taken on an empty stomach 30 minutes before a meal unless gastrointestinal side effects necessitate taking it with food. Noticeable improvements in mood are sometimes achieved as soon as 3–7 days from the start of treatment.

Case reports suggest that the antidepressant efficacy of SAMe is sustained over time; however, long-term data are not available. Higher oral doses probably have an equivalent efficacy to that of lower doses administered parenterally. Clinical case reports suggest that SAMe is an effective augmentation strategy when used with serotonergic antidepressants, including selective serotonin reuptake inhibitors (SSRIs).

Safety

SAMe is a safe and well-tolerated substance that naturally occurs in the human body and has no known medical risks. Doses as high as 3,600–5,000 mg/day have been studied over extended periods of time in nonpsychiatric populations with no reports of adverse events. Mild transient adverse effects may include headache, loose stools or constipation, nausea, vomiting, anxiety, agitation, insomnia, jitteriness, dry mouth, reduced appetite, heart palpitations, sweating, and dizziness. Interactions with conventional drugs have not been reported; however, formal studies have not ruled out interactions with monoamine oxidase inhibitors (MAOIs). There have been no published case reports of serotonin syndrome when SAMe is combined with serotonergic antidepressants, nor is there evidence that SAMe changes the results of common laboratory tests, vital signs, weight, or electrocardiographic findings. As with conventional antidepressants, there are case reports of SAMe causing mania in bipolar patients. Clinicians should use the same cautions in prescribing SAMe for bipolar disorder patients that they would with conventional antidepressants. Case reports suggest that SAMe is safe in pregnant women; however, this has not been established by controlled studies. Tests by ConsumerLab.com have verified 11 of 12 brands for quality and label accuracy, including the least expensive ones carried by the major warehouse stores.

Discussion

In view of the positive findings of the three large multicenter trials summarized above, there is sufficient evidence to conclude that in the treatment of outpatients with nonpsychotic unipolar major depression, SAMe (oral and intramuscular) and TCAs have equal efficacy. Head-to-head studies comparing SAMe and SSRIs are lacking, although a study comparing SAMe with venlafaxine (Effexor) is ongoing (Papakostas et al. 2003). Because SSRIs and TCAs are generally accepted as having equivalent antidepressant efficacy, SAMe probably compares favorably with SSRIs. Further studies are needed to determine adequate dosing strategies, drug interactions, and efficacy when SAMe is used to augment conventional antidepressants. Consistently positive findings combined with a benign risk profile support the use of SAMe in this population.

The superior tolerability of SAMe compared with TCAs is no great selling point in view of the long list of TCA-induced side effects. Evidence of the superior tolerability of SAMe compared with SSRIs is supported by anecdotal reports. The fact that SAMe has a benign side-effect profile and is a molecule that naturally occurs in the body suggests that SAMe will likely outperform SSRIs in terms of tolerability. The absence of sexual side effects alone makes SAMe an important choice on the menu of currently available antidepressants.

Perhaps the most significant issue that has prevented SAMe from assuming a more prominent position in the antidepressant market is the high cost of effective doses. Even through the most inexpensive sources (generally through warehouse clubs or online outlets), oral SAMe costs roughly $1 for each 400-mg dose. A therapeutically effective dose (800–1,600 mg/day) runs $60–$120/month, which, while comparable with the price of SSRIs, is out of reach for most patients who rely on third-party reimbursement to cover medication costs. As is true for conventional antidepressants, underdosing SAMe to cut costs may contribute to misconceptions about its antidepressant efficacy.

FOLATE

Folic acid (or folate) is a water-soluble vitamin that is plentiful in the diet but easily inactivated in food by cooking or processing. Many essential nutrients are involved in a complex series of reactions that convert folate to its biologically active form, 5-methyltetrahydrofolate (methylfolate). Folate's vulnerability to destruction along with its requirement for extensive processing in the body contribute to making folate deficiency one of the most common nutritional deficiencies in humans. Unlike folate, methylfolate is readily transported across the blood-brain barrier, explaining a central nervous system (CNS) concentration that is threefold higher than serum levels (Kelly 1998). In rat brain, the areas of highest methylfolate concentrations also have the highest density of serotonergic neurons. In humans, low folate levels are correlated with low levels of serotonin metabolites in depressed patients.

Neurological and psychiatric syndromes resulting from folate deficiency include dementia, insomnia, irritability, forgetfulness, depression, organic psychosis, peripheral neuropathy, myelopathy, and restless legs syndrome. Two-thirds of patients with megaloblastic anemia secondary to vitamin B_{12} or folate deficiency have some neuropsychiatric symptoms, most commonly reversible mood disorders. Numerous studies have demonstrated a consistent correlation between folate deficiency and depressed mood, fatigue, apathy, irritability, forgetfulness, anxiety, and cognitive slowing.

Although fewer than 5% of psychiatric patients have vitamin B_{12} deficiency, 10%–33% have folate deficiency compared with fewer than 10% of control subjects. An even larger discrepancy is found in geriatric populations, where folate deficiency may reach 90%. In one study of geriatric patients, only 22% of general medical admissions were found to have deficient folate levels compared with 67% of psychiatric admissions at the same hospital (Hurdle and Williams 1966). Folate deficiency is prevalent in patients with all psychiatric diagnoses but is most commonly found in those with depression and dementia.

The mechanism of action that links folate deficiency and depressed mood is unclear. Impaired nutritional intake due to appetite loss may be at fault, but studies have not supported this hypothesis. Depressed inpatients have been found to be more folate deficient compared with schizophrenic or other psychiatric inpatients on the same hospital diet. It has been suggested that depressed patients have elevated folate requirements.

One cause of folate deficiency is a known genetic defect that impairs the body's ability to manufacture methylfolate from folic acid. Methylenetetrahydrofolate reductase (MTHFR) catalyzes the final step in the conversion of inactive folate to active methylfolate. A common mutation of the *MTHFR* gene (the T677 allele) results in the production of a defective MTHFR enzyme that has less than half the normal activity in synthesizing active folate. This mutation (homozygous T677) was significantly more common in 297 patients with schizophrenia (odds ratio = 1.9) and 32 patients with depression (odds ratio = 2.8) compared with control subjects (Arinami et al. 1997).

Folate deficiency can also be caused by medications that lower folate levels, including the anticonvulsants phenytoin (Dilantin), carbamazepine (Tegretol),

valproic acid (Depakote), and phenobarbital. Folate supplementation may interfere with the antiseizure efficacy of phenytoin (Dilantin) and phenobarbital.
Conclusive information regarding potential interactions with newer anticonvulsants is not available at the time of this writing. Anticonvulsant-induced folate
deficiency may play a role in the psychiatric complications of epilepsy.

Botez et al. (1979) have proposed that folate deficiency associated with depression is part of a syndrome that includes neurological, psychiatric, and gastrointestinal symptoms, with restless legs syndrome as the primary clinical expression of folate deficiency. Malabsorption resulting in folate deficiency and
chronic constipation are the gastrointestinal symptoms of this syndrome. Neurological symptoms include permanent muscular and mental fatigue, restless
legs, decreased ankle reflexes, impaired vibrational sensation in the legs, and
stocking-type sensation loss. Folate supplementation at 5–10 mg/day for 6–12
months may eliminate or reduce the severity of these symptoms. No studies assessing folate absorption in psychiatric patients have been published.

The degree of folate deficiency appears to correlate with the severity of psychiatric symptoms. Even among individuals with normal folate levels, higher
levels are correlated with less severe depression and later age at onset. In individuals presenting for a dementia workup, higher folate levels correlate with
higher scores on the Mini-Mental State Exam. Furthermore, depressed patients
with higher folate levels are more likely to respond fully to conventional treatment, in contrast to depressed individuals with folate deficiency, whose depression is more likely to be treatment resistant.

Methylfolate donates a methyl group in the one-carbon cycle responsible for
the production of SAMe and the remethylation of homocysteine to methionine.
This is one link between folate and monoamine neurotransmitter synthesis
(Bottiglieri et al. 2000). This cycle is also thought to link folate deficiency and
elevated homocysteine levels with coronary, cerebral, and peripheral vascular
disease and depression. Folate and homocysteine levels are inversely correlated
regardless of the cardiac or psychiatric status of the individual.

Evidence for Use

Recent evidence has confirmed earlier findings of the relevance of folate levels to
major depression. Two studies measured folate, B_{12}, and homocysteine levels in
outpatients with major depression who had been treated for 8 weeks with fluoxetine 20 mg/day and assessed for responsiveness. In one study, the 71 subjects
who responded to fluoxetine were followed on maintenance fluoxetine 20 mg/
day for 26 weeks (Papakostas et al. 2004b). The 7 subjects with low folate levels
had a 43% relapse rate, and the 64 with normal folate levels had a 3% relapse rate;
B_{12} and homocysteine levels were not associated with risk of relapse. The 55 subjects who did not respond to treatment were then randomized to receive lithium

augmentation, desipramine augmentation, or increased fluoxetine in a double-blind fashion (Papakostas et al. 2004a). Among these 55 subjects, a response to any of the three further treatments was seen in 7% of the 14 subjects with low folate levels, compared with 45% of the 38 subjects with normal folate levels; there were no correlations between response rates and serum B_{12} or homocysteine levels.

Several studies have assessed the benefits of folate supplementation in the treatment of depression. In a retrospective survey (Carney and Sheffield 1970), total time in the hospital and overall social recovery were significantly improved in psychiatric patients receiving supplemental folic acid compared with those in whom low folate levels were not treated. Coppen et al. (1986) conducted a long-term double-blind study in which 70 subjects whose disorder was stable while they were taking maintenance lithium (53 with unipolar depression, 17 with bipolar disorder) were randomized to folic acid 200 µg/day versus placebo for 1 year in addition to ongoing medications. Plasma folate levels were significantly reduced in patients taking lithium at baseline and were increased twofold in the folate group. Overall, significant differences in outcome measures that were clinically stable at baseline were not found between the two groups. Among folate-deficient patients whose levels responded to folate supplementation, there was a significant decrease in the severity of mood symptoms during the year. Among unipolar patients in the folate group, there was a significant correlation between higher final serum folate levels and lower final depression scores. Because only the patients with the highest posttrial folate levels experienced clinical benefit, the authors suggest that higher doses (300–400 µg/day) should be routinely administered to patients taking prophylactic lithium.

Godfrey et al. (1990) found that 33% of 123 patients admitted for in- or outpatient psychiatric treatment were folate deficient, even though none were alcohol dependent or taking a medication known to decrease folate levels. They assigned 41 subjects with major depression ($n=24$) or schizophrenia ($n=17$) to receive methylfolate 15 mg/day versus placebo for 6 months in a double-blind fashion in addition to ongoing treatment. Clinical improvement was measured at 1, 3, and 6 months. In both the depressed and schizophrenic groups, subjects taking folate had more significant improvements in clinical symptoms and overall social functioning than those taking placebo. The depressed group taking folate had improved significantly at 3- and 6-month follow-up; the schizophrenia group taking folate improved significantly after 6 months. The magnitude of clinical improvement increased over time, consistent with the idea that the CNS responds slowly to folate supplementation.

Godfrey et al. (1992) published a 6-week double-blind study of 31 depressed outpatients, most with normal red blood cell (RBC) folate levels, comparing monotherapy with methylfolate 50 mg/day versus amitriptyline 150 mg/day. Depression scores were equally reduced in each treatment arm. Two of the 3 subjects who did not respond to amitriptyline and crossed over to methylfolate improved. Within the folate group, those who responded showed a dramatic in-crease in RBC folate levels compared with those who did not respond. In re-viewing the evidence for folate supplementation in psychiatric disorders, Crellin et al. (1993) concluded that supplementation is beneficial either as a monother-apy or as an adjunct to conventional drugs.

Coppen and Bailey (2000) reported on 127 patients with unipolar major de-pression (Ham-D score ≥ 20) who were randomly assigned to receive 500 μg/day folate versus placebo in addition to 20 mg/day fluoxetine for 10 weeks. Flu-oxetine was started concurrently with the folate or placebo. Folate and homocys-teine levels were measured at baseline and after 10 weeks of treatment. Patients receiving folate showed a significant increase in plasma folate, although this effect was less in men than in women. Homocysteine levels were significantly de-creased in women but not in men. The group receiving folate in addition to flu-oxetine showed more significant improvement compared with the group receiv-ing fluoxetine alone, with this difference being more marked in women. In the folate group, 94% of women responded compared with 61% in the placebo group. Significantly fewer patients in the folate group (13%) reported side effects compared with the placebo group (30%). The authors concluded that men may require a higher dose of folate to achieve clinical response and that dosing should be sufficient to decrease plasma homocysteine to normal levels.

Alpert et al. (2002) studied 22 subjects with major depression who had partial or no response after at least 4 weeks of treatment with an SSRI and who had normal RBC folate levels at baseline. In an 8-week open trial, leucovorin, which is metabolized to methylfolate (see "Guidelines for Use" section below), was added to the SSRI at 15 mg/day for 2 weeks and then at 30 mg/day for 6 weeks. The results indicated that 33% of patients improved and 19% achieved full re-mission. Response rates may be higher in subjects with folate deficiency, but these findings suggest that folate supplementation improves treatment response even in those with normal folate levels. Given the lack of a placebo group in this trial, it is unclear how many subjects would have achieved remission if they had taken the SSRI for a longer period. The authors noted that many of those who did not respond had also failed to respond to previous medication trials.

Wesson et al. (1994) took the converse approach by looking at the effect of successful antidepressant treatment on folate status. RBC folate was measured before and after a 5-week trial of desipramine (mean dose 150 mg/day, range 75–225 mg/day) in 99 unmedicated outpatients with nonpsychotic, unipolar depression who had been medication free for at least 2 weeks; 8% of the subjects were folate deficient. Baseline folate levels were inversely correlated with de-pression severity (patients with higher levels had less severe symptoms) and pos-itively correlated with age at onset (patients with higher levels had later onset of their first depression episode). Compared with those who did not respond, those who did had higher baseline folate levels and higher posttreatment folate levels, even though they had not received folate supplementation. At 5 weeks, the percent change in depression scores was significantly correlated with the percent change in folate levels. The greater the increase in RBC folate levels, the greater the improvement in affective symptoms. The change in folate status was independent of weight change before or during the trial and was not thought to be due to improved nutritional status. Significantly more of those who responded had increased RBC folate levels compared with those who did not respond. Successful antidepressant treatment was correlated with improved folate status. An increased serum folate level was either a marker for the biochemical shift taking place during the antidepressant response or was required for that response.

Guidelines for Use

Folate supplements can be given as folic acid, folinic acid, or methylfolate. Folinic acid, also known as calcium folinate or leucovorin calcium (leucovorin), is metabolized to methylfolate, the biologically active form of folate (Kelly 1998). Although head-to-head studies using different forms of folate have not been reported, the consensus is that supplementation with methylfolate or its precursor, leucovorin, is preferable to supplementing with folic acid. This approach bypasses a complex series of steps required to convert folic acid to methylfolate in vivo. Supplementation with leucovorin or methylfolate is believed to result in an equivalent antidepressant response (Whitehead et al. 1972).

Studies of folate supplementation in psychiatric disorders report a wide range of doses from 200 μg/day to 50 mg/day. The daily recommended intake (DRI)—the minimum dosage recommended to avoid deficiency—is 400 μg/day (see Chapter 11, "Nutrition"). There is evidence to suggest that patients with affective disorders and schizophrenia may have higher requirements. Given the benign nature of supplementation with this water-soluble vitamin, a conservative recommendation for patients with a psychiatric disorder is 1 mg/day. This is 2½ times the DRI but still within the upper limit. To avoid masking a B_{12} deficiency, folate should be taken with at least the DRI of vitamin B_{12} (2.4 μg/day). Clinical results may require treatment over a number of months.

Recommendations are mixed regarding routine screening of psychiatric patients for folate deficiency. Although research findings suggest that folate-deficient patients are more likely to respond to supplementation compared with those with normal folate levels, even patients with normal folate status appear to benefit, making screening unnecessary. In some cases, tangible evidence of deficiency may increase patient compliance with supplementation. Genotyping (offered by Great Smokies Diagnostic Laboratory, among others) for the T677 *MTHFR* mutation can confirm elevated folate requirements in a particular patient. Folate deficiency does not correlate well with anemia or macrocytosis; therefore, screening for those hematological abnormalities is insufficient. Serum folate fluctuates with recent oral intake. An RBC folate level provides a more accurate measurement of a person's folate status over the preceding 3 months. Because folate reduces homocysteine levels, plasma homocysteine levels may indicate the degree of functional folate deficiency. One treatment strategy suggests gradually increasing the folate dosage until homocysteine levels are reduced to desirable levels.

Safety

Supplemental folate is generally well tolerated with no adverse effects. Side effects are typically mild and may include disturbed sleep, gastrointestinal distress, and concentration difficulties. Vitamin B_{12} should be added when using folate adjunctively, as folate supplementation alone can mask potentially dangerous B_{12} deficiency. Pancreatic enzymes may impair folate absorption, so these supplements should be taken at different times during the day. There is no evidence that folate supplementation impairs zinc absorption. Folate may reduce the antiseizure efficacy of phenytoin (Dilantin) and phenobarbital. Data on newer anticonvulsants are not available at the time of this writing; however, clinicians should use caution in patients with seizure disorders. We have no data to determine whether folate supplements interfere with the psychiatric benefits of anticonvulsant medications. Some have suggested that the sleeplessness, hyperactivity, increased anxiety, and poor concentration sometimes seen with folate supplementation do not represent side effects of folate but instead hyperarousal and even hypomania due to folate's antidepressant effect.

Certain drugs may interfere with folate activity. Cimetidine, antacids, and sulfasalazine reduce folate absorption; aminopterin, methotrexate, pyrimethamine, trimethoprim, and triamterene act as folate antagonists; and anticonvulsants, antitubercular agents, alcohol, lithium, and oral contraceptives lower serum folate levels.

Discussion

Although the relation between folate metabolism and affective disorders is clear, larger prospective studies on the benefits of folate supplementation in affective disorders, either as monotherapy or augmentation, are unavailable. More data are needed on the benefits of different forms and doses of folate in different psychiatric disorders, the time course of response, and the relation of the response to baseline deficiency. Meanwhile, the available evidence supports recommending folate supplementation to all patients with a history of depression or current depression and especially to those with a history of nonresponse to conventional treatment. Because the costs and risks of supplementation are small, folate should also be routinely recommended to patients with other affective disorders, schizophrenia, and dementia. Findings suggest that a large number of patients may improve with folate supplementation.

MULTIVITAMINS AND MINERALS

Vitamins are essential nutrients that cannot be synthesized either at all or in sufficient quantities by the body, making dietary intake essential for maintaining good health. Vitamins are essential factors in neurotransmitter synthesis. Pyridoxine functions as a coenzyme in the synthesis of norepinephrine, serotonin, and γ-aminobutyric acid. Folate and B_{12} are coenzymes that facilitate the synthesis and breakdown of monoamine neurotransmitters. Ascorbic acid is essential for dopamine and norepinephrine synthesis. Thiamin, riboflavin, and nicotinamide assist in the production of glucose, the brain's only energy source. Trace minerals, including zinc, magnesium, and copper, are believed to play important roles in cortical functioning.

Accumulating evidence suggests that vitamin and mineral supplementation may be necessary to maintain not only physical but also mental health. This need to supplement the diet may be due to gradually diminishing nutrient levels in the food supply, increasing nutrient requirements in the population as a whole (i.e., secondary to toxins or stress), or genetic variations in individual vulnerabilities to nutritional deficiencies manifested in disease states.

Mayer (1997) reported that compared with 50 years earlier, vegetables in Britain contained significantly lower levels of calcium, magnesium, copper, and sodium. Most notably, copper levels in vegetables had dropped to less than 20% of previous levels. Fruits were found to contain significantly lower levels of magnesium, iron, copper, and potassium. The etiology of these findings is unknown but may involve modern agricultural practices, which deplete the soil. Processing depletes the nutrient content of food even further.

On the other hand, increasing stress levels raise nutrient requirements because adrenaline and related compounds increase the production of free radicals. Free radicals, in turn, damage DNA and other vital cellular structures, resulting in aging and an increased risk of degenerative diseases, including cancer and heart disease as well as decreased immune functioning and declines in normal cognitive functioning. Essential nutrients fight the detrimental effects of free radicals in the body.

The value of studying multinutrient supplements has been questioned. Critics assert that testing multinutrient preparations instead of individual nutrients does not contribute to attempts to identify precise treatments. Advocates of multinutrients argue that the silver bullet approach is flawed and that broad supplementation is more suited to the in vivo reality of the human body in which many nutrients act synergistically in a dynamic environment governed by tight homeostatic controls. Our increasing understanding of the complexity of the human nervous system is paralleled by growing recognition that the likelihood of discovering a single heroic molecule is remote.

Evidence for Use

Benton et al. (1995) reported the results of a double-blind study of 129 healthy young adults who took a multivitamin or placebo for 1 year. The multivitamin contained 10 times the DRI of nine vitamins (B_1, B_2, B_6, B_{12}, C, E, folate, biotin, and nicotinamide) along with the DRI of vitamin A. Quarterly assessment included the bipolar Profile of Mood States questionnaire with six subscales for evaluating mood, the General Health Questionnaire (a measure of overall psychiatric health), and laboratory determination of serum vitamin levels. Although serum vitamin levels reached a plateau at 3 months, statistically significant changes in mood were found after only 12 months of multivitamin treatment. At 12 months, ratings on the agreeable (versus the hostile) subscale were significantly improved in subjects of both sexes taking a multivitamin compared with placebo. Enhanced mood was associated with improved riboflavin (B_2) and pyridoxine (B_6) status. Other significant findings were seen in women in the multivitamin group: baseline thiamin (B_1) deficiency was associated with poor mood; improved thiamin status at 3 months was associated with improved mood, and at 12 months, with improved attention; improvement in B_2 and B_6 status was correlated at 12 months with significant improvement on the composed (versus the anxious) subscale and significant improvement in overall mental health; and sleep improvement was associated with improved B_1, B_2, B_6, C, E, and biotin status. No association was found between folate status and mood changes. These data support the hypothesis that vitamins B_1, B_2, and B_6 are important for affect regulation. The delay between reaching improved serum vitamin levels and experiencing significant mood changes suggests that the resolution of chronic nutritional deficiency is responsible for these changes.

Carroll et al. (2000) studied 80 psychiatrically and medically healthy men (ages 18–42 years) who were randomized to receive a multivitamin-multimineral supplement versus placebo for 28 days in double-blind fashion. The supplement (marketed in Britain under the name Berocca) contained B_1, B_2, niacin, pantothenic acid, B_6, biotin, folic acid, B_{12}, C, calcium, magnesium, and zinc. All vitamins were present at up to 12 times the DRI. By day 28, the treatment group had significantly lower anxiety levels compared with the placebo group, a difference confirmed by several standardized measures of anxiety. Severe depression scores were significantly improved in both groups. Perceived stress was significantly lower in the treatment group. Fatigue and ability to concentrate were lower in the treatment group at levels approaching statistical significance.

In an 8-week placebo-controlled study of 1,081 psychiatrically and medically healthy young men, Heseker et al. (1992) compared mood, mental performance, and other psychological variables in groups taking a multivitamin (containing levels close to the DRI of common vitamins) versus placebo. Subjects with chronic nutrient deficiency had heightened irritability, nervousness, fear, depression, and a decreased sense of general well-being. Significant clinical improvements by the end of the study were observed only in subjects who had a deficiency at baseline. In subjects with baseline folate deficiency, supplementation resulted in significant improvements in lability, concentration, extraversion, self-confidence, and mood. In subjects with baseline vitamin C deficiency, supplementation resulted in significantly reduced nervousness, depression, and mood lability. In those with baseline thiamin deficiency, supplementation resulted in significantly improved sociability and sensitivity. The authors of the study concluded that these statistically significant findings supported the hypothesis that nutritional status is correlated with psychological functioning and that even slight deficiencies, if chronic, can result in clinically significant impairment.

Guidelines for Use

There are no definitive guidelines for the use of multivitamins in psychiatry. As discussed in Chapter 11, DRIs are established to prevent deficiency in healthy populations, not to prevent or treat illness. Accumulating evidence suggests that nutritional requirements (especially for the B vitamins) in affective disorders exceed the DRIs. The efficacy of once-a-day multivitamins is limited by the amount of multivitamins that can be contained in one tablet. Multivitamin preparations designed to be taken at 2–6 tablets per day offer more substantial doses of a wide range of important micronutrients.

Safety

There are no reports of serious adverse events or side effects associated with the use of multivitamins in psychiatric patients.

Discussion

There are no studies of general multivitamin supplementation in clinical populations. The results of the above studies on psychiatrically and medically healthy populations show that multivitamin supplementation improves overall psychological functioning and suggest a role for supplementation in all symptomatic patients, even individuals who do not meet criteria for major psychiatric disorders. Additional prospective controlled studies are needed to provide definitive answers regarding multinutrient supplementation in the treatment and prevention of mental illness. In the interim, given the low risk and relatively low cost of this intervention and the mounting evidence suggesting a role for nutrient deficiency in psychiatric illness, supplementation of conventional pharmacological treatment with a multivitamin should be recommended, especially for depressed patients experiencing less than a full remission in response to conventional treatments.

EMPowerPlus

EMPowerPlus is a 36-ingredient micronutrient formula modeled after an agricultural treatment for aggressive behavior in farm animals, including pigs that become violent, biting each other's ears and tails. After hearing of the success of this strategy from David Hardy, an animal nutrition specialist, Anthony Stephan added similar nutrients to the diets of his own children, who were struggling with treatment-resistant bipolar disorder. The results were striking, and the proprietary supplement, developed by TrueHope Nutritional Support, Ltd., has been used in more than 7,000 psychiatric patients. EMPowerPlus, which is recommended for use at high dosages, contains 12 vitamins, 12 chelated minerals, and a proprietary blend of amino acids, herbs, and trace minerals.

Kaplan et al. (2001, p. 942) discussed possible mechanisms of action of EMPowerPlus:

> It is possible that bipolar disorder is an inborn error of metabolism, analogous to others such as phenylketonuria in which metabolic "errors" lead to altered brain function, but whose symptoms become clinically evident long after birth. If this is the case, the fact that a nutritional supplement may partially correct that metabolic error suggests that the predisposing genes are coding for proteins involved in metabolic pathways dependent on some of those nutrients. Many minerals (e.g., zinc) are important in dozens of biochemical pathways vital to brain function, so this observation provokes questions about the specific mechanisms by which predisposing genes might affect mental health.

Evidence for Use

Kaplan et al. (2001) reported a 6-month open trial in which 11 subjects with DSM-IV bipolar disorder (6 with type I, 4 with type II, 1 with bipolar disorder not otherwise specified [NOS]) received EMPowerPlus. The mean time from diagnosis was 7 years; subjects had tried an average of 10 medications before entering the study. Seven subjects had a history of hospitalization, and 3 had required electroconvulsive therapy. Ongoing psychiatric medications were continued during the trial, with the treating psychiatrists being free to change medications as needed. Symptom reduction was reported as early as 2 weeks after adding the supplement. At 6 months, symptoms were reduced by 55%–66%, as measured by the Ham-D, Brief Psychiatric Rating Scale, and Young Mania Scale. The changes on all three outcome measures were statistically and clinically significant. The number of psychiatric medications required decreased by more than 50% from a mean of 2.7 before the study to 1.0 with EMPowerPlus. During the study, two subjects started taking a new medication that may have contributed to their improvement. In some cases, subjects remained well while taking EMPowerPlus alone with no other psychiatric medication. Subjects who were followed for as long as 21 months reported no significant mood symptoms while continuing to take the supplement.

In a companion article commenting on Kaplan's study, Popper (2001) reported on his own observational study of 22 subjects (10 adults, 9 adolescents, and 3 preadolescents) with bipolar disorder treated with EMPowerPlus. He determined that 19 responded positively to the micronutrient formula and, that of those, 10 improved markedly, 7 improved moderately, and 2 experienced mild clinical improvement. Of the 15 subjects who had required psychiatric medication to stabilize their illness before the study, 11 experienced no significant mood symptoms while taking EMPowerPlus without conventional medications over a 6- to 9-month follow-up period.

Kaplan et al. (2002) reported on the results of an open-label pilot study in two medication-free boys, ages 8 and 12 years, with mood lability and explosive rage who were treated with EMPowerPlus. Both boys experienced rapid and significant improvements on measures of mood, anger, and obsessional symptoms. Clinical improvement was monitored with the Conners Parent Rating Scale, the Child Behavior Checklist, and, for one child with atypical obsessive-compulsive disorder, the children's version of the Yale-Brown Obsessive Compulsive Scale. Symptoms remitted with EMPowerPlus supplementation, returned when the supplement was discontinued, and remitted again with retreatment over several cycles of treatment withdrawal and reintroduction.

Simmons (2003) performed an observational study of 19 subjects with bipolar disorder (14 with type I and 5 with type II) taking a mean of 2.7 medications at baseline who were treated with EMPowerPlus. Of the 19 subjects, 15 subjects were determined to have improved: 12 with marked, 3 with moderate, and 1 with mild improvement. Overall, 13 subjects were able to discontinue all medications over a mean period of 5.2 weeks (range 3–10 weeks) and reported that their symptoms remained stable while they were taking EMPowerPlus alone. In all, 11 subjects chose to continue taking EMPowerPlus instead of conventional psychiatric medications and were followed for an average period of 13 months; 4 eventually discontinued EMPowerPlus because of gastrointestinal side effects, 3 discontinued the medication because of recurrent psychiatric symptoms, and 1 was lost to follow-up.

Guidelines for Use

Perhaps the main challenge in treating patients with EMPowerPlus is managing potential interactions with conventional psychiatric medications. Although EMPowerPlus augments the desirable effects obtained with psychiatric medications, it also increases the severity of adverse effects. The distributor of EMPowerPlus recommends decreasing and, when appropriate, discontinuing psychiatric medications when EMPowerPlus is used. Managing the transition is sometimes complicated as Popper (2001, p. 934) reported: "Introducing micronutrients too quickly can increase the adverse effects of medications, including agitation, while withdrawing psychiatric medications too quickly can result in symptom exacerbation." Both complications can take place at the same time. Popper cautioned, "Clinicians who mistakenly approach these new findings as encouragement to combine micronutrients with psychiatric medications may find that they have stepped into a serious quagmire" (p. 934). Treating medication-naïve patients is reportedly less challenging.

EMPowerPlus dosing generally starts at 32 tablets per day (8 tablets qid) and is gradually reduced to a maintenance regimen of 8 tablets per day. The specific ingredients are listed on the distributor's Web site (www.TrueHope.com). To assist in managing the complications involved in adding this supplement to ongoing conventional psychiatric medications and maximize the chances for a good outcome, TrueHope offers live phone support to patients and physicians.

Safety

The adverse effects reported with EMPowerPlus are predominantly gastrointestinal in nature, including nausea (particularly if taken on an empty stomach), diarrhea, vomiting, flatulence, and, less commonly, agitation. There are no reports of serious adverse events with EMPowerPlus. Nutrients in the supplement are present at much higher doses than recommended daily levels. Because it contains high levels of vitamin A, EMPowerPlus should not be used by pregnant or lactating women. The safety of vitamin A supplementation at this level carries an unknown risk. (Nutrient DRIs were developed to prevent deficiency disorders in the general population, not to establish limits of toxicity.) Proponents of EMPowerPlus argue that the risk of toxicity is moderated by the fact that nutrient absorption is impaired in vitamin-deficient individuals.

Discussion

Although the double-blind, placebo-controlled trials currently being conducted have not been completed, early evidence supports the beneficial effects of EMPowerPlus. Popper (2001, p. 933) wrote, "In view of the 50 years of experience with lithium, the notion that minerals can treat bipolar disorder is unsurprising." Further evidence regarding EMPowerPlus and other multinutrient treatment strategies is eagerly awaited. A controlled, double-blind clinical trial of EMPowerPlus is under way in Canada. In the United States, a three-arm double-blind trial comparing EMPowerPlus with placebo and a comparator drug in bipolar patients has received FDA approval and awaits funding.

There has been controversy in Canada surrounding EMPowerPlus and its manufacturers. Consumer advocacy groups opposed to alternative medical practices had applied significant pressure to the Canadian agency responsible for supervising pharmaceutical research, delaying authorization of the study (mentioned above) that is now in progress. That authorization was ultimately granted through a new branch of Health Canada, which is charged with oversight of all natural health products, including research on dietary supplements.

5-HYDROXYTRYPTOPHAN

Two essential amino acids, tryptophan and phenylalanine, are precursors of the monoamine neurotransmitters, which are thought play an important role in the regulation of mood. Tryptophan becomes 5-hydroxytryptophan (5-HTP), a precursor of serotonin, and phenylalanine becomes tyrosine, a precursor of dopamine and norepinephrine. Evidence supporting the use of tyrosine, phenylalanine, or tryptophan in depression is inconclusive. Evidence supporting the use of 5-HTP in mental health care is somewhat stronger and is presented here.

The theoretical basis for using neurotransmitter precursors to treat depression stems from the hypothesis that the depletion or deficiency of certain neurotransmitters leads to depression. The goal of amino acid supplementation is to increase the pool of available neurotransmitter precursors, with the aim of increasing the production, release, and therapeutic effects of the neurotransmitter that is deficient. Amino acid supplementation does not appear to result in increased neurotransmitter production and release, at least in the short term. Meyers (2000), in a review of studies on neurotransmitter precursors in depression, framed the unanswered question of whether the increased neurotransmitter production and release result in long-term, ongoing stimulation of neurotransmitter signaling, creating observable therapeutic effects. Neurotransmitter systems include feedback loops that maintain homeostasis by adapting to changes in nutrition, stress, and physical activity. Conventional antidepressants almost immediately block neurotransmitter reuptake, resulting in rapid increases in neurotransmitter concentration in the synaptic cleft. The fact that clinical improvement is delayed with conventional antidepressants by weeks suggests that something other than the neurotransmitter concentration in the synaptic space is responsible for the beneficial effects of these medications. Therefore, the fact that supplementation with L-tryptophan or 5-HTP acutely increases serotonin release, as demonstrated by the increased concentration of serotonin metabolites in CSF fluid, does not guarantee an antidepressant effect.

Serotonin does not cross the blood-brain barrier and must be produced in the brain from its precursor, 5-HTP, a modified form of tryptophan. Although tryptophan faces competition for absorption from the gut into the bloodstream and for transport across the blood-brain barrier, 5-HTP does not face these obstacles and appears to be a more reliable route for increasing CNS levels of serotonin. A significant percentage of orally administered 5-HTP is converted into serotonin in the peripheral circulation before reaching the CNS, thus reducing its potential clinical efficacy. To facilitate increased efficacy at lower doses of 5-HTP (with a commensurate reduction in nausea), a peripheral decarboxylase inhibitor (e.g., carbidopa) is sometimes administered with 5-HTP to block peripheral conversion into serotonin. Some studies have demonstrated increased blood levels of 5-HTP with carbidopa, but none using this strategy have shown increased clinical benefit or reduced side effects. 5-HTP supplementation results in increased levels of serotonin and its metabolites in the brain. Proponents of amino acid supplementation argue that 5-HTP has significant beneficial effects in the treatment of depression, fibromyalgia, binge eating, headaches, obesity, and insomnia.

Evidence for Use

Byerley and Risch (1987) analyzed the results of six open and seven controlled studies in which 5-HTP was used to treat depression. Within the pooled group of 292 subjects, 29%–69% of subjects responded favorably to 5-HTP. However, these results are of limited use because of the small sample sizes, mixed diagnoses, and uncontrolled study designs. Van Hiele (1980) reported the results of an open study of 99 subjects with refractory depression who had been symptomatic for an average of 9 years and treated with 5-HTP 50–600 mg/day over several months. In all, 43 of the 99 subjects experienced complete recovery and 8 improved significantly. In an open trial of 25 depressed patients, Zmilacher et al. (1988) found no difference in the efficacy of 5-HTP with and without carbidopa. Although a head-to-head comparison was not done, both treatments were considered to have equivalent efficacy to conventional antidepressants.

Many studies have compared 5-HTP with antidepressants in the treatment of depression. In two open, controlled, crossover studies (Nolen et al. 1985, 1988), 5-HTP was not found to be beneficial when compared with MAOIs in depressed patients who had failed to respond to TCAs or SSRIs. Angst et al. (1977) reported no difference between the efficacy of 5-HTP and TCAs in a short-term study of depressed patients. Poldinger et al. (1991) compared 5-HTP 300 mg/day with fluvoxamine 150 mg/day for 6 weeks in a double-blind fashion in 69 nonpsychotic, depressed outpatients and found equivalent efficacy between the two treatments. In two double-blind studies, researchers concluded that augmenting conventional antidepressant therapy with 5-HTP (versus placebo) resulted in significant clinical improvement in depressed inpatients already taking MAOIs (Alino et al. 1976) or TCAs (Nardini et al. 1983).

Kahn and colleagues (Kahn and Westenberg 1985; Kahn et al. 1987) reported the results of two trials of 5-HTP in DSM-III (American Psychiatric Association 1980) anxiety disorders. In an open trial, 10 patients with anxiety disorders who were treated for 12 weeks with carbidopa 50 mg tid and 5-HTP 300 mg/day showed significant reductions in anxiety, as measured using three different anxiety scales (Kahn and Westenberg 1985). In a double-blind study of 45 patients with an anxiety disorder, 5-HTP was compared with clomipramine and placebo. The 5-HTP group experienced a moderate decrease in anxiety but no reduction in depressive symptoms, whereas the clomipramine group experienced significant improvement on all measures (Kahn et al. 1987).

Van Praag and de Hann (1980) examined the efficacy of 5-HTP in preventing depression in a double-blind crossover study comparing 5-HTP with placebo for 1 year each. The authors followed 20 patients, 14 with recurrent unipolar depression and 6 with bipolar depression, over 2 years. There were 7 relapses (1 each in 5 subjects and 2 in 1 subject) during the year of active treatment with 5-HTP, compared with 24 relapses in 17 subjects (more than 1 per person) during the year of placebo administration. Overall, 13 patients from both groups were identified as being "low serotonin producers"; only 1 such patient relapsed while taking 5-HTP, whereas 5 of 7 patients with normal serotonin production relapsed while taking 5-HTP. The authors suggested that patients with impaired serotonin production constitute a distinct subtype of depression. These findings indicate that 5-HTP may be effective in preventing depressive episodes, especially in individuals who have impaired serotonin production. In a later study, van Praag and Lemus (1986) reported that in about 20% of depressed patients who responded to 5-HTP, the antidepressant effects of 5-HTP waned after 1 month of treatment. Although serotonin levels were still increased from baseline at 1-month follow-up, dopamine and norepinephrine levels had fallen. Tyrosine supplementation reportedly restored the antidepressant effect in this subgroup.

Guidelines for Use

Research findings suggest that it is reasonable to begin dosing 5-HTP at 50 mg tid, although the sedation effects of 5-HTP may necessitate starting at a lower dosage. The dosage can be eventually increased to a maximum of 150 mg qid, as tolerated. Because the half-life of 5-HTP is 2–5 hours, it should be taken three to four times daily on an empty stomach, ideally about 20 minutes before meals. Nausea, which is a dose-dependent side effect, is a frequent obstacle to achieving therapeutic doses. Enteric-coated preparations reportedly reduce nausea. Clinical improvement in mood may be evident within 3–14 days. Although many studies report rapid benefits (after 3–5 days) with 5-HTP, one found benefits as late as 2 months into treatment. If the response to 5-HTP wanes, L-tyrosine 500 mg tid and/or DL-phenylalanine 100 mg tid may be added, taken with a protein meal. The appropriate dosing of 5-HTP for insomnia is 100–300 mg taken 30–45 minutes before bedtime. Doses up to 600 mg have been shown to be effective in treating insomnia but may increase the incidence of vivid dreams.

Safety

5-HTP is reasonably well tolerated, with no serious adverse reactions having been reported. The most problematic side effects include nausea and sedation, both of which are dose dependent and diminish with continued treatment. Other less problematic side effects include heartburn, gastrointestinal upset, and, less commonly, headache, insomnia, palpitations, dry mouth, dizziness, and constipation. Study dosages up to 15 times the generally recommended maximum (9,000 mg/day) for up to 3 years have been well tolerated. Serotonin syndrome has not been reported in two studies combining 5-HTP with MAOIs or TCAs; results of studies combining 5-HTP with SSRIs have not been reported. Monitoring for serotonin syndrome is indicated when 5-HTP is combined with conventional serotonergic drugs. There is no evidence to support the safety of 5-HTP in pregnant or lactating women. As with any antidepressant, there is a risk of inducing mania in patients with bipolar disorder.

Despite the fact that 5-HTP is manufactured using a different process than that used for tryptophan, one case of eosinophilic myalgia syndrome has been reported in a patient taking 5-HTP. In this case, the contaminant responsible for the fatal eosinophilia with tryptophan supplementation was identified in the 5-HTP preparation. Clinicians should caution patients to use only reputable suppliers when selecting a 5-HTP supplement. Compounding pharmacies guarantee pure pharmaceutical-grade 5-HTP, which requires a prescription from a physician. There have been reports of anxiety when carbidopa or another peripheral carboxylase inhibitor was combined with 5-HTP.

Discussion

The available research evidence for 5-HTP is of little clinical utility in view of the small sample sizes, uncontrolled study conditions, and heterogeneous patient populations in most of the studies. Large prospective, controlled studies with homogeneous patient populations are required before the antidepressant efficacy of 5-HTP can be determined. The report by van Praag and Lemus (1986) of a 20% relapse rate among 5-HTP responders after the first month of treatment makes the typical short study duration even more of a concern. The finding in this group that norepinephrine and dopamine levels were decreased even as serotonin levels rose with 5-HTP supplementation highlights our incomplete understanding of the complex effects of using amino acids as neurotransmitter precursors for treating depression. Furthermore, nausea and sedation are significant obstacles to achieving potentially therapeutic doses. The most useful role for 5-HTP may be in the treatment of insomnia.

INOSITOL

Inositol is a naturally occurring isomer of glucose present in high concentrations in brain tissue. Unlike amino acid supplements, which are precursors to neurotransmitter synthesis, inositol is a precursor to the phosphatidylinositol (PI) cycle, an important intracellular second-messenger system. The PI cycle relays the message to the cell interior that serotonin, norepinephrine, dopamine, and other neurotransmitters are occupying receptor sites on the cell membrane. Inositol's intracellular action is unique among psychotropic agents that typically act at the cell membrane.

A role for inositol in affective disorders was first suggested by an interaction between lithium and the PI cycle. Patients with unipolar and bipolar depression have been found to have markedly low levels of CSF inositol (Barkai et al. 1978). Dietary supplementation with inositol 12 g/day raises levels by as much as 70%.

Evidence for Use

In a 1997 review of eight controlled studies, Levine (1997) concluded that inositol is beneficial in treating the same spectrum of psychiatric illnesses that respond to SSRIs, including depression, panic disorder, and obsessive-compulsive disorder. Controlled studies of inositol do not support its use in the treatment of schizophrenia, Alzheimer's disease, attention-deficit/hyperactivity disorder, autism, or electroconvulsive therapy–induced memory loss.

Depression

In an open 4-week study (Levine et al. 1993) of 11 patients with treatment-resistant depression taking inositol 6 g/day, 9 of 11 patients improved, with mean Ham-D scores dropping from 32 to 16. In a 4-week double-blind, placebo-controlled study (Levine et al. 1995a), 28 patients with unipolar or bipolar depression who had previously failed conventional treatment were randomized to receive inositol 12 g/day or placebo. The trial was preceded by a 1-week washout of all other psychotropic medication. There was no difference in response rates between the inositol and placebo groups at 2 weeks. However, by 4 weeks, Ham-D scores in the inositol group were significantly lower compared with those in the placebo group. A decrease of 15 points or more on the Ham-D was experienced by 6 of 13 subjects taking inositol and 3 of 15 subjects taking placebo; depressive symptoms worsened in 1 of 13 taking inositol and 6 of 15 taking placebo. The time course of inositol's antidepressant effect was 2–4 weeks; however, no subject achieved clinical remission by 4 weeks. Hypomania was not reported in the inositol group (4 patients had bipolar depression). However, one inositol patient dropped out because of mild psychotic symptoms, although it was unclear whether this was due to inositol or discontinuation of conventional medications. Half of the subjects who responded to inositol relapsed within 8 weeks of discontinuing inositol, a result that supported the validity of inositol's antidepressant effect (Levine et al. 1995b).

Bipolar Disorder

Chengappa et al. (2000) reported the results of a 6-week double-blind study of 22 patients with bipolar disorder (20 with type I and 2 with type II) who received 12 g/day of inositol or placebo in addition to continuing their conventional medications; 10 of the 22 had previously failed a 6-week trial of conventional antidepressants. No statistically significant differences in response based on Ham-D scores were found in these patients. However, significantly more inositol subjects (8 of 12) achieved a 50% or greater reduction in their total Montgomery-Åsberg Depression Rating Scale score compared with patients taking placebo (4 of 12). There were no manic or hypomanic episodes during the study period. Inositol did not alter serum levels of lithium, valproate, or carbamazepine. At the conclusion of the study, 8 subjects (6 who responded to inositol and 2 who were taking placebo) continued inositol in an open-label extension study for up to 24 weeks. Manic episodes occurred in 2 of the 8 subjects during the extension phase (at the 12th and 15th week of taking inositol); both subjects had a history of recent pre-inositol manic episodes, one with a rapid-cycling course. In both subjects, it was impossible to determine the degree to which inositol contributed to the switch to mania. The authors commented that the 25% (2 of 8) switch rate is similar to the observed rate with conventional mood stabilizers (29%).

Levine et al. (1996) reported three cases of possible inositol-induced hypomania, all involving a mood switch within days of beginning or significantly increasing the dosage of inositol. One patient with treatment-resistant depression initially responded to phenelzine 45 mg/day plus inositol 15 g/day but subsequently relapsed. He became hypomanic 7 days after increasing inositol to 27 g/day; his hypomanic symptoms remitted 4 days after the dosage was lowered to 20 g/day. A woman with treatment-resistant depression who had discontinued conventional antidepressants because they were ineffective (an independent risk factor for hypomania) became hypomanic 5 days after starting inositol 9 g/day. Her hypomania remitted 16 hours after inositol was discontinued. A man with bipolar II depression whose symptoms were stable while he was taking fluoxetine and lithium became hypomanic 4 days after adding inositol 3 g/day for seborrheic dermatitis. His hypomania remitted 4 days after the inositol was discontinued. It has been suggested that inositol interferes with the antimanic effects of lithium.

Anxiety Disorders

In a 2-week study (Cohen et al. 1997) of 184 rats given inositol 1.25 g/kg (about five times the human dose), the treated rats spent significantly more time in an open maze compared with the rats given placebo. This change in behavior was interpreted as signifying reduced overall anxiety. A 12-week double-blind, crossover study (Fux et al. 1996) of 13 patients with obsessive-compulsive disorder found that obsessions and compulsions were significantly reduced in patients taking 18 g/day inositol versus those given placebo. The authors noted that the level of improvement was similar to that reported for fluoxetine and fluvoxamine, although a head-to-head comparison had not been done at the time of this writing. An 8-week double-blind crossover study (Benjamin et al. 1995) of 25 patients with panic disorder found that panic scores were significantly lower in patients taking 12 g/day inositol versus those taking placebo, even though the placebo response was quite large.

Eating Disorders

In a 12-week double-blind crossover study of 12 patients with bulimia nervosa or binge-eating disorder who had not responded to previous conventional treatment, Gelber et al. (2001) observed a significantly greater improvement in patients taking inositol 18 g/day versus those taking placebo. Patients with comorbid Axis I disorders were excluded from the study, and conventional psychotropic medications were not allowed. The authors reported that inositol produced a complete remission of symptoms that was maintained over 6 months in one patient with severe bulimia whose symptoms had previously not responded to fluoxetine.

Guidelines for Use

Therapeutic dosing of inositol is thought to be 12–18 g taken in two or three divided doses. This is 10–20 times the average dietary intake of about 1 g/day. Inositol is available as a powder (2 g/teaspoon), which dissolves easily in water or juice. Usual dosing begins at 2 g bid and is gradually increased to 6 g tid. At 12–18 g/day, the daily cost is about $1–$2. Clinical improvement generally occurs over 2–4 weeks.

Safety

Inositol is well tolerated. Common side effects are mild and include flatulence, diarrhea, nausea, and abdominal pain. Inositol dosages of up to 20 g/day have been studied, with no reports of adverse effects or abnormal findings on routine measures of renal, hepatic, or hematological functioning. There have been rare reports of decreased peripheral nerve conduction at high dosages. The risk of inducing uterine contractions makes inositol contraindicated in pregnant women. There have also been several reports of patients switching from depression to hypomania or mania with inositol and of inositol interfering with the actions of lithium; thus, caution is advised in bipolar populations or patients taking lithium. There is no evidence of interactions with conventional drugs; however, few studies combining inositol with conventional medications have been reported.

Discussion

Many small well-designed controlled studies have provided promising evidence to support inositol's therapeutic efficacy in the same spectrum of psychiatric disorders that respond to SSRIs. In one controlled study of inositol in depression, the outcomes were not significant on a number of standardized measures, and patients did not achieve clinical remission as measured by Ham-D scores. This may have been due to the treatment-resistant illness of the study population, the small sample size, or the short (4-week) duration of the study. Most trials of inositol have come out of a single research group (Levine and colleagues). Replication of that group's results by other researchers will add weight to the group's findings. Larger trials with homogeneous diagnostic populations are needed to validate these early data. The fact that inositol, like conventional antidepressants, may cause switching from depression to hypomania in bipolar patients is consistent with its putative antidepressant action. All studies reviewed here examined inositol as a monotherapy. Future augmentation studies will provide valuable information about effective and safe combinations of inositol and conventional medications. In the meantime, in view of the low risks associated with inositol use, it is reasonable to recommend an inositol trial to patients with a mild-to-moderate depressive or anxiety disorder or to those who have failed to respond to standard therapies.

CHROMIUM

Chromium, a trace mineral found in the diet, is an essential micronutrient that plays an important role in glucose and lipid metabolism and impacts monoamine neurotransmitter systems. By increasing the efficiency of insulin utilization, chromium increases insulin sensitivity and can reverse impaired glucose tolerance. In controlled studies, chromium has been found to reduce depression. Insulin resistance and depression are believed to be related; however, the connection is not yet well understood. Patients with diabetes (type 1 or 2) have an elevated risk of depression, and depressed patients show poor utilization of glucose in glucose tolerance tests and decreased hypoglycemic response to insulin. An association between peripheral insulin sensitivity and central serotonergic activity has been demonstrated in humans.

Theories regarding chromium's mechanism of action in depression (Franklin and Odontiatis 2003) include the following:

- The enhanced insulin sensitivity from chromium may facilitate greater noradrenergic and serotonergic activity, resulting in an antidepressant effect.
- An increased availability of neurotransmitter precursors may be responsible for the antidepressant effect of chromium. In rats, chromium increases free (not total) serum and brain levels of tryptophan, serotonin, noradrenaline, and pineal melatonin. The effect is dose dependent and peaks at 2 hours.
- The antidepressant effects of chromium may stem from postsynaptic downregulation of 5-hydroxytryptamine type 2A receptors seen with chromium supplementation in humans.

In addition to aiding insulin sensitivity and improving mood, chromium reportedly enhances athletic performance and stamina, increases lean body mass, reduces addictive behaviors, and improves sleep. To date, the evidence supporting these claims is mixed.

Evidence for Use

Davidson et al. (2003) reported the results of an 8-week placebo-controlled, double-blind, randomized study of 15 patients with atypical depression (unipolar or bipolar II [breakdown not specified]) who received placebo ($n=5$) or chromium picolinate 600 μg/day ($n=10$). Conventional psychotropic medications were washed out for 7–30 days before the study began, depending on the drug. At 8 weeks, 70% (7 of 10) of the subjects had responded and 60% (6 of 10) were in remission in the chromium group, compared with none in the placebo group. Although these results were statistically significant, the Ham-D score reduction did not achieve significance, perhaps because of the small sample size. In those subjects who responded, the clinical improvement was robust. Partial improvement (50% drop in Ham-D score) was evident by week 2 in 50% (5 of 10) in the chromium group versus 20% (1 of 5) in the placebo group. Overeating, a common symptom in atypical depression, disappeared in 4 of 8 patients in the chromium group who reported that symptom at baseline, versus 1 of 5 patients in the placebo group. Symptoms of fatigue also improved significantly. No significant adverse effects were reported. Hypomanic symptoms were not reported in the bipolar II depressed patients.

McLeod and Golden (2000) reported on the cases of eight patients with a refractory mood disorder (two with bipolar II depression, two with unipolar depression, three with dysthymia, and one with depression NOS) with a seasonal pattern. The subjects were given chromium monotherapy (400–600 μg/day). All subjects had a long history of a mood disorder refractory to multiple conventional drugs; most had atypical features, including carbohydrate cravings and increased appetite. All experienced rapid and persistent clinical remission without significant residual symptoms. Of the three subjects who were followed for up to 16 months after the study ended, two remained in remission while continuing to take chromium. One subject (with depression NOS) who had experienced full remission discontinued chromium at 4 months and remained in remission at 16-month follow-up. One subject with comorbid type 2 diabetes noted improved control of blood glucose levels. Hypomania was not reported in the two bipolar II subjects, including one who continued taking chromium for 16 months.

McLeod et al. (1999) published five compelling single-blind case reports of chromium augmentation in dysthymic disorder. Five patients with a long-standing history of dysthymia that was refractory to conventional antidepressants underwent a series of 1- to 4-week trials. They were given either chromium picolinate 200–400 μg/day or other nutrients (including vitamin C, guarana, ginseng, selenium, and B$_{12}$ capsules) in an alternating, single-blind fashion in addition to continuing their ongoing antidepressant medication (nortriptyline in one case and sertraline in four other cases). In all cases, chromium therapy resulted in a complete or near-complete remission of dysthymic symptoms within 1 week; symptoms promptly recurred on discontinuation of chromium therapy. In two patients, sertraline was discontinued and chromium alone produced remission, with the remission being maintained in one of these patients through 15 months of follow-up. The combination of sertraline and chromium was required in another patient to sustain a remission that was not produced by sertraline alone. A fourth patient achieved remission of long-standing premenstrual symptoms with chromium as well as sustained improvement in depressed mood.

Guidelines for Use

Dietary chromium preparations contain trivalent chromium, reportedly one of the least toxic nutrients. Hexavalent chromium, present in industrial chemicals, is an oxidizing agent with significant toxicity. Trivalent chromium supplements are available as chromium picolinate, chromium nicotinate (or polynicotinate), and high-chromium brewer's yeast. The recommended daily intake for chromium is 50–200 µg. The precise therapeutic dose in mood disorders has not yet been established; study dosages have ranged from 200 to 600 µg/day in divided doses.

Safety

Chromium is well tolerated. Initial insomnia caused by chromium can be addressed by avoiding bedtime dosing. Another side effect, increased vivid dreaming, has been reported to remit after 2 weeks. Mild side effects include tremor and "caffeine-like" psychomotor agitation.

One report described flushing and orthostasis in three patients taking chromium polynicotinate that remitted when the patients were switched to chromium picolinate. Multiple studies have reported the absence of toxic effects of chromium supplementation up to dosages of 1 mg/day (1,000 µg/day). As further evidence of its safety, the Institute of Medicine chose not to designate a tolerable upper limit for trivalent chromium. However, rare cases of adverse effects have been anecdotally reported, including systemic contact dermatitis due to allergic sensitivity; renal failure in two cases, one with high-dosage chromium (1,200–2,400 µg/day for 4 months) and another with 600 µg/day taken in combination with other nephrotoxic medications (Crone et al. 2001); and uric acid renal stones (one case) after 1 year of taking chromium 600 µg/day. The stones reportedly did not recur after 1 year once the patient was switched to a different (unspecified) chromium preparation (McLeod et al. 1999). The results of an in vitro study of hamster cells in culture suggested that the picolinate form of chromium may damage DNA. The relevance of this finding to human supplementation is unknown. The effect is thought to be specific to the picolinate form and not to trivalent chromium itself.

Discussion

Although, to date, there have been no findings from controlled studies that support the use of chromium in mood disorders, the available data from open trials and observational studies are compelling. In a number of cases, the treatment response has been robust. Large prospective, controlled studies are needed to validate chromium's antidepressant effect. The potential benefits of chromium treatment appear to outweigh the minimal safety risks for patients with a mood disorder who cannot tolerate or who fail to respond to conventional treatments. The available evidence suggests that chromium supplementation can be used as a monotherapy or as an adjunct therapy with conventional antidepressants.

ACETYL-L-CARNITINE

Acetyl-L-carnitine (ALC) is a modified form of L-carnitine made from lysine and methionine with the help of vitamin C that is synthesized in the brain, kidney, and liver. Orally administered ALC readily crosses the blood-brain barrier and has two mechanisms of action. Structurally similar to acetylcholine, it has a cholinomimetic effect that increases cholinergic neural transmission. This is the theoretical basis for the finding that ALC supplementation may partially correct the cholinergic neurotransmission deficits characteristic of Alzheimer's disease and some cases of depressed mood. ALC is also a metabolic cofactor that improves neuronal energetics and repairs mechanisms by facilitating mitochondrial function, especially fat metabolism. ALC stimulates protein and phospholipid synthesis and exerts a general neuroprotective effect at the mitochondrial level by preventing excessive neuronal death.

Depressed patients often have increased total cortisol levels and disrupted circadian rhythms of cortisol secretion, likely because of the activation of the hypothalamic-pituitary-adrenal (HPA) axis. It has been suggested that ALC modulates overall HPA activity in animals, resulting in lower cortisol levels. This, in turn, may be responsible for the observed improvements in depressive symptoms. Studies support the use of ALC in moderate-to-severe depression, especially in geriatric populations. ALC is also reportedly beneficial in treating Alzheimer's disease, ischemia and reperfusion of the brain, diabetic neuropathy, and cognitive impairment related to chronic alcohol abuse.

Evidence for Use

Bella et al. (1990) reported the results of a double-blind, placebo-controlled 60-day study of 60 patients (ages 60–80 years) with dysthymic disorder who were treated with ALC 3 g/day after a 7-day washout of conventional medications. The ALC group experienced significantly reduced depressive symptoms and significantly improved quality of life compared with the placebo group. The ALC group also improved significantly compared with placebo on over a dozen measures of cognitive function. Tempesta et al. (1987) studied 24 institutionalized elderly patients with depression in a 2-month open, randomized, placebo-controlled crossover study. ALC was significantly superior to placebo in reducing depressive but not anxiety symptoms. It was especially effective in patients with more severe symptomatology. Garzya et al. (1990) presented the results of a 60-day double-blind, placebo-controlled crossover study of 28 depressed patients (ages 70–80 years) who received ALC 500 mg tid. Depression, cognitive function, memory, fatigue, and general feelings of well-being were all significantly improved in patients receiving ALC treatment versus those given placebo. Finally, Gecele et al. (1991) conducted a double-blind, placebo-controlled study of 28 patients (ages 69–79 years) with severe depression who were treated with ALC 500 mg qid for 40 days after a 15-day washout of all conventional medications. They reported that 43% (6 of 14) of the ALC group achieved full remission as measured by Ham-D scores, compared with none in the placebo group. Serum cortisol levels, which had been elevated at baseline, were normalized in the ALC group, although this did not correlate with clinically significant antidepressant effects. Anxiety scores did not change for either group.

Guidelines for Use

The typical starting dosage of ALC is 500 mg/day; ALC can be gradually increased to a maximum of 1–3 g/day in three to four divided doses.

Safety

ALC is well tolerated and is considered safe for long-term use at dosages of 1–3 g/day. Studies have reported no subjects dropping out because of side effects, no serious adverse events, and no interactions with conventional drugs. The safety profile of ALC is especially attractive in elderly patient populations, who are more sensitive to side effects and drug interactions than younger adults. The most common side effects are mild symptoms of nausea, vomiting, and agitation.

Discussion

ALC may be especially helpful for treating atypical depression and as therapy for elderly depressed patients who have dementia. Large controlled, prospective trials are needed to further substantiate the antidepressant efficacy of ALC, determine optimal dosing strategies, and identify the beneficial and safe integrative strategies that combine ALC with conventional antidepressants.

REFERENCES

Alino J, Gutierrez J, Iglesias M: 5-Hydroxytryptophan (5-HTP) and an MAOI (niala-mide) in the treatment of depressions: a double-blind controlled study. Int Pharma-copsychiatry 11:8–15, 1976

Alpert J, Mischoulon D, Rubenstein G, et al: Folinic acid (Leucovorin) as an adjunctive treatment for SSRI-refractory depression. Ann Clin Psychiatry 14:33–38, 2002

American Psychiatric Association: Diagnostic and Statistical Manual of Mental Disorders, 3rd Edition. Washington, DC, American Psychiatric Association, 1980

American Psychiatric Association: Diagnostic and Statistical Manual of Mental Disorders, 4th Edition. Washington, DC, American Psychiatric Association, 1994

Angst J, Woggon B, Schoepf J: The treatment of depression with L-5-hydroxytryptophan versus imipramine: results of two open and one double-blind study. Archiv Psychi-atr Nervenkr 224:175–186, 1977

Arinami T, Yamada N, Yamkawa-Kobayahsi K, et al: Methylenetetrahydrofolate reduc-tase variant and schizophrenia/depression. Am J Med Genet 74:526–528, 1997

Barkai I, Dunner D, Gross H, et al: Reduced myo-inositol levels in cerebrospinal fluid from patients with affective disorder. Biol Psychiatry 13:65–72, 1978

Bell K, Potkin S, Plon L, et al: S-adenosylmethionine blood levels in major depression: changes with drug treatment. Acta Neurol Scand 154:15–18, 1994

Bella R, Biondi R, Raffaele R, et al: Effect of acetyl-L-carnitine on geriatric patients suf-fering from dysthymic disorders. Int J Clin Pharmacol Res 10:355–360, 1990

Benjamin J, Levine J, Fux M, et al: Double-blind, placebo-controlled crossover trial of inositol treatment for panic disorder. Am J Psychiatry 152:1084–1086, 1995

Benton D, Haller J, Fordy J: Vitamin supplementation for 1 year improves mood. Neuro-psychobiology 32:98–105, 1995

Botez M, Botez T, Leveille J, et al: Neuropsychological correlates of folic acid deficiency: facts and hypotheses, in Folic Acid in Neurology, Psychiatry, and Internal Medi-cine. Edited by Botez M, Reynolds E. New York, Raven, 1979, pp 435–461

Bottiglieri T, Laundy M, Crellin R, et al: Homocysteine, folate, methylation, and monoamine metabolism in depression. J Neurol Neurosurg Psychiatry 69:228–232, 2000

Bressa G: S-adenosyl-L-methionine (SAMe) as antidepressant: meta-analysis of clinical studies. Acta Neurol Scand 154:7–14, 1994

Byerley W, Risch S: Depression and serotonin metabolism: rationale for neurotransmit-ter precursor treatment. J Clin Psychopharmacol 5:191–206, 1985

Carney M, Sheffield B: Associations of subnormal serum folate and vitamin B_{12} values and effects of replacement therapy. J Nerv Ment Dis 150:404–412, 1970

Carroll D, Ring C, Suter M, et al: The effects of an oral multivitamin combination with cal-cium, magnesium, and zinc on psychological well-being in healthy young male volun-teers: a double-blind placebo-controlled trial. Psychopharmacology 150:220–225, 2000

Chengappa K, Levine J, Gershon S, et al: Inositol as an add-on treatment for bipolar de-pression. Bipolar Disord 2:47–55, 2000

Cohen H, Kotler M, Kaplan Z: Inositol has behavioral effects with adaptation after chronic administration. J Neural Transm 104:299–305, 1997

Crone C, Gabriel G, Wise T: Non-herbal nutritional supplements: the next wave. Psychosomatics 42:285–299, 2001

Coppen A, Bailey J: Enhancement of the antidepressant action of fluoxetine by folic acid: a randomized, placebo controlled trial. J Affect Disord 60:121–130, 2000

Coppen A, Chaudhry S, Swade C: Folic acid enhances lithium prophylaxis. J Affect Disord 10:9–13, 1986

Crellin R, Bottiglieri T, Reynolds E: Folates and psychiatric disorders: clinical potential. Drugs 45:623–636, 1993

Davidson J, Abraham K, Connor K, et al: Effectiveness of chromium in atypical depression: a placebo-controlled trial. Biol Psychiatry 53:261–264, 2003

Delle Chiaie R, Pancheri P, Scapicchio P: Efficacy and tolerability of oral and intramuscular S-adenosyl-L-methionine 1,4-butanedisulfonate (SAMe) in the treatment of major depression: comparison with imipramine in 2 multicenter studies. Am J Clin Nutr 76 (suppl):1172S–1176S, 2002

Franklin M, Odontiatis J: Effects of treatment with chromium picolinate on peripheral amino acid availability and brain monoamine function in the rat. Pharmacopsychiatry 36:176–180, 2003

Fux M, Levine J, Aviv A, et al: Inositol treatment of obsessive-compulsive disorder. Am J Psychiatry 153:1219–1221, 1996

Garzya G, Corallo D, Fiore A, et al: Evaluation of the effects of L-acetylcarnitine on senile patients suffering from depression. Drugs Exp Clin Res 16:101–106, 1990

Gecele M, Francesetti G, Meluzzi A: Acetyl-L-carnitine in aged subjects with major depression: clinical efficacy and effects on the circadian rhythm of cortisol. Dementia 2:333–337, 1991

Gelber D, Levine J, Belmaker R: Effect of inositol on bulimia nervosa and binge eating. Int J Eat Disord 29:345–348, 2001

Godfrey P, Toone B, Carney M, et al: Enhancement of recovery from psychiatric illness by methylfolate. Lancet 336:392–395, 1990

Godfrey P, Crellin R, Toone BK, et al: Enhancement of recovery from psychiatric illness by methylfolate. Br J Psychiatry 161:126–127, 1992

Goodwin J, Tangum M: Battling quackery: attitudes about micronutrient supplements in American academic medicine. Arch Intern Med 158:2187–2191, 1998

Heseker H, Kubler W, Puel V, et al: Psychological disorders as early symptoms of mild-to-moderate vitamin deficiency. Ann N Y Acad Sci 669:352–357, 1992

Hurdle A, Williams T: Folic-acid deficiency in elderly patients admitted to hospital. BMJ 5507:202–205, 1966

Kahn R, Westenberg H: L-5-Hydroxytryptophan in the treatment of anxiety disorders. J Affect Disord 8:197–200, 1985

Kahn R, Westenberg H, Verhoeven W, et al: Effect of a serotonin precursor and uptake inhibitor in anxiety disorders: a double blind comparison of 5-hydroxytryptophan, clomipramine and placebo. Int Clin Psychopharmacol 2:33–45, 1987

Kaplan B, Simpson S, Ferre R, et al: Effective mood stabilization with a chelated mineral supplement: an open-label trial in bipolar disorder. J Clin Psychiatry 62:936–944, 2001

Kaplan B, Crawford S, Gardner B, et al: Treatment of mood lability and explosive rage with minerals and vitamins: two case studies in children. J Child Adolesc Psychopharmacol 12:203–218, 2002

Kelly G: Folates: supplemental forms and therapeutic actions. Altern Med Rev 3:208–220, 1998

Levine J: Controlled trials of inositol in psychiatry. Eur Neuropsychopharmacol 7:147–155, 1997

Levine J, Gonsalves M, Babur I, et al: Inositol 6 gm daily may be effective in depression but not in schizophrenia. Human Psychopharmacology 8:49–53, 1993

Levine J, Barak Y, Gonzalves M, et al: Double-blind, controlled trial of inositol treatment of depression. Am J Psychiatry 152:792–794, 1995a

Levine J, Barak Y, Kofman O, et al: Follow-up and relapse of analysis of an inositol study of depression. Isr J Psychiatry Relat Sci 32:14–21, 1995b

Levine J, Witztum E, Greenberg B, et al: Inositol-induced mania? Am J Psychiatry 153:839, 1996

Mayer A: Historical changes in the mineral content of fruits and vegetables. British Food Journal 99:207–211, 1997

McLeod M, Golden R: Chromium treatment of depression. Int J Neuropsychopharmacol 3:311–314, 2000

McLeod M, Gaynes B, Golden R: Chromium potentiation of antidepressant pharmacotherapy for dysthymic disorder in 5 patients. J Clin Psychiatry 60:237–240, 1999

Meyers S: Use of neurotransmitter precursors for treatment of depression. Altern Med Rev 5:64–71, 2000

Nardini M, DeStefano R, Iannuccelli M, et al: Treatment of depression with L-5-hydroxytryptophan combined with chlorimipramine: a double-blind study. Int J Clin Pharmacol Res 3:239–250, 1983

Nolen W, van de Putte J, Dijken W, et al: L-5-HTP in depression resistant to re-uptake inhibitors: an open comparative study with tranylcypromine. Br J Psychiatry 147:16–22, 1985

Nolen W, van de Putte J, Dijken W, et al: Treatment strategy in depression, II: MAO inhibitors in depression resistant to cyclic antidepressants; two controlled crossover studies with tranylcypromine versus L-5-hydroxytryptophan and nomifensine. Acta Psychiatr Scand 78:676–683, 1988

Pancheri P, Racagni G, Delle Chiaie R, et al: Recent experimental and clinical findings on the efficacy and safety of ademetionine (SAM-e) in the pharmacological treatment of depression. Giornale Italiano di Psicopatologia 3:1–23, 1997

Pancheri P, Scapicchio P, Chiaie RD: A double-blind, randomized parallel-group, efficacy and safety study of intramuscular S-adenosyl-L-methionine 1,4-butanedisulphonate (SAMe) versus imipramine in patients with major depressive disorder. Int J Neuropsychopharmacol 5:287–294, 2002

Papakostas G, Alpert J, Fava M: S-Adenosyl-methionine in depression: a comprehensive review of the literature. Curr Psychiatry Rep 5:460–466, 2003

Papakostas G, Petersen T, Mischoulon D, et al: Serum folate, vitamin B_{12}, homocysteine in major depressive disorder, 1: predictors of clinical response in fluoxetine-resistant depression. J Clin Psychiatry 65:1090–1095, 2004a

Papakostas G, Petersen T, Mischoulon D, et al: Serum folate, vitamin B$_{12}$, homocysteine in major depressive disorder, 2: predictors of relapse during the continuation phase of pharmacotherapy. J Clin Psychiatry 65:1096–1098, 2004b

Poldinger W, Calanchini B, Schwarz W: A functional-dimensional approach to depression: a serotonin deficiency as a target syndrome in a comparison of 5-hydroxytryptophan and fluvoxamine. Psychopathology 24:53–81, 1991

Popper C: Do vitamins or minerals (apart from lithium) have mood-stabilizing effects? J Clin Psychiatry 62:933–935, 2001

Simmons M: Nutritional approach to bipolar disorder. J Clin Psychiatry 64:338, 2003

Tempesta E, Casella L, Pirrongelli C, et al: L-Acetylcarnitine in depressed elderly subjects: a crossover study vs placebo. Drugs Exp Clin Res 13:417–423, 1987

Van Hiele L: L-5-Hydroxytryptophan in depression: the first substitution therapy in psychiatry? The treatment of 99 outpatients with "therapy-resistant" depressions. Neuropsychobiology 6:230–240, 1980

van Praag H, de Hann S: Depression vulnerability and 5-hydroxytryptophan prophylaxis. Psychiatry Res 3:75–83, 1980

van Praag H, Lemus C: Monoamine precursors in the treatment of psychiatric disorders. Nutrition and the Brain 7:89–139, 1986

Wesson V, Levitt A, Joeffe R: Change in folate status with antidepressant treatment. Psychiatry Res 53:313–322, 1994

Whitehead V, Pratt R, Viallet A, et al: Intestinal conversion of folinic acid to 5-methyltetrahydrofolate in man. Br J Haematol 22:63–72, 1972

Zmilacher K, Battegay R, Gastpar M: L-5-Hydroxytryptophan alone and in combination with a peripheral decarboxylase inhibitor in the treatment of depression. Neuropsychobiology 20:28–35, 1988

ADDITIONAL READING

Mischoulon D, Rosenbaum J (eds): Natural Medications for Psychiatric Disorders: Considering the Alternatives. Philadelphia, PA, Lippincott Williams & Wilkins, 2002

Shannon S (ed): Handbook of Complementary and Alternative Therapies in Mental Health. New York, Academic Press, 2002

7

Omega-3 Essential Fatty Acids

James Lake, M.D.

This chapter reviews the putative mechanism of action of omega-3 essential fatty acids, also known as omega-3 polyunsaturated fatty acids, and current research findings pertaining to their use in mental health care.

IMPORTANCE OF FATTY ACIDS TO PHYSICAL AND MENTAL HEALTH

It has been established since the 1930s that certain fatty acids are required for normal human fetal and neonatal development (Uauy et al. 1996) and that an inadequate supply of these essential fatty acids (EFAs) during critical developmental periods results in pathological changes in immune function; degenerative changes in the lungs, liver, and kidneys; and abnormalities in central nervous system (CNS) maturation. It has been hypothesized that chronic deficiencies in dietary EFAs may also result in an increased incidence of multiple sclerosis, arthritis, enteritis, immune system dysfunction, heart disease, cancer, schizophrenia, bipolar disorder, diabetes, and many other diseases (Rudin 1982).

Essential fatty acids are highly unsaturated molecules (containing many carbon-carbon double bonds) that play an important role in normal cellular metabolism, growth, muscle physiology, and CNS maturation and functioning. Fatty acids are named according to the position of double bonds. For example, in omega-3 EFAs, the first double bond is three carbons from the terminal, or in the "omega" position on the carbon chain—hence the term *omega-3 fatty acid*. Omega-3 and omega-6 EFAs are the two classes of EFAs of greatest relevance to the understanding of normal and pathological processes in the human body. Omega-3 EFAs are concentrated in two principal sources: deep-dwelling, cold-water fish, such as salmon and halibut, and products of cold-adapted plants, including flaxseed oil. In contrast, omega-6 EFAs are concentrated in products of heat-adapted plants, including olive, peanut, safflower, and sunflower oils. By definition, EFAs cannot be manufactured de novo by the human body and must be acquired directly through diet or in the form of their parent fatty acids, linoleic acid (LA) and α-linolenic acid (ALA). LA and ALA are available from many plant and animal sources and are metabolically transformed into longer chain fatty acids (the omega-3 and omega-6 EFAs) in the liver with the aid of many cofactors, including insulin, zinc, and several vitamins. Omega-3 and omega-6 EFAs subsequently enter the circulation and are diffused across the blood-brain barrier, where they are incorporated into nerve cell membranes. At several points in their synthesis or supply to the brain, EFAs are susceptible to oxidative damage, cortisol-associated metabolic stress, puberty- or menopause-related hormonal changes, viral infection, and other factors that can interfere with the availability of EFAs to the brain, heart, lungs, and other organs, and become manifest in a range of medical and psychiatric disorders.

ESSENTIAL FATTY ACIDS IN NORMAL BRAIN DEVELOPMENT AND FUNCTION

To clearly understand the role of EFAs in brain structure and function, it is important to briefly review phospholipid metabolism. Phospholipids are comprised of a three-carbon glycerol backbone with a terminal phosphorus group. The final step in the synthesis of phospholipids in nerve cell membranes is the attachment of highly unsaturated fatty acids by phospholipases to the glycerol molecule. The four EFAs that are the normal structural elements of brain phospholipids are the omega-6 EFAs, dihomo-γ-linolenic acid and arachidonic acid (AA), and the omega-3 EFAs, eicosapentaenoic acid (EPA) and docosahexanoic acid (DHA).

DHA is an omega-3 fatty acid that is essential to normal fetal and neonatal maturation of the brain, where it is synthesized into phospholipids that are fundamental components of nerve cell membranes. Infants who do not receive adequate amounts of the necessary EFAs in utero or during the neonatal period are at risk for numerous medical complications, including peripheral neuropathy, abnormal visual development, and reduced slow-wave sleep, if the deficiency is not corrected early. If the required EFAs are not present in adequate amounts, other fatty acids will be incorporated into nerve cell membranes, thereby possibly predisposing the infant to a range of medical and psychiatric disorders. Preterm infants are especially at risk, as they do not receive intrauterine DHA during the third trimester; if they are not breast-fed or provided formula containing DHA, they will be susceptible to many disorders. The other omega-3 fatty acid, EPA, is also essential for normal brain functioning. EPA plays a central role in the maintenance of nerve cell membranes from early development through adulthood.

Fatty acids are precursors of prostaglandins, the body's principal regulatory molecules. A consequence of this fact is that a diet consisting of relatively more omega-6 than omega-3 EFAs will adversely affect the balance of opposing processes in normal human physiology. The omega-6 EFAs are crucial to the synthesis of cytokines that mediate inflammation, including several interleukins, tumor necrosis factor-α, and interferon-γ (Maes et al. 1997b), whereas diets high in the omega-3 EFAs are correlated with reduced production of proinflammatory cytokines (Caughey et al. 1996). Factors that increase levels of proinflammatory cytokines include infection, trauma, allergens, and toxins (Logan 2003). The anti-inflammatory role of omega-3 EFAs has been well documented, and research findings suggest that DHA and EPA suppress cell-mediated immune responses (Logan 2003; Simopoulos 2002). The potent immunomodulatory activities of the omega-3 EFAs affect the type and amount of eicosanoids (inflammatory precursors) manufactured in the body, act on intracellular signaling pathways, and influence transcription factor activity and gene expression (Simopoulos 2002). In this context, omega-3 EFAs obtained from fish oil are believed to be more biologically potent than those obtained from flaxseed oil and other plant sources (Simopoulos 2002).

POSSIBLE ROLE OF PHOSPHOLIPIDS IN THE PATHOGENESIS OF PSYCHIATRIC DISORDERS

Two models have been developed to explain the role of phospholipids or their absence in the development of schizophrenia and other psychiatric disorders.

Phospholipid Deficiency Hypothesis

It has been suggested (Rudin 1982) that the widespread deficiencies in omega-3 EFAs in industrialized countries have resulted from trends in dietary preferences and food processing methods dating back to the early 1900s and that increased prevalence rates of numerous medical and psychiatric disorders in industrialized countries are a direct consequence of these dietary changes. The *phospholipid deficiency hypothesis* states that increases in the ratio of omega-6 to omega-3 EFAs in the average industrialized diet have resulted from increased consumption of plant-derived products high in omega-6 EFAs concurrent with reduced consumption of food sources rich in omega-3 EFAs. According to the hypothesis, the relative shift in fatty acid consumption has resulted in the increased prevalence of medical and psychiatric disorders mediated by chronic inflammatory changes, including heart disease and major depressive disorder (Severus 1999). The pathophysiology of depression, schizophrenia, and other psychiatric disorders may be associated with excessive production of proinflammatory cytokines, including interleukin-1B, -2, and -6; interferon-γ; and tumor necrosis factor-α (see above). These cytokines have direct and indirect effects on the CNS by lowering the availability of neurotransmitter precursors and altering biosynthetic pathways of neurotransmitters implicated in psychiatric disorders (Logan 2003; Simopoulos 2002). Epidemiological findings suggest that many disorders result from the pathological effects of chronic EFA deficiencies on phospholipid metabolism that affect cell membrane function in the brain and other major organs (Horrobin 1996; Rudin 1982; Severus 1999). The hypothesis asserts that disorders resulting from deficiencies of dietary EFAs mimic a general deficiency in the B vitamins (especially B_6, pyridoxine) because many B vitamins are essential cofactors required for the conversion of EFAs into prostaglandins. Thus the same medical and psychiatric symptoms that potentially result from chronic B vitamin deficiencies are postulated consequences of chronic EFA deficiencies. Disorders associated with B vitamin deficiencies include neuropathies, dermatoses, enteritis, diabetes, immune system dysfunction, and numerous psychiatric syndromes, including schizophrenia and depressed mood.

Membrane Phospholipid Hypothesis

Horrobin (1996, 1998) has proposed a membrane phospholipid model of schizophrenia that argues that abnormal metabolism of phospholipids resulting from genetic and environmental factors manifests as symptoms of chronic psychosis and possibly other severe psychiatric disorders. This model may provide a unifying conceptual framework for understanding not only schizophrenia but also bipolar disorder and possibly dyslexia, schizotypal personality disorder, other schizophrenia-like syndromes, and other psychiatric disorders. This hypothesis is compatible with the dominant paradigm in contemporary biological psychiatry that ascribes the etiology of psychiatric disorders to dysfunction at the level of neurotransmitters and their receptors. The synthesis and breakdown of phospholipids in the brain are integral to the normal growth of axons and dendrites as well as to the formation of new synapses and the pruning of old ones. Phospholipids comprise approximately 25% of the dry weight of the human brain, and AA and DHA together account for roughly half of total brain phospholipids. Brain phospholipids are essential for fluidity of nerve cell membranes and provide the physicochemical environment in which cell membrane–associated proteins are embedded, influencing their tertiary structure and therefore their capacity to function as neurotransmitter receptors. Abnormal phospholipid metabolism in nerve cell membranes indirectly affects the functional integrity of neurotransmitter receptors and intraneuronal signaling systems that are believed to be centrally involved in the pathogenesis of schizophrenia, bipolar disorder, and other psychiatric disorders. According to the membrane phospholipid hypothesis, an inadequate dietary supply of EFAs or metabolic factors interfering with the normal conversion of parent EFAs (LA or ALA) into DHA or EPA restrict the supply of omega-3 EFAs to the brain for incorporation into nerve cell membranes, resulting in abnormal phospholipid composition and suboptimal functioning of a range of membrane-based neurotransmitter systems.

According to the hypothesis, a spectrum of psychiatric syndromes is associated with structural and functional abnormalities in neuronal membranes, and the specific symptoms and their severity are expressions of the magnitude and type of metabolic errors leading to abnormal phospholipid metabolism. Severe psychiatric syndromes such as schizophrenia develop when genetic errors of metabolism resulting in chronic brain deficiencies of dietary EFAs are combined with other metabolic abnormalities that result in errors of EFA incorporation into phospholipid membranes or abnormally high rates of removal of EFAs from nerve cell membranes by phospholipases. Less severe psychiatric syndromes may result from chronic dietary EFA deficiencies or metabolic errors interfering with the normal biosynthetic pathways that incorporate EFAs into nerve cell membranes. Examples of the latter include dyslexia (Richardson et al. 1999), which is often associated with schizotypal personality (a mild schizophrenia-like syndrome), and possibly attention-deficit/hyperactivity disorder (ADHD; Stevens et al. 1995).

In contrast to disorders resulting from abnormalities of phospholipid synthesis, bipolar disorder may result from an abnormally high rate of remodeling of nerve cell membranes, which affects the functional integrity of specific neurotransmitter receptors or cell-signaling systems. According to this hypothesis, remodeling errors are mediated by excess activity of phospholipase A2, the enzyme that removes EFAs from nerve cell membranes.

The following research findings are consistent with the membrane phospholipid hypothesis (Horrobin 1996, 1998):

- Increased blood levels in schizophrenic patients of an enzyme (phospholipase A2) that is known to remove EFAs from phospholipids in nerve cell membranes
- Reduced levels of AA and DHA in red cell membranes of schizophrenic patients
- Relatively increased rates of phospholipid breakdown in the brains of schizophrenic patients who have never been medicated, as evidenced by functional magnetic resonance imaging
- Reduced electroretinogram response in schizophrenic patients, an indicator of reduced retinal DHA
- The ability of clozapine to increase red blood cell phospholipid AA and DHA levels, indicating clozapine and other atypical antipsychotic drugs may achieve their efficacy through this mechanism of action as well as by blocking dopamine

- The ability of clozapine to act like a prostaglandin E analogue, which may relate to its antipsychotic mechanism of action in regulating neuronal membrane lipid metabolism
- The location of the gene for lipoprotein lipase, the enzyme that regulates supply of EFAs to the brain, on chromosome 8, where there is evidence for a gene predisposing individuals to schizophrenia; the activity of this enzyme is typically diminished during puberty, which is often the period of onset of schizophrenia and other psychotic syndromes
- Reduced blood concentrations of EFAs required for normal brain development frequently found in children diagnosed with ADHD

RESEARCH ON OMEGA-3 ESSENTIAL FATTY ACIDS IN MENTAL HEALTH CARE

Depressed Mood

Food preferences that influence the consumption of EFAs may be directly related to observed differences in the rate of depression when industrialized countries are compared with those in more traditional cultures. Countries where fish is a mainstay of the average diet are characterized by significantly lower rates of major and postpartum depression (Hibbeln 1998). Epidemiological data suggest an inverse relation between the consumption of food sources rich in omega-3 fatty acids and the prevalence of major depression. Cross-national studies show a decrease in the prevalence of major depression, postpartum depression, and depressive symptoms as the per capita consumption of fish increases (Hibbeln 2002). In Japan, where fish consumption is very high, only 0.12% of the population experiences depressed mood in a given year. In contrast, New Zealanders, who consume relatively little fish, reported a 6% annual rate of depression and a high suicide rate. Most epidemiological data are consistent with the hypothesis that fish consumption has a general protective effect on mood (Silvers and Scott 2002; Tanskanen et al. 2001); however, some studies have not confirmed this association (Hakkarainen et al. 2004). Although epidemiological studies show apparent correlations between dietary preferences and prevalence rates of depression, definitive proof of a causal association between low levels of the EFAs found in fish oil or other foods and depression can only be obtained through controlled studies.

Accumulating laboratory evidence suggests a plausible link between the dietary ratio of omega-6 to omega-3 EFAs and the incidence of depression. One study found a positive correlation between the severity of depression and the ratio of AA (an omega-6 fatty acid) to EPA in erythrocytes (Adams et al. 1996). Another study reported increased production of proinflammatory cytokines in the initial acute phase of major depression (Maes et al. 1996). The clinical significance of these findings is supported by the observation that direct administration of the same cytokines into the brain causes a dysregulation in serotonin metabolism that is consistent with changes observed in depressed individuals. Furthermore, both tricyclic antidepressants and selective serotonin reuptake inhibitors are known to suppress the release of certain proinflammatory cytokines by immune cells, consistent with the hypothesis that conventional antidepressants perform a similar function in the brain, thereby positively affecting depressed mood (Maes et al. 1997a). The finding that omega-3 EFAs reduce the incidence of coronary artery disease by modulating the production of proinflammatory cytokines in the heart may help to explain the observed relation between the risk of heart disease and major depressive disorder (Hibbeln 1995).

Findings to date from randomized, controlled trials on omega-3 EFAs in the treatment of depression are inconsistent. A published case report claimed rapid dramatic improvement in a severely depressed, suicidal patient whose depression had been refractory to multiple antidepressant trials, including lithium augmentation (Puri et al. 2002). That patient showed sustained improvement in mood over a 9-month period while taking EPA (4 g/day) alone. No adverse effects were reported.

Three controlled studies have yielded promising results for pure EPA in the form of ethyl ester EPA as an adjunctive treatment in refractory major depressive disorder. A small double-blind study ($n=36$) comparing monotherapy with DHA 2 g/day and placebo for 6 weeks showed no statistical difference in depression response rates (Marangell et al. 2003). However, three other double-blind, placebo-controlled trials found that purified ethyl ester EPA or combinations of purified EPA and DHA resulted in significant improvement in the severity of depressed mood compared with placebo (Nemets et al. 2002; Peet and Horrobin 2002; Su et al. 2003). One study demonstrated significant improvements in depressed mood in response to combinations of EPA and DHA at dosages as high as 9.6 g/day (Su et al. 2003). Researchers in another small double-blind trial concluded that depressed patients taking EPA 1 g/day were more likely to improve compared with a placebo group, but that higher doses of EPA did not result in an improved response (Peet and Horrobin 2002). Another controlled trial compared two groups of adults with uncomplicated depression (i.e., no comorbid medical or psychiatric disorders) treated with a placebo versus purified ethyl ester EPA (2 g/day) while continuing their antidepressant medications (Nemets et al. 2002). No patients included in the study met criteria for refractory depression, and all but one had experienced complete remission with previous trials of conventional antidepressants. Ratings using the Hamilton Rating Scale for Depression (Ham-D) were taken at the start of the study and weekly thereafter. Average baseline scores were 18 or higher. By week 2, Ham-D scores were significantly different between the placebo and EPA groups, and by the end of the study, EPA-treated patients showed a mean reduction of 12.4

points, compared with only 1.6 points in patients receiving a placebo. Overall, 6 of the 10 patients assigned to the EPA group showed a 50% reduction in Ham-D scores, compared with only 1 of 10 patients in the placebo group. EPA had a significant effect on several core depressive symptoms, including insomnia and feelings of guilt and worthlessness. There were no reports of significant adverse effects in either group, and only one patient dropped out (placebo group) because of worsening depression. The authors noted that the results did not clarify whether EPA had an independent antidepressant effect or augmented antidepressants via second-messenger systems in a manner similar to the postulated mechanism for lithium augmentation. Confirmation of the significance of a primary antidepressant effect and clarification of the mechanism of action of EPA will require long-term, prospective studies that include arms assigned to receive antidepressants alone, omega-3 fatty acids alone, or combined antidepressants and omega-3 fatty acids and a broader range of depression subtypes.

A trial is currently being conducted that will determine whether adding EPA to citalopram (Celexa) will accelerate treatment response ("PUFA Augmentation in Treatment of Major Depression," available at: www.clinicaltrials.gov/ct/show/NCT00067301?order=1). All patients in the study ($N = 60$) will receive citalopram, and one-half will be randomized to EPA or placebo. The study is expected to be completed in mid-2006.

Bipolar Disorder

Case reports and the findings of one small double-blind trial suggest that omega-3 EFAs improve depressive and manic symptoms in bipolar patients, possibly by inhibiting the activity of CNS phospholipases and thereby reducing the release of unsaturated EFAs from nerve cell phospholipids and by limiting the production of specific prostaglandins (e.g., prostaglandin E_1) that are known to be associated with mania or depression. It has been postulated that lithium, dopamine antagonists, and serotonin-blocking agents are effective in treating mania through a similar mechanism of action that corrects overactivity in cell membrane signal transduction processes.

Until now there have been no large studies on the efficacy of omega-3 EFAs in the treatment of bipolar disorder, and all studies conducted to date have been designed to assess the efficacy of omega-3 EFAs in combination with mood-stabilizing medications and not alone. However, findings from one small double-blind study (Stoll et al. 1999) suggest that bipolar disorder patients taking omega-3 fatty acids alone remained in remission significantly longer than matched patients receiving only a placebo. In this 4-month placebo-controlled, double-blind study, 30 bipolar patients were treated with a combination of omega-3 EFAs (6.16 g EPA plus 3.36 g DHA for a total dosage of 9.5 g/day) or placebo (olive oil) in combination with their usual mood-stabilizing medications (including lithium, valproic acid, carbamazepine, and others). Post hoc analysis determined that 4 out of 8 patients who took only omega-3 fatty acids remained in remission significantly longer than 3 patients who received only placebo. Furthermore, among the remaining 22 patients taking mood-stabilizing drugs, those treated with omega-3 EFAs performed significantly better on all outcome measures compared with patients in the placebo arm. In another 4-month double-blind, placebo-controlled study, 120 bipolar patients were randomized to omega-3 EFAs (ethyl ester EPA) 6 g/day or placebo in combination with their conventional mood stabilizers (Keck et al. 2002). The response rates in the omega-3 EFA and placebo groups were not significantly different.

Schizophrenia

Case reports (Puri et al. 2002; Su et al. 2001) and small double-blind trials (Laugharne et al. 1996; Mellor et al. 1995; Peet et al. 1996) have demonstrated sustained improvements in positive and negative symptoms in chronic schizophrenic patients who consume certain omega-3 EFAs and are not being treated with conventional antipsychotic medications. Findings of a small 4-month open study suggest that combining EPA and DHA with antioxidant vitamins reduces the severity of positive and negative symptoms and improves overall quality of life (Arvindakshan et al. 2003). Findings of studies evaluating the putative antipsychotic efficacy of omega-3 EFAs as an adjunctive treatment for schizophrenia have been inconsistent. In a 12-week controlled trial, schizophrenic patients randomized to adjunctive EPA experienced greater reductions in psychotic symptoms compared with those who received only DHA or placebo while continuing on a conventional antipsychotic (Peet et al. 1996). All patients remained on conventional antipsychotics throughout the study. In a large 3-month controlled study ($n=115$), patients with schizophrenia refractory to conventional antipsychotics were randomized to ethyl ester EPA 1, 2, or 4 g/day or placebo while remaining on conventional drugs (Peet et al. 2002). Those taking EPA 2 g/day concurrently with clozapine experienced the most significant and sustained improvements; however, a differential effect was not observed in patients who combined EPA with other antipsychotic drugs. The finding of a specific augmentation effect with clozapine is consistent with Horrobin's membrane phospholipid hypothesis (see above). In another controlled study, sustained reductions in psychotic symptoms and tardive dyskinesia were observed after 3 months of augmentation with purified EPA (ethyl ester EPA 3 g/day) (Emsley et al. 2002). However, another double-blind, placebo-controlled study found no differences in response between EPA (3 g/day) and placebo in a group of 87 schizophrenic patients concurrently taking antipsychotic medications (Fenton et al. 2001). In contrast to the studies discussed earlier, these patients were treated for residual psychotic symptoms and were not treated while in the early, acute phase of illness.

OTHER EMERGING USES OF OMEGA-3 ESSENTIAL FATTY ACIDS IN PSYCHIATRY

Dementia and Mild Cognitive Impairment in Elderly Individuals

It has been postulated that high dietary intake of omega-6 EFAs, including LA, contributes to increased oxidative stress in the brain, thereby promoting athero-sclerosis and thrombosis, which manifest as incremental declines in cognitive functioning (Kalmijn et al. 1997a). Conversely, high intake of foods rich in omega-3 EFAs may reduce oxidative stress and associated atherosclerotic changes in the brain. Animal studies suggest that increased consumption of omega-3 EFAs improves general cognitive performance (de Wilde 2002). Low brain levels of omega-3 EFAs may be a marker of Alzheimer's disease (Corrigan et al. 1998). Emerging evidence suggests that regular intake of omega-3 EFAs may reduce the risk of developing dementia or cognitive impairment or reduce the rate of cognitive decline in nondemented elderly individuals; however, ep-idemiological data on the relation between dementia risk and omega-3 EFA consumption are inconsistent. A large epidemiological study (Kalmijn et al. 1997b) compared cognitive impairment scores over a 3-year period in two groups of elderly men (ages 69–89 years) with different dietary preferences. The initial findings suggested that high intake of foods rich in omega-6 EFAs was as-sociated with higher rates of cognitive decline and that high fish consumption was protective against the risk of cognitive impairment with aging. However, subsequent findings from the same study failed to support those findings (Engel-hart et al. 2002). A prospective observational study found that regular consump-tion of fish was associated with significantly reduced risk of developing Alzhe-imer's disease (Morris et al. 2003).

Violent and Impulsive Behavior

Observational studies (Hibbeln et al. 1998a, 1998b) suggest that low plasma DHA levels may increase the predisposition of some individuals to violent or impulsive behavior. This effect appears to be larger in certain groups, especially boys who develop alcohol dependence before age 20 years. One proposed ex-planation is that genetic abnormalities in EFA metabolism result in a higher turnover rate of serotonin in the CNS that is associated with higher cerebrospi-nal fluid 5-hydroxyindoleacetic acid levels. A placebo-controlled, double-blind study (Hamazaki et al. 1996) compared DHA (1.8 g/day) with placebo in matched cohorts of Japanese students. A significant rate of "aggression against others" was reported in the placebo group at times of peak academic stress. Stu-dents taking DHA did not exhibit increased aggressive behavior. A small ($n=30$) placebo-controlled study reported reduced hostility in individuals diagnosed with borderline personality disorder treated with EPA (1 g/day) (Zanarini and Frankenburg 2003). Supplementation with omega-3 EFAs may also reduce violent behavior in prison populations (Gesch et al. 2002).

Attention-Deficit/Hyperactivity Disorder and Learning Disabilities

Certain behavioral and learning problems in children may be associated with low plasma levels of omega-3 fatty acids (Bekaroglu et al. 1996; Stevens et al. 1995). To date, findings of placebo-controlled studies are inconsistent. The results of two studies suggest that combining DHA with a conventional drug does not improve symptoms of ADHD (Hirayama et al. 2004; Voigt et al. 2001). However, children exhibiting ADHD-like symptoms taking a mixture of DHA, EPA, and two omega-6 EFAs but no conventional drug experienced significant improvements in impulsivity and hyperactivity (Richardson and Puri 2002). In a descriptive study, parents and teachers assessed the behavior of 100 boys ages 6–12 years using standardized scales measuring conduct, impulsivity-hyperactivity, anxiety, psychosomatic complaints, and learning problems (Stevens et al. 1996). Boys found to have lower plasma omega-3 EFA levels were also reported to have higher frequencies of symptoms associated with fatty acid deficiencies, including increased thirst and dry skin. Boys with lower total omega-3 EFA levels consistently had higher scores on behavior scales measuring anxiety, hyperactivity, and impulsivity. Lower serum omega-3 EFA levels also correlated with more frequent temper tantrums and problems going to sleep and getting up in the morning. Teacher ratings of overall academic ability were significantly lower for boys with lower omega-3 EFA serum levels, but there were no significant differences in the reading or writing ability between boys with normal omega-3 EFA levels and those with low levels. A subsequent placebo-controlled trial ($N=50$) found that children diagnosed with ADHD experienced significant beneficial changes in inattention and disruptive behavior with a mixture of omega-3 (EPA and DHA) and omega-6 (AA and γ-linolenic acid) EFAs and vitamin E (Stevens et al. 2003).

Dyslexia

Two randomized, double-blind studies on the effects of omega-3 fatty acids in dyslexia are currently under way. At the time of this writing, data analysis has not been completed. However, anecdotal reports of improvements in dyslexia with DHA supplementation have long suggested that abnormal phospholipid metabolism is associated with this disorder. This view is consistent with Horrobin's theory (Horrobin et al. 1995) relating abnormalities in phospholipid metabolism to neurodevelopmental disorders in general, including schizophrenia.

Findings of several case studies along with a detailed discussion of the two on-going studies mentioned above are reviewed in Richardson et al. (1999).

SAFETY CONSIDERATIONS WHEN RECOMMENDING OMEGA-3 ESSENTIAL FATTY ACIDS

Several case reports have suggested that some fish oil supplements can result in hy-pervitaminosis A (Grubb 1990) or that individuals who consume large amounts of omega-3 EFA–containing supplements have an increased incidence of hyperten-sion and stroke (Kenny 1990); however, controlled studies have not confirmed these risks. Some patients complain of gastrointestinal distress when taking flaxseed oil or fish oil products. Omega-3 EFAs alone or in combination with aspirin do not adversely affect bleeding time (Eritsland et al. 1995; Mueller et al. 1991). In a small double-blind, placebo–controlled trial (Stoll et al. 1999), 8 of 13 (62%) pa-tients taking omega-3 EFAs reported mild gastrointestinal side effects compared with 8 of 15 (53%) subjects receiving placebo. This difference was not statistically significant, and no other adverse effects were reported frequently.

Case reports suggest that a high intake of some EFAs is associated with re-duced glycemic control in type 2 diabetic patients (Glauber et al. 1988). High doses of omega-3 EFAs may induce increased liver enzyme activity, thereby po-tentially affecting metabolic clearance of some medications. Cases of high doses of omega-3 EFAs causing hypomania have been reported (Kinrys 2000; Stoll and Damico 2000), including 10 cases in a series of more than 300 patients treated with different open-label preparations of flaxseed or fish oil (Stoll 2000). Most cases of apparent hypomania induction were associated with flaxseed but not fish oil. This effect was first noticed more than 20 years ago (Rudin 1981) and, at that time, was also associated with high doses of flaxseed oil but not fish oil products. The mechanism of action for this effect remains unclear, but in view of known metabolic pathways that transform EFAs in the human body, it may be related to the relatively higher content of ALA in flaxseed oil, which results in significant increases in serum EPA but not DHA levels. It has been suggested that the high amounts of ALA in flaxseed oil might predispose susceptible depressed or bipolar patients to hypomania by causing a reduced ratio of DHA to EPA in the serum and presumably also in the CNS (Stoll and Damico 2000). The resulting imbal-ance could trigger hypomania in genetically susceptible individuals.

RECOMMENDATIONS FOR USE OF OMEGA-3 ESSENTIAL FATTY ACIDS IN MENTAL HEALTH CARE

The following recommendations are based on a critical analysis of the peer-reviewed medical literature on omega-3 EFAs. At this time, the research evidence does not support the use of omega-3 EFAs in place of conventional medications in patients who have been diagnosed with a major psychiatric disorder. These general recommendations are based on current findings and will probably continue to change in light of future basic or clinical research.

Treatment Recommendations

Dietary recommendations pertaining to EFAs are especially important because of established links between cardiovascular disease and mental illness. The adult diet should include at least two meals containing fish every week. Most research findings to date support the use of omega-3 EFAs as adjunctive treatments of psychiatric disorders but not as monotherapy. Effective dosages range from 1 to 9.6 g/day, depending on the study and disorder being treated. Based on available evidence, it is appropriate to use EPA or a combination of EPA and DHA as an adjunctive treatment for medication-refractory major depression and schizophrenia; however, research findings at this time do not support the use of omega-3 EFAs as a monotherapy for major psychiatric disorders. EPA is probably more effective than DHA as an adjunctive treatment to conventional antipsychotics. A combination of EPA, DHA, and omega-6 EFAs may be an effective monotherapy for ADHD symptoms.

Specific omega-3 EFA treatment recommendations must be carefully considered. Large doses of EPA, DHA, or combination formulas may result in an imbalance in the body's EFA profile that is not optimal for good physical or mental health. In patients who are chronically deficient in EFAs, at least 3 months of dietary supplementation are required to restore the normal EFA balance in the CNS. Omega-3 EFA supplements are generally well tolerated, and no adverse effects are associated with increased fish consumption. The following treatment guidelines are based on a critical review of the literature on omega-3 EFAs:

- Chronically depressed individuals, schizophrenic patients, or patients diagnosed with disorders of attention or impulse control should take an omega-3 EFA supplement (1 g/day) consisting of a combination of EPA and DHA.
- Dosages of omega-3 EFAs up to 9 g/day may be beneficial for patients with both major depressive disorder and bipolar disorder. Individuals taking daily omega-3 EFA supplements at dosages over 3 g/day should be monitored by a physician.

Research Recommendations

Current research findings supporting the use of omega-3 EFAs in the treatment of psychiatric disorders are promising but not compelling. Large double-blind, placebo-controlled studies designed to determine optimum doses and combinations of omega-3 (or omega-6) EFAs in specific psychiatric disorders are needed.

Continued basic research on omega-3 EFAs will help clarify the putative mechanism(s) of action of specific fatty acids and differentiate between the relative contributions of genetic predisposition versus dietary deficiencies in the pathogenesis of disparate psychiatric syndromes. An important clinical research issue is the putative mitigating role of omega-3 EFAs on type 2 diabetes and elevated serum triglycerides associated with atypical antipsychotic agents. Finally, additional epidemiological studies are needed to clarify the putative benefits of omega-3 EFA supplementation begun in early childhood as a primary intervention aimed at the prevention of many psychiatric disorders.

REFERENCES

Adams PB, Lawson S, Sanigorski A, et al: Arachidonic acid to eicosapentaenoic acid ratio in blood correlates positively with clinical symptoms of depression. Lipids 31(suppl):S157–S161, 1996

Arvindakshan M, Ghate M, Ranjekar PK, et al: Supplementation with a combination of omega-3 fatty acids and antioxidants (vitamins E and C) improves the outcome of schizophrenia. Schizophr Res 62:195–204, 2003

Bekaroglu M, Aslan Y, Gedik Y, et al: Relationships between serum free fatty acids and zinc, and attention deficit hyperactivity disorder: a research note. J Child Psychol Psychiatry 37:225–227, 1996

Caughey GE, Mantzioris E, Gibson RA, et al: The effect on human tumor necrosis factor alpha and interleukin 1 beta production of diets enriched in omega-3 fatty acids from vegetable oil or fish oil. Am J Clin Nutr 63:116–122, 1996

Corrigan F, Horrobin D, Skinner E, et al: Abnormal content of omega-6 and omega-3 long-chain unsaturated fatty acids in the phosphoglycerides and cholesterol esters of parahippocampal cortex from Alzheimer's disease patients and its relationship to acetyl CoA content. Int J Biochem Cell Biol 30:197–207, 1998

de Wilde MC, Farkas E, Gerrits M, et al: The effect of omega-3 polyunsaturated fatty acid-rich diets on cognitive and cerebrovascular parameters in chronic cerebral hypoperfusion. Brain Res 947:166–173, 2002

Emsley R, Myburgh C, Oosthuizen P, et al: Randomized, placebo-controlled study of ethyl-eicosapentaenoic acid as supplemental treatment in schizophrenia. Am J Psychiatry 159:1596–1598, 2002

Engelhart M, Geerlings M, Ruitenberg A, et al: Diet and risk of dementia: does fat matter? The Rotterdam Study. Neurology 59:1915–1921, 2002

Eritsland J, Arnesen H, Seljeflot I, et al: Long-term effects of omega-3 polyunsaturated fatty acids on haemostatic variables and bleeding episodes in patients with coronary artery disease. Blood Coagul Fibrinolysis 6:17–22, 1995

Fenton WS, Dickerson F, Boronow J, et al: A placebo-controlled trial of omega-3 fatty acid (ethyl eicosapentaenoic acid) supplementation for residual symptoms and cognitive impairment in schizophrenia. Am J Psychiatry 158:2071–2074, 2001

Gesch CB, Hammond SM, Hampson SE, et al: Influence of supplementary vitamins, minerals and essential fatty acids on the antisocial behaviour of young adult prisoners. Randomised, placebo-controlled trial. Br J Psychiatry 181:22–28, 2002

Glauber H, Wallace P, Griver K, et al: Adverse metabolic effect of omega-3 fatty acids in non-insulin dependent diabetes mellitus. Ann Intern Med 108:663–668, 1988

Grubb B: Hypervitaminosis A following long-term use of high-dose fish oil supplements. Chest 97:1260, 1990

Hakkarainen R, Partonen T, Haukka J, et al: Is low dietary intake of omega-3 fatty acids associated with depression? Am J Psychiatry 161:567–569, 2004

Hamazaki T, Sawazaki S, Itomura M, et al: The effect of docosahexaenoic acid on aggression in young adults: a placebo-controlled double-blind study. J Clin Invest 97:1129–1133, 1996

Hibbeln J: Dietary polyunsaturated fatty acids and depression: when cholesterol does not satisfy. Am J Clin Nutr 62: 1–9, 1995

Hibbeln J: Fish consumption and major depression. Lancet 351:1213, 1998

Hibbeln JR: Seafood consumption, the DHA content of mothers' milk and prevalence rates of postpartum depression: a cross-national, ecological analysis. J Affect Disord 69:15–29, 2002

Hibbeln JR, Linnoila M, Umhau JC, et al: Essential fatty acids predict metabolites of serotonin and dopamine in cerebrospinal fluid among healthy control subjects, and early- and late-onset alcoholics. Biol Psychiatry 44:235–242, 1998a

Hibbeln JR, Umhau JC, Linnoila M, et al: A replication study of violent and nonviolent subjects: cerebrospinal fluid metabolites of serotonin and dopamine are predicted by plasma essential fatty acids. Biol Psychiatry 44:243–249, 1998b

Hirayama S, Hamazaki T, Terasawa K: Effect of docosahexaenoic acid–containing food administration on symptoms of attention-deficit/hyperactivity disorder: a placebo-controlled double-blind study. Eur J Clin Nutr 58:467–473, 2004

Horrobin D: Schizophrenia as a membrane lipid disorder which is expressed throughout the body. Prostaglandins Leukot Essent Fatty Acids 55:3–7, 1996

Horrobin D: The membrane phospholipid hypothesis as a biochemical basis for the neurodevelopmental concept of schizophrenia. Schizophr Res 30:193–208, 1998

Horrobin DF, Glen AI, Hudson CJ: Possible relevance of phospholipid abnormalities and genetic interactions in psychiatric disorders: the relationship between dyslexia and schizophrenia. Med Hypotheses 45:605–613, 1995

Kalmijn S, Feskens EJ, Launer LJ, et al: Polyunsaturated fatty acids, antioxidants, and cognitive function in very old men. Am J Epidemiol 145:33–41, 1997a

Kalmijn S, Launer L, Ott A, et al: Dietary fat intake and the risk of incident dementia in the Rotterdam Study. Ann Neurol 42:776–782, 1997b

Keck P, Freeman M, McElroy S, et al: A double-blind, placebo-controlled trial of eicosapentaenoic acid in rapid cycling bipolar disorder. Bipolar Disord 4 (suppl 1):26–27, 2002

Kenny D: Adverse effects of fish oil. Arch Intern Med 150:1967, 1971, 1990

Kinrys G: Hypomania associated with omega-3 fatty acids. Arch Gen Psychiatry 57:715–716, 2000

Laugharne JD, Mellor JE, Peet M: Fatty acids and schizophrenia. Lipids 31 (suppl):S163–S165, 1996

Logan AC: Neurobehavioral aspects of omega-3 fatty acids: possible mechanisms and therapeutic value in major depression. Altern Med Rev 8:410–425, 2003

Maes M, Smith R, Christophe A, et al: Fatty acid composition in major depression: decreased omega 3 fractions in cholesteryl esters and increased C20:4 omega 6/C20:5 omega 3 ratio in cholesteryl esters and phospholipids. J Affect Disord 38:35–46, 1996

Maes M, Bosmans E, De Jongh R, et al: Increased serum IL-6 and IL-1 receptor antagonist concentrations in major depression and treatment resistant depression. Cytokine 9:853–858, 1997a

Maes M, Smith R, Christophe A, et al: Lower serum high-density lipoprotein cholesterol (HDL-C) in major depression and in depressed men with serious suicidal attempts: relationship with immune-inflammatory markers. Acta Psychiatr Scand 95:212–221, 1997b

Marangell LB, Martinez JM, Zboyan HA, et al: A double-blind, placebo-controlled study of the omega-3 fatty acid docosahexaenoic acid in the treatment of major depression. Am J Psychiatry 160:996–998, 2003

Mellor JE, Laugharne JD, Peet M: Schizophrenic symptoms and dietary intake of n-3 fatty acids. Schizophr Res 18:85–86, 1995

Morris M, Evans D, Bienias J, et al: Consumption of fish and omega-3 fatty acids and risk of incident Alzheimer disease. Arch Neurol 60:940–946, 2003

Mueller B, Talbert R, Tegeler C, et al: The bleeding time effects of a single dose of aspirin in subjects receiving omega-3 fatty acid dietary supplementation. J Clin Pharmacol 31:185–190, 1991

Nemets B, Stahl Z, Belmaker RH: Addition of omega-3 fatty acid to maintenance medication treatment for recurrent unipolar depressive disorder. Am J Psychiatry 159:477–479, 2002

Peet M, Horrobin DF: A dose-ranging study of the effects of ethyl-eicosapentaenoate in patient undergoing depression despite apparently adequate treatment with standard drugs. Arch Gen Psychiatry 59:913–919, 2002

Peet M, Laugharne JD, Mellor J, et al: Essential fatty acid deficiency in erythrocyte membranes from chronic schizophrenic patients and the clinical effects of dietary supplementation. Prostaglandins Leukot Essent Fatty Acids 55:71–75, 1996

Peet M, Horrobin DF, E-E Multicentre Study Group: A dose-ranging exploratory study of the effects of ethyl-eicosapentaenoate in patients with persistent schizophrenic symptoms. J Psychiatr Res 36:7–18, 2002

Puri BK, Counsell SJ, Richardson AJ, et al: Eicosapentaenoic acid in treatment-resistant depression. Arch Gen Psychiatry 59:91–92, 2002

Richardson A, Puri B: A randomized double-blind, placebo-controlled study of the effects of supplementation with highly unsaturated fatty acids on ADHD-related symptoms in children with specific learning difficulties. Prog Neuropsychopharmacol Biol Psychiatry 26:233–239, 2002

Richardson AJ, Easton T, McDaid AM, et al: Essential fatty acids in dyslexia: theory, experimental evidence and clinical trials, in Phospholipid Spectrum Disorder in Psychiatry, 2nd Edition. Edited by Peet M, Glen I, Horrobin DF. Carnforth, UK, Marius Press, 1999, pp 225–241

Rudin D: The major psychoses and neuroses as omega-3 essential fatty acid deficiency syndrome: substrate pellagra. Biol Psychiatry 16:837–850, 1981

Rudin D: The dominant diseases of modernized societies as omega-3 essential fatty acid deficiency syndrome: substrate beriberi. Medical Hypotheses 8:17–47, 1982

Severus W: Omega-3 fatty acids: the missing link? Arch Gen Psychiatry 56:380–382, 1999

Silvers KM, Scott KM: Fish consumption and self-reported physical and mental health status. Public Health Nutr 5:427–431, 2002

Simopoulos AP: Omega-3 fatty acids in inflammation and autoimmune diseases. J Am Coll Nutr 21:495–505, 2002

Stevens LJ, Zentall SS, Deck JL, et al: Essential fatty acid metabolism in boys with attention-deficit hyperactivity disorder. Am J Clin Nutr 62:761–768, 1995

Stevens LJ, Zentall SS, Abate ML, et al: Omega-3 fatty acids in boys with behavior, learning, and health problems. Physiol Behav 59:915–920, 1996

Stevens L, Zhang W, Peck L, et al: EFA supplementation in children with inattention, hyperactivity, and other disruptive behaviors. Lipids 38:1007–1021, 2003

Stoll A, Damico K: Are omega-3 fatty acids beneficial in depression but not mania? Arch Gen Psychiatry 57:716–717, 2000

Stoll AL, Severus WE, Freeman MP, et al: Omega 3 fatty acids in bipolar disorder: a preliminary double-blind, placebo-controlled trial. Arch Gen Psychiatry 56:407–412, 1999

Su KP, Shen WW, Huang SY: Omega-3 fatty acids as a psychotherapeutic agent for a pregnant schizophrenic patient. Eur Neuropsychopharmacol 11:295–299, 2001

Su KP, Huang SY, Chiu CC, et al: Omega-3 fatty acids in major depressive disorder: a preliminary double-blind, placebo-controlled trial. Eur Neuropsychopharmacol 13:267–271, 2003

Tanskanen A, Hibbeln JR, Hintikka J, et al: Fish consumption, depression and suicidality in a general population. Arch Gen Psychiatry 58:512–513, 2001

Uauy R, Peirano P, Hoffman D, et al: Role of essential fatty acids in the function of the developing nervous system. Lipids 31 (suppl):S167–S176, 1996

Voigt R, Llorente A, Jensen C, et al: A randomized, double-blind, placebo-controlled trial of docosahexaenoic acid supplementation in children with attention-deficit/hyperactivity disorder. J Pediatr 139:189–196, 2001

Zanarini M, Frankenburg F: Omega-3 fatty acid treatment of women with borderline personality disorder: a double-blind, placebo-controlled pilot study. Am J Psychiatry 160:167–169, 2003

8

Chinese Medical Treatments

Julia Thie, L.Ac., Dipl.Ac., Dipl.CH.

Treatments used in Chinese medicine include acupuncture, herbs, moxibustion heat therapy, tuina tissue manipulation, and qigong (see Chapter 17). This chapter reviews the evidence for using acupuncture in the treatment of common psychiatric disorders. The use of compound herbal preparations in Chinese medicine presents many complicated pharmacological and safety issues for Western-trained mental health practitioners, which are not reviewed here.

Chinese medicine affords patients the opportunity to understand and control factors in the environment that promote health and "balance." Physiological and diagnostic descriptions of illness in Chinese medicine provide a sense of manageability to Western psychiatric patients, contributing to improved coherence in healing. When a Western patient is told that he or she is experiencing symptoms due to an imbalance in brain chemistry, the patient frequently has little recourse other than to passively rely on pharmacotherapy. In contrast to this therapy-centered approach, Chinese medicine is a patient-centered approach that attempts to explain symptoms to patients in the context of concepts that are widely understood in China and other Asian countries, including qi, yin, and yang.

Chinese medical physiology is based on the premise that the human body and its processes are a microcosm of the exterior phenomenal world. Descriptions of illness refer to complementary pairs of natural qualities like hot and cold and dampness and dryness. According to Chinese medical theory, all disease is attributable to a loss of harmony between one's inner and outer worlds. Thus, illness is an indication that a person's lifestyle needs to be altered in a manner that brings life back into harmony with the natural principles that surround that person.

HISTORY AND PHILOSOPHY OF TRADITIONAL CHINESE MEDICINE

Historical records of treatments using acupuncture, herbs, and other methods of traditional Chinese medicine date back more than 2,000 years. The earliest known compendium of Chinese medical theory, the *Huang-Di Neijing* (*The Yellow Emperor's Classic of Internal Medicine*) was compiled in approximately 100 B.C.E. It is possible to examine an historical bibliography of Chinese medicine, showing an unbroken chain of evolving concepts, within the classical literature.

Chinese medicine is based on Taoist philosophy and the interdependence between people and the environment. Yin and yang, the eight principles, and the five phases are the fundamental concepts of traditional Chinese medicine. This philosophical perspective pervades all aspects of Asian life, including understandings of health and illness. Although treatment protocols vary among different geographical areas, the historical and scientific foundations of traditional Chinese medicine are similar among Japanese, Korean, Taiwanese, Vietnamese, and Chinese practitioners.

Through careful observation of the environment, ancient practitioners determined that the body was a reflection of the natural elements and energies they could experience and observe. Using terminology that describes these phenomena within the human body, a system of treatment was developed with the goal of preventing or eliminating pathology caused by energetic imbalances. In Chinese medicine, the energetic principle embodied in spirit, mind, or consciousness is called *shen*. The condition of the shen is determined by an individual's capacity to respond to the inner and outer environment in ways that are adaptive. The presence of mental illness frequently connotes a disturbance of the shen due to deficiencies or excess amounts of other energetic elements in the body. Jing, qi, and shen comprise the *three treasures*. This is an ancient concept that quantifies energy and matter. *Jing,* or "essence," is the most material quality and is used to build, nourish, and replicate biological structures in the body. *Qi* is an animating force and is regarded as the intermediary between matter and thought. The *shen* is the most rarefied element and is regarded as the decision-making principle. None of these essential qualities of the body can function without the others.

When treating mental and emotional symptoms, traditional Chinese medicine practitioners consider the balance between the physical and energetic elements of the body. Diagnoses reveal energetic patterns that frequently correspond to conventional Western medical diagnoses. For example, in the Chinese system, depressed mood and other mental and emotional problems are symptom patterns not discrete disorders. Emphasizing symptoms over disorders permits traditional Chinese medicine practitioners to effectively use thousands of years of historical information about the energetic causes and treatments of physical and mental illness.

Practitioners of Chinese medicine use acupuncture together with other modalities such as nutritional prescriptions, body work therapies known as *tuina* or *shiatsu-anma,* energy manipulation techniques known as *qigong,* and varied compound herbal formulas. In recent decades, traditional Chinese medicine has adapted to modern times and Western culture and has been consolidated into a coherent body of theory and clinical methods.

FUNDAMENTAL CONCEPTS OF CHINESE MEDICAL THEORY

Different theories in Chinese medicine are used to understand the causes of symptoms and formulate appropriate acupuncture treatment protocols. Before selecting acupuncture points and techniques for needle manipulation or other energetic treatments, a clear differential diagnosis is necessary. Manipulation techniques include reducing, reinforcing, stimulation, indirect or direct moxibustion, warming needles, cupping, bleeding, pressure techniques, and electrical stimulation. The specific clinical approach to be applied is selected on the basis of the pathogenic agent(s) identified and inferences about associated energetic imbalances in the patient. In Chinese medicine, diagnoses are established principally on the basis of empirical findings that are interpreted as a "pattern discrimination" of energetic imbalances. Methods used to obtain information about symptoms include the patient interview; observation of the tongue, eyes, body, smells, and sounds; and palpation of nine radial pulse locations, the abdomen, and the meridians. "The Doctor of Chinese Medicine widens his or her view to assess changes in a broad range of common bodily functions such as urination, defecation, sweating, thirst and so on. Furthermore...the Doctor of Chinese Medicine takes into account many clinical manifestations ranging from certain facial and bodily signs to psychological and emotional traits" (Maciocia 1989, p. 175).

Chinese medicine describes phenomena or attributes that are believed to cause energetic imbalances and are manifested as physical or mental illness (e.g., dry, damp, hot, cold, and wind). The concept of *blood* in Chinese medical terminology is much more complex than it is in conventional Western medicine; it encompasses the idea that blood is the liquid that nourishes and maintains organs and is a yin substance. Although blood is regarded as principally moving through the blood vessels, certain aspects of blood are also believed to move along the meridians. Furthermore, the various organs in Chinese medicine describe functional or energetic states of the body and not discrete physical organs, as they are understood in Western medicine. In Chinese medical theory, each organ has particular tasks and functions that sometimes overlap with conventional Western understandings of physiology. The clinician asks questions and examines the patient in an effort to ascertain how and where these attributes accumulate. Many acupuncture points along the meridians are believed to stimulate the elimination of pathogenic factors and restore the body to its optimum balance. Movement of qi, the elemental energetic principle, is stimulated by acupuncture treatment, which signals the body's self-healing capacity.

Meridians, sometimes described as channels or vessels, are analogous with bio-electrical fields and have specific patterns and functions, such as moving the qi and connecting the physical components of the body. Smaller vessels that act as connectors to these fields and other structures are called *collaterals.* In Chinese medical theory, each organ (or dynamic principle) is connected to one or more of the 12 main surface meridians, which are named after internal organs. The channels and collaterals form an intricate web among physical parts of the body, functional patterns described as organs, and other meridians. Acupuncture points are selected on the basis of their energetic function within this web, their location on the meridian and in the body, and their effects in terms of facilitating internal actions that cause the flow of qi to be regulated in beneficial ways. In many instances, several points are associated through the meridians or collaterals with the same organ or dynamic energetic pattern, and stimulating these in a coordinated manner is thus more beneficial than stimulating only one or few points.

Another important concept in Chinese medicine is the *zang fu theory,* or the distinction between solid (or *zang*) and hollow (or *fu*) organs. A zang fu diagnosis is generally used when formulating herbal prescriptions; however, this approach also facilitates the selection of acupuncture points by providing an overall picture of the body. Once the zang fu diagnosis is clear, the most appropriate acupuncture protocol can be selected on the basis of meridian theory. Figure 8–1 shows complementary organ pairings according to zang fu theory.

Zang, solid Yin type	Liver	Heart	Pericardium	Spleen	Lung	Kidney
Fu, hollow, Yang type	Gall-bladder	Small intestine	Triple energizer	Stomach	Large intestine	Urinary bladder

FIGURE 8–1.   Zang fu organ pairings.

Starting from zang fu theory, in Chinese medical diagnoses, the energetic quality of a symptom is characterized according to *the eight principles,* which, like the organs in zang fu theory, are arranged in complementary pairs (Figure 8–2). A further characterization of the dynamic energetic organization of the body is based on the *six-stage theory.* Exterior and interior aspects of the body are assigned to one of six stages in relation to the depth and location of their corresponding meridians. Table 8–1 illustrates the stages of pathogenic progression that eventually manifest as physical or psychiatric symptoms, according to six-stage theory.

Yang	Exterior	Repletion/Excess	Hot
Yin	Interior	Vacuous/Deficient	Cold

FIGURE 8–2. The eight principles for characterizing the energetic quality of a symptom.

TABLE 8–1. The six stages of pathogenic progression and corresponding meridians

Six levels	Meridians (foot, hand)	Depth
Greater yang (Tai Yang)	Urinary bladder, small intestine	Most exterior yang level
Lesser yang (Shao Yang)	Gallbladder, triple energizer	Half exterior/half interior
Bright yang (Yang Ming)	Stomach, large intestine	Pivotal point before going into the internal organs
Greater yin (Tai Yin)	Spleen, lung	Most exterior yin level
Lesser yin (Shao Yin)	Kidney, heart	Deficient patterns apparent
Reverting yin (Jue Yin)	Liver, pericardium	Most interior

An additional important framing concept in Chinese medicine is the *five-phase theory,* also called the *five-element theory.* This approach provides valuable insights when mental and emotional symptoms are being evaluated and treated. Specific practice using five-element theory is considered a specialty, and some schools teach this style of treatment as a primary focus. Table 8–2 shows the principal energetic characteristics of the emotions and mental attributes as well as their relation to the principal organs, phases, and pathogenic influences. The associations among the various elements or phases are of fundamental importance when a Chinese medical practitioner is evaluating a patient and formulating a treatment plan. For example, the heart is regarded as the yin organ ruled by the element of fire. The fire element, in turn, is controlled by the water element and is engendered or strengthened by the wood element. Thus, specific acupuncture points are selected in accordance with these principles when treating symptoms attributable to the heart/mind. Figure 8–3 illustrates possible generating and controlling dynamic influences or cycles that exist among the five elements.

TABLE 8–2. Emotions and mental attributes in the five-element theory

Phase	Organ system (yin aspect)	Component	Governing attribute	Related pathogen
Metal	Lung	Po	Sensitivity, grief	Dryness
Water	Kidney	Zhi	Will	Cold
Wood	Liver	Hun	Anger, creativity	Wind
Fire	Heart	Shen	Spirit, consciousness	Heat or fire
Earth	Spleen	Yi	Thinking	Dampness

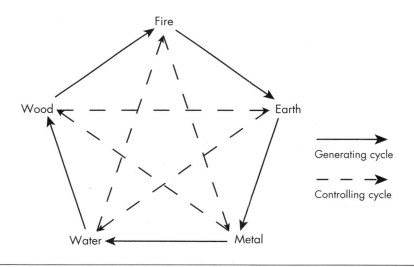

FIGURE 8–3. The controlling and generating cycles according to the five-element theory.

In addition to the 12 main meridians described above, Chinese medical theory describes eight extraordinary vessels that are also important meridians. With the exception of the conception (or *ren*) and governing (or *du*) meridians, the extraordinary vessels do not follow external meridian pathways but overlap with several internally located meridians. The eight extraordinary vessels control and provide nourishment for the 12 main meridians by means of a reservoir of qi and blood. The practitioner may choose to stimulate many points along these channels; however, in clinical practice, acupuncture needles are generally inserted in pairs on opposite sides of the body, as described by Yitian Ni, O.M.D.:

Clinically, when one point is selected on the right side (e.g., Sp 4), its paired point (P 6) will usually be treated on the left side. Frequently, two pairs will be used together, further expanding the area of influence of the treatment, and creating an energetic circulation from left to right, and upward and downward, as symbolized in the Pa Gua (Eight Trigrams) and the Tai Ji (Yin/Yang symbol). (Ni 1996, p. 134)

Table 8–3 shows the names, opening points, and paired channels of the eight extraordinary vessels.

TABLE 8–3. Eight extraordinary vessels

Channel	Opening	Paired channel	Opening
Dai	GB 41	Yang Wei	SJ 5
Yin Qiao	P 6	Chong	Sp 4
Ren	Lu 7	Yin Wei	K 6
Du	SI 3	Yang Qiao	UB 62

The *du channel* regulates all the yang (external) meridians and sense organs. Along with the yin qiao and yang qiao, the du channel is believed to directly regulate brain function and is often used to treat symptoms of schizophrenia or other psychotic syndromes. Stimulation of the *yin qiao* is indicated in cases of apathy and somnolence, whereas stimulation of points along the *yang qiao* is beneficial when the therapeutic goal is to reduce symptoms of agitation or hyperactivity. Stimulation of the *yang wei* helps to balance the emotions and is commonly done in efforts to stabilize manic-depressive mood swings or reduce symptoms of excessive anger. The *chong channel* regulates circulation of qi and blood along the 12 main meridians. In clinical practice, this vessel is stimulated when the therapeutic goal is to regulate "rebellious" qi manifesting as anxiety attacks, palpitations, or endocrinological imbalances that are detrimental to mental harmony. The *ren channel* regulates all yin channels and is believed to facilitate the circulation of blood, essence, and body fluids. Stimulation of ren channel points is beneficial for symptoms of anxiety or depression when there is an underlying deficiency of these substances.

The *five transporting points* on the 12 main channels are frequently selected when treating psychiatric symptoms. These points are located on the forearms and lower legs and are assigned to the elements according to their location. Stimulation of these points is performed to optimize the energetic relations among the meridians. Table 8–4 provides an overview of the five transporting points and their attributes.

TABLE 8–4.   The five transporting points

Transporting point	Location	Action	Examples
Jing/Well	End points of fingers and toes	Strong, fast-moving; dynamic effect on mental state	K 1 (YongQuan): subdues empty heat, calms the mind, clears the brain
Ying/Spring	Proximal to web of fingers and toes	Swift; eliminates pathogens, especially heat	SJ 3 (ZhongZhu): clears heat and wind, regulates qi, lifts the mind
Shu/Stream/ Transporting	Distal to junction of metacarpals and metatarsals	Defensive qi gathered here; eliminates painful obstruction, especially dampness	Ht 7 (ShenMen): source point, calms the mind, nourishes heart blood, opens the orifices
Jing/River/ To pass through	One-third of the distance from wrist to elbow or ankle to knee	Large current, less quick; able to divert pathogens to joints; affects the chest	P 5 (JianShi): resolves phlegm in the heart, regulates heart qi, opens the chest; ghost point
He/Sea/Joining	Knees and elbows	Slower to act; connects to circulation of body and affects internal organs	St 36 (ZuSanLi): tonifies qi and blood, raises yang, strengthens the body

Other important categories of points that are frequently used when treating mental and emotional symptoms are listed below, including specific clinical examples. Some points fall into more than one category and may serve multiple functions.

- *Connecting (Luo) points* interact with the collaterals. St 40 (FengLong) influences the brain and resolves phlegm.
- *Source points* are primarily used to tonify yin organs. Ren 15 (JiuWei) is the source point for all yin organs. Stimulation of this point can have a strong effect on calming the mind.

- *Lower Yang He (Sea) points* give more influence to the internal yang organs than the arm He (Sea) points. St 37 (ShangJuXu), the lower He (Sea) of the large intestine, strongly eliminates damp heat in the stomach and intestines and facilitates resolution of food and phlegm retention.
- Certain points on the urinary bladder channel known as *Back (Shu) transporting points* are beneficial when treating chronic illnesses. Each Back Shu point is related to a specific organ or body part, and its stimulation affects the corresponding organ. UB 15 (XinShu) is the Back transporting point for the heart and is useful when treating many mental disorders, because stimulation of this point is believed to be beneficial for brain functioning as well as for facilitating removal of excess heat from the heart. Stimulation with needles and/or cupping of the XinShu is frequently used when treating cases of uncontrolled laughter or chronic anxiety.
- Each organ has a *Front (Mu)* or *collecting point* that is used to diagnose and treat acute or chronic illnesses. St 25 (TianShu) is the mu point of the large intestine channel. This point is often stimulated when phlegm (fire) in the stomach is believed to be influencing the heart.
- The 12 main meridians and the eight extraordinary vessels have *Xi cleft (accumulation) points* where qi gathers. These are used mostly when treating acute pain conditions. P 4 (XiMen) regulates the heart rhythm and removes stasis. Stimulation of this point strengthens the mind and provides relief when palpitations and other symptoms of acute anxiety are brought on by fear.
- The points referred to as the *gathering* (or *influential*) *points* are believed to affect certain tissues and organs as well as energy and blood. Ren 17 (ShanZhong) is the influential point for qi and is directed at alleviating tightness in the chest accompanying insomnia, anxiety, depression, and palpitations.
- *Ghost points* are 13 points used to treat a range of mental disorders. Although few modern texts discuss these points, many practitioners continue to use them. UB 62 (ShenMai) is both a ghost point and the opening point of the yang qiao. Stimulation of this point clears the mind and eliminates excess interior wind.

In Chinese medical theory, mental disorders arise from a variety of factors, including "rebellious" or excessive qi, "hyperactive" yang, and excess phlegm, all of which obscure and obstruct the senses. Symptoms of mental illness are sometimes believed to be caused by a depression pattern or a "spasm" pattern. Treatment of symptoms caused by "depression" requires clearing the channels of repressed emotion and resolving "congealed phlegm." Treating symptoms caused by "spasm" generally requires opening the yang channels to drain "heat" (Shanghai College of Traditional Medicine 1981, pp. 628–629). Mixed symptom patterns fall into an intermediate category in which both treatment principles are applied together, depending on the relative severity of different symptoms. In such cases, treating only the *Biao* (*branch*) *conditions* that manifest outwardly will result in superficial improvements and benefit the patient in a limited way. In contrast, treating the *Ben* (or underlying *root*) *condition* together with the Biao will result in deeper changes in energetic imbalances and thus greater and more enduring clinical improvement.

CURRENT USAGE OF TRADITIONAL CHINESE MEDICINE

In 1996, an expert consensus panel of the National Institutes of Health identified medical and psychiatric disorders that are effectively treated using acupuncture. An excerpt from the panel's report summarizes the current uses of acupuncture in the United States:

> Acupuncture as a therapeutic intervention is widely practiced in the United States. Although there have been many studies of its potential usefulness, many of these studies provide equivocal results because of (problems in) design, sample size, and other factors. The issue is further complicated by inherent difficulties in the use of appropriate controls, such as placebos and sham acupuncture groups. However, promising results have emerged, for example, showing efficacy of acupuncture in adult postoperative and chemotherapy nausea and vomiting and in postoperative dental pain. There are other situations, such as addiction, stroke rehabilitation, headache, menstrual cramps, tennis elbow, fibromyalgia, myofascial pain, osteoarthritis, low back pain, carpal tunnel syndrome, and asthma, in which acupuncture may be useful as an adjunctive treatment or an acceptable alternative or be included in a comprehensive management program. Further research is likely to uncover additional areas where acupuncture interventions will be useful. ("NIH consensus conference: acupuncture" 1998)

In the United States, acupuncture is used in approximately 300 government-funded and private clinics as an adjunctive treatment for abuse and dependence on many substances, including opiates, cocaine, tobacco, and alcohol (Brewington et al. 1994). Most of these protocols are based on a successful program at New York City's Lincoln Hospital conducted in the 1970s (Smith and Khan 1988). Acupuncture treatment programs are also being widely instituted in prisons to treat substance abuse (Brumbaugh 1993). The National Acupuncture Detoxification Association (NADA) promotes acupuncture as a treatment for addictions and administers an examination that qualifies practitioners to be certified as acupuncture detoxification specialists.

TRAINING REQUIREMENTS FOR PRACTITIONERS

According to the Accreditation Commission for Acupuncture and Oriental Medicine (www.acaom.org), 53 traditional Chinese medicine schools are currently accredited by the U.S. government to provide 4-year graduate training programs in Chinese medicine. Colleges of traditional Chinese medicine offer training in many specialized styles of acupuncture and are tasked with ensuring their graduates have acquired the level of clinical competency that is needed for successful completion of the examination administered by the National Certification Commission for Acupuncture and Oriental Medicine (www.nccaom. org). Each state has unique licensing requirements and privileges for Chinese medical practitioners, including conventionally trained physicians who have completed specialized courses in acupuncture. The American Academy of Medical Acupuncture (www.medicalacupuncture.org) maintains certification for physicians interested in practicing acupuncture. Some states allow physicians to practice acupuncture after completing abbreviated training programs without requiring them to pass a national examination.

Guidelines issued in 1996 by the World Health Organization (WHO) indicate that clinical competency in acupuncture requires approximately 2,500 hours of training for nonphysicians and 1,500 hours for physicians or professional Western medical practitioners, although this minimum is not met in most physician training programs at this time. Training should cover basic theory, core acupuncture techniques, and clinically supervised practice. WHO recommends that training for nonphysicians include 500 hours of basic science courses similar to theory taught in Western medical schools and familiarity with the language and concepts of Western clinical methods (World Health Organization 1999). All licensed acupuncturists are required to successfully perform the clean needle technique as put forth by the Occupational Safety & Health Administration and the Centers for Disease Control and Prevention. In 1996, the U.S. Food and Drug Administration reclassified acupuncture needles from class III (for investigational use only) to class II (for general use by qualified practitioners) medical devices, subject to requirements governing material biocompatibility, single use, and sterility (in the United States, only disposable, sterile needles are permitted to be used).

EVIDENCE FOR MENTAL HEALTH BENEFITS OF ACUPUNCTURE

Research on Chinese medicine treatments of psychiatric disorders has yielded promising results; however, methodological flaws limit the significance of most findings, and a great deal of evidence is in the form of case reports. Flaws and Lake (2001) recently completed a comprehensive review of the evidence base supporting the use of acupuncture, herbal medicines, and other traditional Chinese medicine treatments in mental health care.

The challenges associated with methodology in acupuncture research are currently being addressed by the Society for Acupuncture Research (www.

acupunctureresearch.org) and are frequently discussed in the society's *Journal of Alternative and Complementary Medicine*. Recent research in all areas of Chinese medicine has been in the form of randomized, controlled studies in which acupuncture point selection is dictated by described protocols and a control group receives treatment at sham acupuncture points. Another research paradigm that is gaining popularity is the "pragmatic randomized controlled trial" in which point selection is determined on the basis of the individual's unique energetic diagnosis, with the control group being treated with an established intervention generally used for the symptom pattern in question rather than with sham acupuncture (MacPherson 2000). It is likely that future clinical trials evaluating the efficacy of acupuncture according to the standards of Western medical research will result in more useful clinical findings compared with earlier studies that did not follow rigorous research methodologies (Hammerschlag 1998).

Depression

The findings of many sham–controlled trials suggest that electroacupuncture is as effective as amitriptyline for patients with moderate depressed mood (Luo et al. 1985). In one small 5-week study, two points on the scalp and forehead were stimulated using electroacupuncture 1 hour/day for 6 days a week. The comparison group received three daily doses of amitriptyline for 1 week, after which the dosage was increased depending on the subject's response. The results showed that 70% of the group receiving electroacupuncture achieved complete remission or marked improvement compared with 65% in the comparison group. In another comparison study, additional points were stimulated using electroacupuncture for 6 weeks; approximately 90% of the patients treated with acupuncture or amitriptyline experienced significant clinical improvement (Yang et al. 1994). After 6 weeks of electroacupuncture treatment, slow-wave delta activity decreased and fast-wave alpha increased. These changes are similar to changes in electrical brain activity that occur when depressed patients respond to conventional medications. In two studies conducted at the Institute of Mental Health in Beijing, China, the researchers concluded that electroacupuncture was the preferred treatment among patients who were unable to tolerate the anticholinergic side effects of tricyclic antidepressants (Luo et al. 1998). The initial study and subsequent multicenter trials found that the efficacy of 6 weeks of electroacupuncture was comparable with that of amitriptyline in managing anxiety, somatization, and cognitive symptoms in depressed patients and had fewer adverse effects.

A comparison study found similar relapse rates in patients diagnosed with major depressive disorder treated with acupuncture or a conventional antidepressant (Gallagher et al. 2001). At the end of an 8-week course of acupuncture, 17 of 33 subjects achieved full remission of depressive symptoms. At 6-month follow-up, 4 of those had relapsed. Longer trials are needed to determine whether ongoing acupuncture therapy results in sustained improvements in depressed patients. In a large open study, acupuncture was evaluated as a stand-alone treatment in a heterogeneous population of 167 patients with a history of severe depression who had been diagnosed with bipolar disorder or schizophrenia (Poliakov 1987). Some patients who had previously been nonresponsive to conventional antidepressants improved with acupuncture. The researchers determined that the antidepressant mode of action associated with acupuncture resembles that of conventional antidepressants.

Schizophrenia

In a large study conducted in China, 213 adolescents with schizophrenia were treated using a combination of herbal therapy, body acupuncture, and ear acupressure based on pattern discrimination (Tiecheng 1994). Three cycles of ear acupressure treatment were administered using small metallic seeds that adhere to the ears and elicit sensation. Each 10-day treatment cycle included 1 minute/day of acupressure, with patients resting 5 days between cycles. Body acupuncture using patient-specific points was performed twice a week with 20 minutes of needle retention after stimulation. Herbal therapy consisted of a compound formula known as Jia Wei Shao Yao Tang, a formula that reportedly has beneficial effects in cases of depressed mood and is believed to move liver qi, nourish blood, and clear heat. At the end of treatment, 19.2% of the patients were described as being "cured," 29.1% as being markedly improved, 47.4% as being moderately improved, and 4.4% as having not changed. A small control group consisting of 11 patients who received acupuncture and moxibustion reportedly experienced a similar combined rate of clinical improvement.

The findings of the Tiecheng (1994) study are difficult to interpret because of the study's serious methodological shortcomings. The diagnosis of schizophrenia was not confirmed according to conventional Western criteria, outcomes were not measured using standardized instruments, the control group was very small in comparison with the active treatment group, and individuals in the control group also received traditional Chinese treatments addressing the target symptoms. Furthermore, no study arm received conventional antipsychotic medications for comparison, and there was no wait-list group that received no treatment. Future methodologically sound studies using similar acupuncture protocols are needed.

Anxiety Disorders

Many studies have examined acupuncture in the treatment of anxiety. In a sham-controlled study conducted in Germany, the electrocardiographically measured effects of acupuncture treatment on resting heart activity in 36 patients diagnosed with "minor depression" or "minor anxiety" were evaluated

(Agelink et al. 2003). The verum acupuncture group experienced a significant decrease in the mean resting heart rate and a significant decrease in the ratio of low-frequency to high-frequency heart electrical activity. In the verum acupuncture group, acupuncture needles were applied at classical acupuncture points, including ShenMen (He 7), NeiGuan (Pe 6), BaiHui (GV 20), ShenMai (UB 62), and extra point 6 (Ex 6). A sham control group was treated with epidermal needles applied at nonacupuncture points. Both groups underwent standardized electrocardiographic measurements of 5-minute resting heart rate variability before the first and after the ninth acupuncture session of a series and three times during the third acupuncture session (before the treatment started and 5 and 15 minutes after needle application). The results of this German study suggest that in patients with minor depression or anxiety, needling specific acupuncture points causes an increase in parasympathetic activity of the heart, thereby reducing patients' overall heart rate.

Another German study using the same acupuncture protocol demonstrated significant clinical improvement in 43 patients diagnosed with mild symptoms of anxiety and depression and 13 patients with generalized anxiety disorder after 10, but not after only 5, acupuncture sessions (Eich et al. 2000). After 10 sessions, 60.7% of the acupuncture group versus 21.4% of the sham control group had improved significantly based on a standardized rating scale. In those patients diagnosed with a generalized anxiety disorder, 87.5% showed significant clinical improvement. The findings of this study demonstrate that total acupuncture sessions and the specific protocol used are significant determinants of clinical response.

Dementia

A study on the effects of acupuncture combined with the inhalation of herbal medicines and oxygen was performed in 50 elderly patients diagnosed with "senile dementia" in a hospital setting in China (Geng 1999). A control group of 50 patients was treated parenterally with an unspecified brain tissue extract believed to be beneficial in dementia. The group receiving combined acupuncture and inhalation herbal therapy showed clinical improvements in symptoms of cognitive functioning superior to those of the control group, and the researchers claimed a 96% overall response rate. Acupuncture points were divided into two groups: the reducing method was applied to group 1 (SiShenCong [EX-HN1], BaiHui [GV 20], ShenMen [He 7], FengLong [St 40], NeiGuan [Pe 6]) and the reinforcing method was applied to group 2 (GanShu [UB 18], ShenShu [UB 23], ZuSanLi [St 36]). The general treatment strategy was to supplement kidney, resolve phlegm, remove blood stasis, and restore consciousness.

The Geng (1999) study was unique in its comprehensive point selection and needle manipulation techniques; however, the significance of the findings is limited by the study's methodological problems. It is unclear what criteria were used to diagnose the enrolled subjects, and it is probable that these criteria did not correspond to conventional Western diagnostic criteria. Therefore, it is impossible to infer the type and severity of cognitive impairments treated in the study. Because no group was treated with acupuncture alone, the observed clinical improvements cannot be ascribed to acupuncture alone. A sham acupuncture protocol or other described treatment protocol was not used as a control condition, and there was no effort to follow clinical changes after the study ended. It is possible that cognitively impaired individuals responded to the oxygen with transient cognitive improvements. Future well-designed studies are needed to verify the possible beneficial effects of acupuncture on dementia and other forms of cognitive impairment.

Drug, Alcohol, and Nicotine Addiction

Many studies have investigated ear acupuncture (auriculotherapy) and ear electroacupuncture as treatments for alcohol abuse and drug addiction.

Illicit Drugs

An early study reported that prolonged ear acupuncture for 8 days lessened withdrawal symptoms in chronic opium users (Wen and Cheung 1973). The researchers noted that psychosocial rehabilitation was required after detoxification. In a study on auricular acupuncture for craving reduction in cocaine-addicted patients, 82 patients on methadone maintenance were randomly assigned to receive true acupuncture, sham acupuncture, or regular relaxation training (Avants et al. 2000). Acupuncture treatments were administered five times each week for 8 weeks. Random urine toxicology screens confirmed that patients in the acupuncture group were significantly less likely to use cocaine compared with both control groups. In another study on acupuncture in patients addicted to prescription narcotics, the researchers reported that 12 out of 14 patients were successfully withdrawn from the narcotic using ear acupuncture alone when treated for 60 minutes per day (Kroening and Oleson 1985). Acupuncture may lessen the severity of withdrawal symptoms during detoxification in heroin addicts but may have limited efficacy in cases of severe chronic heroin addiction (Severson et al. 1977).

Alcohol

Acupuncture in combination with carbamazepine shows promise in the management of alcohol withdrawal after chronic heavy drinking. In a 2-week single-blind, sham-controlled study, 34 alcoholic patients were randomly assigned to receive acupuncture to the ear and the body versus sham acupuncture over 10 sessions (Karst et al. 2002). Patients assigned to acupuncture showed a tendency toward improved overall outcomes and reported significantly fewer withdrawal symptoms by the end of the study. In a pilot study, 54 patients with chronic alcohol abuse were randomly assigned to a sham acupuncture control group versus a protocol believed to lessen alcohol withdrawal consisting of three true ear points and two points on each wrist (Bullock et al. 1987). Treatments were administered daily for the first week, thrice weekly for the next month, and twice weekly for the next 45 days (30 treatments in total). Significantly more patients completed treatment in the acupuncture group compared with in the control group, and these patients reported significantly fewer alcohol cravings, relapses, and hospital admissions for detoxification during the study. A larger study using a similar protocol was subsequently conducted in a population of 80 individuals with a history of severe chronic alcohol abuse and multiple treatment failures (Bullock et al. 1989). Acupuncture treatments were administered daily for 1 week, thrice weekly for 2 weeks, and twice weekly for 2 weeks (15 treatments in total). Follow-up interviews at 1, 3, and 6 months showed significant group differences in favor of acupuncture. The readmission rate to detoxification centers was significantly lower for the acupuncture group.

In a study in rats, acupuncture stimulation of ear regions that correspond to the pylorus, lung, trachea, stomach, esophagus, endocrine, and heart in Chinese meridian theory resulted in increased satiety and reduced cravings for alcohol (Asamoto and Takeshige 1992). Animal studies have also shown that stimulation of these points is associated with a reduction in body weight in contrast to no change in eating behavior or weight when other acupuncture points are stimulated. It has been suggested that acupuncture stimulation reduces withdrawal symptoms by stimulating the release of endorphins (Cheng et al. 1980). Future research may point to possible beneficial clinical effects of auricular acupuncture on overeating and binge eating.

Nicotine

Compared with the outcome of acupuncture treatment for narcotics craving and alcohol withdrawal, there is less evidence for beneficial effects of acupuncture on nicotine craving. A systematic review of 22 studies of smoking cessation indicated that the response rate to acupuncture treatment was not greater than that to placebo (White et al. 2002). Early studies reported outcomes that were equivalent to conventional interventions aimed at smoking cessation; however, subsequent studies have consistently failed to confirm this effect. The findings of a large prospective study suggest that acupuncture and nicotine gum have comparable efficacy in reducing nicotine craving and helping individuals to quit smoking (Clavel et al. 1985). In that study, 651 volunteers were randomly assigned to an acupuncture protocol believed to reduce nicotine craving, nicotine gum treatment, or a control group. Acupuncture sessions lasted 30 minutes (the total number of treatments was not given). The researchers reported that the percentages of ex-smokers in the groups receiving acupuncture and nicotine gum were similar (19% and 22%, respectively) compared with only 8% in the control group. At 13-month follow-up, former smokers accounted for 8% of the acupuncture group, 12% of the nicotine gum group, and 3% of the no-treatment control group.

LIMITATIONS OF FINDINGS TO DATE, AND FUTURE DIRECTIONS IN ACUPUNCTURE RESEARCH

The significance of research findings on acupuncture is limited by many factors. As mentioned above, different diagnostic criteria are used in China and Western countries to identify target symptoms and evaluate clinical progress in study populations. Thus, rigorous comparisons of outcomes from different Chinese and Western studies using similar acupuncture protocols are difficult or impossible to conduct. Until recently, relatively few studies on acupuncture or other Chinese medical treatment approaches have used what Western-trained researchers would consider controlled conditions, making it difficult to separate effects of different factors and conditions on outcomes. For example, many studies combine acupuncture with Chinese herbal treatments, moxibustion, and massage (tuina), thereby confounding efforts to determine specific beneficial effects of a particular acupuncture protocol. These issues are complicated by basic differences in research methodologies used to design studies conducted in China, the United States, and other countries where acupuncture is being investigated.

In addition, basic differences between Western psychiatry and Chinese medicine in categories of emotional or cognitive dysfunction regarded as symptoms or disorders implicitly bias the clinical information that is collected and evaluated by researchers as well as the instruments used to obtain descriptive data and measure clinical improvement in target symptoms. Few Western studies on acupuncture remark on the qualifications of practitioners or other personal factors that enter into assessment or treatment planning, characteristics that a Chinese researcher or medical practitioner would probably consider highly relevant and important to clinical results.

Another issue in conventional Western research studies of acupuncture is the concept of sham acupuncture treatment. It has been established that stimulation of sham acupuncture points sometimes results in therapeutic responses (Cheng et al. 1980). Furthermore, the same sham protocol used by different practitioners may result in substantially different outcomes. There is also limited empirical information about the putative biophysical or energetic mechanism of action of acupuncture in its various forms. Electroacupuncture, computer-controlled electroacupuncture, and laser acupuncture may produce beneficial results through similar or different mechanisms of action.

The design of future studies on acupuncture will benefit substantially from deeper understandings of basic principles. Basic concepts must be addressed at a theoretical level before it will be possible to compare the traditional form of acupuncture with novel innovations that use electrical current and computer-controlled feedback. Future prospective controlled studies that include a no-treatment group and a group receiving conventional psychiatric drugs are needed to confirm the clinical benefits of acupuncture for mental health problems and compare acupuncture with conventional treatments. In 2001, with these goals in mind, a prominent international group of acupuncturists and researchers compiled a list of priorities for future acupuncture research—the Standards for Reporting Interventions in Controlled Trials of Acupuncture, or the STRICTA recommendations—with the goals of improving research designs and more accurately reporting clinical findings (MacPherson et al. 2002).

SAFETY ISSUES

Safety of Traditional Chinese Medicine Treatments

When Chinese medicine is practiced skillfully, adverse effects are relatively infrequent. This has been ascribed to the fact that Chinese medical practitioners are trained to find a specific treatment that will restore each patient to his or her individual state of balance. Even when acupuncture is applied by a low-skilled practitioner, the individualized treatment approach of acupuncture means that the few potential side effects are rarely serious. Training for acupuncturists emphasizes the importance of avoiding errors in practice that might result in side effects or complications, including hematomas or pneumothorax. However, cases of pneumothorax have been reported, and patients seeking acupuncture treatment should be advised of these risks. Few safety issues arise when acupuncture is administered by a well-trained practitioner (NIH Technology Assessment Workshop on Alternative Medicine 1996). In a recent review of surveys on acupuncture safety, the most common adverse effects were needle pain after treatments, tiredness, and bleeding (Ernst and White 2001). Reports of light-headedness and fainting were uncommon, and feelings of deep relaxation were reported by as many as 86% of patients. Pneumothorax was extremely rare, occurring only twice in nearly a quarter of a million treatments. The review concluded that the incidence of minor adverse effects of acupuncture is relatively high but that serious adverse events are rare. The results of other surveys are in agreement with these findings (White et al. 1997, 2001).

A measure of the safety of acupuncture is the gradual decrease in malpractice insurance premiums for licensed acupuncturists because of infrequent claims. Although adverse effects sometimes follow acupuncture, this ancient healing technique is arguably one of the safest medical interventions when administered by a skilled practitioner (MacPherson et al. 2001).

Most Chinese herbal medicines are not as pharmacologically potent as Western drugs because they are compounded from unrefined herbs or other natural products. Chinese medicinals are typically prescribed as compound formulas designed to mitigate side effects. They are individually prescribed on the basis of each person's subjective pattern. Thus, when prescribed by a professional practitioner, Chinese medicinals are not standard formulas for presumed average disorders. Because of this, professionally prescribed Chinese medicines typically have few or no side effects. Chinese medical practitioners are generally trained to continue rethinking and refining a patient's herbal prescription until the desired effects are achieved with few or no side effects. Significant advances continue to take place in the development of Chinese medicinals (Lee 2000).

Despite their strong safety record, side effects and cases of fatal toxicities have been reported with Chinese herbal medicines (Chan 2002; Deng 2002; Wang and Yang 2003; Zhu 2002). Chinese medical practitioners attribute most safety problems to excessive doses of a particular herb or herbal formula, improper preparation of formulas, or erroneous substitution of a particular herbal ingredient in a compound herbal formula (Ferguson et al. 1997; Stengel and Jones 1998; Tomlinson et al. 2000). There have also been reports of the adulteration of Chinese medicinals with synthetic drugs, including steroids, nonsteroidal anti-inflammatory drugs, heavy metals, and other substances (Chan and Critchley 1996; Tomlinson et al. 2000).

Importance of Disclosing Concurrent Conventional and Traditional Chinese Medical Treatments

Western biomedicine and Chinese medicine are presently the two most widely practiced systems of medicine in the world. Even as acupuncture is becoming more accepted as an alternative approach to more conventional medical care in many Western countries, biomedicine is being increasingly embraced in Asia. Most Western patients come to a Chinese medical practitioner with a preestablished biomedical diagnosis, and many are concurrently taking conventional prescription medications or are undergoing other biomedical treatments. Western patients under the care of a Chinese medical practitioner often fail to disclose their alternative treatments to their conventionally trained physicians, including psychiatrists, who are treating them for similar complaints. At the same time, patients receiving Western psychiatric treatment often fail to disclose such personal information to a Chinese medical practitioner treating them for related complaints. Reasons for nondisclosure include patients' reluctance or embarrassment to be seen as naïve or misinformed. Many patients regard each kind of medical treatment as an unrelated or independent matter that does not warrant disclosure to the other health care provider. The negative consequences of nondisclosure include the risk of misdiagnosis or a missed diagnosis, resulting in inappropriate treatment and the possibility of drug–drug or drug–procedure (e.g., acupuncture or moxibustion) interactions.

At the time of this writing, there are limited data on specific clinical methods in which particular acupuncture or herbal therapies and conventional biomedical treatments are combined or on the safety or efficacy of combining these treatments. The combination of Chinese medicine and conventional psychiatric medications raises many important safety issues, and the integration of these two types of treatment should be considered only when the patient provides informed consent after discussing the benefits and risks of the combined therapies. In addition, it is important for the conventionally trained physician and Chinese medical practitioner to obtain the patient's consent to communicate so that they may minimize the risk of safety problems. Combined treatment should be pursued only when the treating psychiatrist and Chinese medical practitioner are in agreement about the appropriateness of concurrent use of both kinds of treatment (Lake 2004).

CASE STUDIES

The two cases discussed in this section describe patients who reported severe anxiety and wished to discontinue conventional medications. The same Chinese medical practitioner treated the patients using different acupuncture protocols based on the unique pattern discriminations and circumstances of each patient. In the clinical practice of acupuncture, point selection generally varies widely even when the same subjective symptoms and pattern discrimination are being treated. These variations reflect different traditions and practice styles in Chinese medicine. In contrast to the fixed protocols used in acupuncture research, in the clinical practice of acupuncture point selection, the duration, number, and frequency of treatments vary widely and take into account personal and financial factors. In China and other Asian countries where acupuncture is widely practiced, mental symptoms are generally treated daily or every other day. In Western countries this is seldom feasible because of financial constraints.

Case 1

A 53-year-old woman complained of chronic insomnia and ongoing anxiety for 20 years. Her symptoms had recently been exacerbated after she discontinued alprazolam (Xanax). The woman had a slight physical build, a quiet voice, and an anxious affect. Her current medications were trazodone, citalopram, buspirone, hydroxyzine, gemfibrozil, atorvastatin (Lipitor), atenolol, and oxcarbazepine (Trileptal). She did not disclose her medication doses to her Chinese medical practitioner.

On examination, her tongue was scarlet and swollen and had no coating. Her pulse was rapid and superficial. Based on her symptoms and the above findings, there were two Chinese medical diagnoses: internal wind generated by fire and chronic liver blood deficiency from stagnation due to emotional trauma.

For the initial treatment session, the acupuncturist selected a protocol directed at expelling wind and restoring deficient liver blood (Table 8–5). The approach was intended to provide mild stimulation using an even acupuncture needling technique. Needles were retained for 35 minutes.

TABLE 8–5. Case 1: Treatment 1

Location	Meridian	Point
Right side	Leg: Jue Yin; Arm: Shao Yang	Lv 8, Lv 3, TE 5, TE 10
Left side	Leg: Shao Yang; Arm: Jue Yin	GB 34, GB 41, Pe 7, Pe 3
Bilateral	Expel wind	GB 20
Auricular	NADA protocol	Neurogate, sympathetic, liver, kidney, lung 2

When no improvement was observed after 3 days, a revised protocol, also directed at expelling wind and involving several new points, was used for the second, third, and fourth treatments (Table 8–6). During the second treatment, the patient's body was observed to shake strongly during treatment, suggesting that wind was being successfully expelled. The acupuncture needles were removed after 15 minutes. After this treatment, the patient's symptoms of anxiety, shakiness, and insomnia improved markedly. The patient underwent the third treatment 3 days later using the same protocol, with the needles being retained for 30 minutes. The two final treatments were administered at 4-day intervals. After the fourth treatment, the patient reported good sleep with trazodone and oxcarbazepine. After the fifth treatment, the patient was able to achieve restful sleep on a reduced dosage of trazodone and had discontinued the oxcarbazepine. At 3-month follow-up, the patient reported experiencing mild anxiety with an occasional need for medication and that she continued to sleep well.

TABLE 8–6. Case 1: Treatments 2–5

Location	Meridian	Point
Right side	Yin Hand: Jing/Well; Yang Foot: Ying/Spring	Lu 11, Pe 9, Ht 9, UB 65, St 43, GB 41
Left side	Yang Hand: He/Sea; Yin Foot: Shu/Stream	LI 11, SI 8, TE 10, Sp 6, K 7, Lv 5
Auricular	NADA protocol	Neurogate, sympathetic, liver, kidney, lung 2

For this patient, a different protocol was tried when the initial protocol failed to achieve the desired changes. The points chosen for the second protocol were based on the work of Richard Te-Fu Tan, Doctor of Oriental Medicine (Tan 2003). Acupuncture points on the arms and legs were mildly stimulated at either the Yin Well (Jing), Yang Spring (Ying), Yin Stream (Shu), or Yang Sea (He) points. This protocol used points on each of the 12 main meridians. Needle placement was intended to create a dynamic balance between yin and yang. The protocol also involved several points included in the NADA auricular protocol in which needles are retained between sessions using subdermal tacks. In the absence of financial or other practical constraints, treatment would ideally continue over many additional sessions with the goal of reversing this patient's energetic imbalances caused by prolonged use of prescription medications. However, in this case, the principal treatment goals were achieved, and the patient decided to discontinue acupuncture therapy.

Case 2

A 60-year-old woman reported having experienced chronic symptoms of generalized anxiety for 6 years. Her family physician had prescribed buspirone (BuSpar) 3 months earlier because of the patient's almost daily panic attacks, which worsened in the evening. The patient reported some improvement with the medication but also stated that her symptoms persisted. Her other symptoms included gastrointestinal distress, with belching, nausea, and excessive hunger, especially in the morning. She reported a gradual loss of her sense of smell. She was motivated to be treated and reported that she had driven over 2 hours to come to her appointment.

On physical examination, the patient had some "swelling" and there were signs of congestion in the chest and sinuses. Her tongue was a pale purple hue in the center and red on the sides and tip. Her pulse was moderately strong and "full" in the central region. On the basis of her self-reported history and physical findings, her diagnosis was qi stagnation in the middle *jiao* (middle area of the body, including the digestive organs) and upward flaring of fire due to vacuity of water. A treatment protocol (Table 8–7) was chosen with the goal of correcting the patient's presumed energetic imbalances manifesting as her physical and psychological symptoms.

TABLE 8–7.   Case 2: Treatments 1–5

Location	Meridian	Point
Right side	Leg: Shao Yin; Arm: Shao Yang	K 10, K 3, TE 5, TE 10
Left side	Leg: Shao Yang; Arm: Shao Yin	Ht 3, Ht 7, GB 34, GB 41
Bilateral	Open nasal orifice, regulate spleen	Bi Tong (an "extra point" at nasolabial fold), Ren 12
Auricular	—	Neurogate, sympathetic

The acupuncturist used mild needle stimulation and an even technique. Needles were retained for 35 minutes. The patient was encouraged to perform daily qigong exercises between treatments. At the consultation 5 days after the initial treatment, the patient reported that she was less nauseous but continued to experience anxiety in the evenings. She had been practicing calming qigong exercises as instructed. Her second treatment was administered 15 days after the first session. At that time, the patient reported that her symptoms improved. On examination, her tongue was red throughout the center region and her pulse was thin and slightly rapid. The third treatment was given 10 days later. The patient reported that she had lowered the dose of buspirone. Her symptoms continued to improve, but she still experienced some anxiety in the evenings. By the time of her fourth treatment, the patient had stopped taking buspirone and reported only mild nighttime anxiety. She no longer experienced nausea, and her sense of smell continued to improve. At the time of her final treatment (7 weeks after the first appointment), she had been withdrawn from conventional medications for 2 months and reported no ongoing anxiety. Maintenance treatment goals were discussed with her, including continued qigong exercises.

After the patient's stagnation of the middle jiao was alleviated, the changes in her tongue and pulse demonstrated a desirable clinical response. The dusky central region of the tongue subsequently transformed into an entirely red tongue. This permitted the acupuncturist to diagnose underlying heat caused by blood and yin deficiency, a pattern that is commonly seen in postmenopausal women. The acupuncturist then stimulated points on the Shao Yin meridians to strengthen the fire and water relationship and applied needles along the Shao Yang meridians to facilitate the expulsion of heat. Between appointments, the patient benefited from self-directed qigong exercises aimed at consolidating beneficial energetic changes achieved through acupuncture. The skillful combination of acupuncture and qigong exercises resulted in therapeutic changes in qi, and the patient was able to discontinue a conventional medication (buspirone) without experiencing adverse effects of medication withdrawal or a recurrence of anxiety symptoms.

REFERENCES

Agelink MW, Sanner D, Eich H, et al: Does acupuncture influence the cardiac autonomic nervous system in patients with minor depression or anxiety disorders? Fortschr Neurol Psychiatr 71:141–149, 2003

Asamoto S, Takeshige C: Activation of the satiety center by auricular acupuncture point stimulation. Brain Res Bull 29:157–164, 1992

Avants SK, Margolin A, Holford TR, et al: A randomized controlled trial of auricular acupuncture for cocaine dependence. Arch Intern Med 160:2305–2312, 2000

Brewington V, Smith M, Lipton D: Acupuncture as a detoxification treatment: an analysis of controlled research. J Subst Abuse Treat 11:289–307, 1994

Brumbaugh AG: Acupuncture: new perspectives in chemical dependency treatment. J Subst Abuse Treat 10:149–159, 1993

Bullock ML, Umen AJ, Culliton PD, et al: Acupuncture treatment of alcoholic recidivism: a pilot study. Alcohol Clin Exp Res 11:292–295, 1987

Bullock ML, Culliton PD, Olander TR: Controlled trial of acupuncture for severe recidivist alcoholism. Lancet 1(8652):1435–1439, 1989

Chan TY: Incidence of herb-induced aconitine poisoning in Hong Kong: impact of publicity measures to promote awareness among the herbalists and the public. Drug Saf 25:823–828, 2002

Chan TY, Critchley JA: Usage and adverse effects of Chinese herbal medicines. Hum Exp Toxicol 15:5–12, 1996

Cheng R, Pomeranz B, Yu G: Electroacupuncture treatment of morphine-dependent mice reduces signs of withdrawal without showing cross-tolerance. Eur J Pharmacol 68:477–481, 1980

Clavel F, Benhamou S, Company-Huertes A, et al: Helping people to stop smoking: randomized comparison of groups being treated with acupuncture and nicotine gum with control group. BMJ 291:1538–1539, 1985

Deng JF: Clinical and laboratory investigations in herbal poisonings. Toxicology 181–182:571–576, 2002

Eich H, Agelink MW, Lehmann E, et al: Acupuncture in patients with minor depressive episodes and generalized anxiety: results of an experimental study. Fortschr Neurol Psychiatr 68:137–144, 2000

Ernst E, White AR: Prospective studies of the safety of acupuncture: a systematic review. Am J Med 110:481–485, 2001

Ferguson JE, Chalmers RJ, Rowlands DJ: Reversible dilated cardiomyopathy following treatment of atopic eczema with Chinese herbal medicine. Br J Dermatol 136:592–593, 1997

Flaws B, Lake J: Chinese Medical Psychiatry: A Textbook and Clinical Manual. Boulder, CO, Blue Poppy Press, 2001

Gallagher SM, Allen JJ, Hitt SK, et al: Six-month depression relapse rates among women treated with acupuncture. Complement Ther Med 9:216–218, 2001

Geng J: Treatment of 50 cases of senile dementia by acupuncture combined with inhalation of herbal drugs and oxygen. J Tradit Chin Med 19:287–289, 1999

Hammerschlag R: Methodological and ethical issues in clinical trials of acupuncture. J Altern Complement Med 4:159–171, 1998

Karst M, Passie T, Friedrich S, et al: Acupuncture in the treatment of alcohol withdrawal symptoms: a randomized, placebo-controlled inpatient study. Addict Biol 7:415–419, 2002

Kroening RJ, Oleson TD: Rapid narcotic detoxification in chronic pain patients treated with auricular electroacupuncture and naloxone. Int J Addict 20:1347–1360, 1985

Lake J: The integration of traditional Chinese Medicine (TCM) and Western biomedicine with emphasis on the treatment of psychiatric disorders. Integrative Medicine, August/September 2004

Lee KH: Research and future trends in the pharmaceutical development of medicinal herbs from Chinese medicine. Public Health Nutr 3:515–522, 2000

Luo H, Jia Y, Zhan L: Electroacupuncture vs. amitriptyline in the treatment of depressive states. J Tradit Chin Med 5:3–8, 1985

Luo H, Meng F, Jia Y, et al: Clinical research on the therapeutic effect of the electro-acupuncture treatment in patients with depression. Psychiatry Clin Neurosci 52 (suppl): S338–S340, 1998

Maciocia G: Foundations of Chinese Medicine. London, Churchill Livingstone, 1989

MacPherson H: Out of the laboratory and into the clinic: acupuncture research in the real world. Clinical Acupuncture and Oriental Medicine 1:97–100, 2000

MacPherson H, Thomas K, Walters S, et al: The York acupuncture safety study: prospective survey of 34,000 treatments by traditional acupuncturists. BMJ 323:486–487, 2001

MacPherson H, White A, Cummings M, et al: Standards for reporting interventions in controlled trials of acupuncture: the STRICTA recommendations. J Altern Complement Med 8:85–89, 2002

Ni Y: Navigating the Channels of Traditional Chinese Medicine. San Diego, CA, Oriental Medicine Center, 1996

NIH consensus conference: acupuncture. JAMA 280(17):1518–1524, 1998

NIH Technology Assessment Workshop on Alternative Medicine: Acupuncture. Gaithersburg, MD, April 21–22, 1994. J Altern Complement Med 2:1–256, 1996

Poliakov SE: Acupuncture in the treatment of patients with endogenous depression. Zh Nevropatol Psikhiatr Im S S Korsakova 87:604–608, 1987

Severson L, Merkoff RA, Chun HH: Heroin detoxification with acupuncture and electrical stimulation. Int J Addict 12:911–922, 1977

Shanghai College of Traditional Medicine: Acupuncture: A Comprehensive Text. Seattle, WA, Eastland Press, 1981, pp 628–629

Smith MO, Khan I: An acupuncture program for the treatment of drug-addicted persons. Bull Narc 40:35–41, 1988

Stengel B, Jones E: End-stage renal insufficiency associated with Chinese herbal consumption in France [in French]. Nephrologie 19:15–20, 1998

Tan R: Dr. Tan's Strategy of Twelve Magical Points: Advanced Principles and Techniques. San Diego, CA, R. Tan, 2003

Tiecheng D: The treatment of adolescent schizophrenia by the ear pressure method. Gan Su Chinese Medicine 7:25, 1994

Tomlinson B, Chan TY, Chan JC, et al: Toxicity of complementary therapies: an eastern perspective. J Clin Pharmacol 40:451–456, 2000

Wang XP, Yang RM: Movement disorders possibly induced by traditional Chinese herbs. Eur Neurol 50:153–159, 2003

Wen HL, Cheung SYC: Treatment of drug addiction by acupuncture and electrical stimulation. Asian J Med 9:138–141, 1973

White AR, Hayoe S, Ernst E: Survey of adverse events following acupuncture. Acupunct Med 15:67–70, 1997

White A, Hayhoe S, Hart A, et al: Adverse events following acupuncture: prospective survey of 32,000 consultations with doctors and physiotherapists. BMJ 323:485–486, 2001

White AR, Rampes H, Ernst E: Acupuncture for smoking cessation. Cochrane Database Syst (2):CD000009, 2002

World Health Organization: Guidelines on Basic Training and Safety in Acupuncture. Geneva, Switzerland, World Health Organization, 1999

Yang X, Liu X, Luo H, et al: Clinical observation on needling extrachannel points in treating mental depression. J Tradit Chin Med 14:14–18, 1994

Zhu YP: Toxicity of the Chinese herb mu tong (*Aristolochia manshuriensis*): what history tells us. Adverse Drug React Toxicol Rev 21:171–177, 2002

ADDITIONAL READING

Discovering Chi: Energy Exercises for Emotional Vitality (videotape). Los Angeles, CA, Terra Entertainment, 2000

Kaptchuk T: The Web That Has No Weaver. Chicago, IL, Cogden & Weed, 1983

Liu C-T, Zheng-Cai L, Hua K: A Study of Daoist Acupuncture. Boulder, CO, Blue Poppy Press, 1999

Maciocia G: Diagnosis in Chinese Medicine. London, Churchill Livingstone, 2004

Ni M (transl): The Yellow Emperor's Classic of Medicine. Boston, MA, Shambala, 1995

Stux G, Berman B, Pomeranz B: Basics of Acupuncture. New York, Springer, 2003

Wiseman N, Ellis N (transl): Fundamentals of Chinese Medicine (Zhong Yi Xue Ji Chu). Brookline, MA, Paradigm, 1995

9

Homeopathy

Iris R. Bell, M.D., M.D.(H.), Ph.D.
Pamela A. Pappas, M.D., M.D.(H.)

Patients with combined medical and psychiatric symptoms have long challenged physicians' best efforts. As documented by several researchers (Eisenberg et al. 1998; Kessler et al. 2001a), patients frequently seek medical care from alternative practitioners or treat themselves through alternative modalities, especially when conventional care fails to relieve their symptoms. Similar trends exist in psychiatric care (Druss and Rosenheck 2000; Kessler et al. 2001a, 2001b; Unutzer et al. 2000). When seeking treatment, many patients desire holistic approaches that address the larger spiritual meaning of their lives as well as the symptoms themselves (Astin 1998).

An artificial conceptual split between mind and body still permeates the architecture of many modern hospitals, where psychiatric units are often placed physically far away from medical and surgical ones. The recent approval of psychosomatic medicine (formerly consultation-liaison psychiatry) as a subspecialty (Kornfeld 2002; Lipsitt 2001; Stone et al. 2004) marks an advance in medicine's appreciation of patients' multidimensional aspects and the impact of these factors on health care outcomes. In this context, it is informative to review homeopathy—a branch of medicine that has from its outset respected patients' mental, physical, emotional, and spiritual unity. This chapter explores the principles, clinical use, research efforts, and current developments within classical homeopathy, a field whose tenets overlap those of modern complex systems and network science more than those of conventional medical reductionism (Bell et al. 2002a; Bellavite 2003; Hyland and Lewith 2002).

Homeopathy is one of the most popular forms of complementary and alternative medicine (CAM) in the world, especially in Great Britain, where more than 40% of physicians refer patients to homeopaths; in France, where 30%–40%

of physicians prescribe homeopathic medicines; and in Germany, where 20% of physicians follow this practice (Ullman 2002). The World Health Organization described homeopathy as one of the systems of traditional medicine that should be integrated worldwide with conventional medicine in order to provide adequate global health care by the year 2000 (Bannerman et al. 1983). India, with over 100,000 homeopathic physicians and approximately 120 homeopathic medical colleges, seems to be the country contributing the most toward this mandate.

In the United States, a survey showed that between 1990 and 1997, the use of homeopathic medicine increased by fivefold and was chosen by 6.7 million adults or 3.4% of the population (Eisenberg et al. 1998). More than 82% of these users, or 5.5 million people, were self-treating rather than visiting homeopathic practitioners. Eisenberg et al. (1998) also reported that most patients were not telling their conventional physicians about their use of homeopathy or other complementary therapies. In a survey of 1,500 people in 1998, Landmark Healthcare, a company that provides services for the delivery and management of physical medicine benefits in California, found that 5% of those surveyed were using homeopathy, with most (73%) using it in combination with traditional medical treatments (Carlston 2003).

Multiple observational studies in primary care settings suggest that 70%–80% of patients report moderate or greater benefit from homeopathic treatment, including when used to treat psychological and psychiatric disorders (Riley et al. 2001; Spence et al. 2005; Van Wassenhoven and Ives 2004; Witt et al. 2005a, 2005b). The data also indicate that homeopathy is generally safe and can reduce the need for conventional pharmaceutical agents. In addition, the biopsychosocial systems orientation of homeopathic theory (Vithoulkas 1980) parallels similar concepts in psychiatric writings, such as Engel's biopsychosocial model (Engel 1977) and other conceptual models in the field (Davidson 1994).

HISTORY AND BASIC PRINCIPLES OF HOMEOPATHY

Classical homeopathy is a controversial system of medicine founded over 200 years ago by the German physician Samuel Hahnemann, a pioneer in the field of psychosomatic medicine. A contemporary of Dr. Phillippe Pinel, who in 1793 broke the chains of insane patients at the Bicêtre Hospital, Hahnemann was also one of the first to humanely treat mentally ill patients (Winston 1999). In fact, Dr. Charles Frederick Menninger, psychiatrist and founder of the Menninger Clinic, wrote, "Homeopathy is wholly capable of satisfying the therapeutic demands of this age better than any other system or school of medicine" (Menninger 1897, p. 430).

During the period when Dr. Hahnemann lived (1755–1843), the treatment of patients included purging with mercury and arsenic, bleeding, and blistering

(Carlston 2003). Considering these methods barbaric (Hahnemann 1843/1996), Hahnemann proposed an entirely different approach based on individualized treatment for each patient (Shalts 2004). He felt that only by understanding each patient's totality of characteristics and peculiarities could appropriate treatment be given. In finding remedies to alleviate suffering, Hahnemann determined that a patient's personal experience of health and illness was far more important than his or her pathological diagnosis (the method so intensely explored in conventional medicine today.)

Law of Similars

Although homeopathic principles are at least as old as Hippocrates, Hahnemann was the first to use the term *homeopathy*. The root Greek words *homoios* ("same") and *pathos* ("suffering") reflect one of homeopathy's cornerstones, the Law of Similars. Hahnemann discovered through personal experimentation that a person taking cinchona (Peruvian bark, source of the medicine quinine) experienced the same fevers, chills, palpitations, and rigors that appeared with malaria, the disease the medicine was supposed to treat. He further noted that mercury, the treatment for syphilis, caused similar bone destruction, gingivitis, and salivation as the disease itself—in fact, conventional physicians of his era used the salivation to signify that the appropriate mercury dose had been taken. The Law of Similars states that a substance producing a characteristic set of symptoms in a healthy person can, when given in a small dose, cure an ill person suffering similar symptoms. The defining principle of "similar suffering" leads homeopaths to prescribe medicines that act in concert with the patient's symptoms, thereby encouraging the patient's perturbed natural defenses to reestablish homeostasis and evoking self-healing. In contrast, the *allopath*, Hahnemann's term for physicians whose treatments produce suffering "other" than that related to the cause of illness, might suppress those symptoms with antidepressants, antibiotics, and antipyretics or use completely unrelated methods (Carlston 2003). Hahnemann was passionate in his views that allopathic treatments were generally off the mark, bearing little relation to the patient's clinical situation. *Antipathic* ("opposite" suffering) medications, such as antianxiety agents, correspond at least partially to the disease's symptoms by being their opposite; Hahnemann felt that both antipathic and allopathic treatments led to deeper overall illness in the patient.

A careful examination of the Law of Similars shows compatibility with many modern biomedical observations (Merrell and Shalts 2002). For example, Merrell and Shalts noted that a therapeutic dose of aspirin can lower body temperature, whereas as a toxic dose produces hyperthermia. Also, some medications can have effects that are opposite to their expected therapeutic activities, such as benzodiazepines producing agitation rather than sedation in some patients. In addition, *hormesis* is a well-documented biological and chemical observation in the conventional field of pharmacological toxicology. Hormesis involves interactions between the agent and host that stimulate homeostatic compensations in the host. As a result, nonlinear, often bidirectional, differential effects of the same substance can occur depending on dose of the substance (Calabrese and Baldwin 2001). For example, scientists have observed hormesis at low levels of various agents, typically either below the lowest-observed-adverse-effect dose or under appropriate sampling intervals relative to the half-life of the host's adaptation to a given exposure regimen (Rozman and Doull 2003). Conventional scientists object to linking homeopathy with hormesis (Calabrese 2005), but the phenomenological overlap remains an empirical question.

Several other principles of homeopathy also bear discussion for their relevance to the field of psychiatry: the vital force, the Law of Minimum Dose, provings, totality of symptoms, and the Laws of Cure.

Vital Force

Like medical systems, such as Ayurveda and traditional Chinese medicine, classical homeopathy posits a life energy that animates all organisms (Oschman 2000). Known as *prana* or *qi* in these other systems, this animating energy is called the *vital force* in homeopathy (Vithoulkas 1980). According to Hahnemann, this force combines the soul and emotions of humans with more physical energies (Bailey 2002) and dynamically responds to change:

> In the healthy human state, the spirit-like life force (autocracy) that enlivens the material organism as dynamis governs without restriction and keeps all parts of the organism in admirable, harmonious, vital operation, as regards both feelings and functions, so that our indwelling rational spirit can freely avail itself of this living, healthy instrument for the higher purposes of our existence. (Hahnemann 1843/1996, p. 65 [Aphorism 9])

Hahnemann's understanding of the vital force's operation mirrors what modern physiologists know of homeostasis: organisms are constantly and simultaneously adjusting to maintain a healthy equilibrium in response to myriad perturbations on multiple levels. When the organism is healthy, all levels function freely and smoothly, with resilience to internal and external stress. If, however, the organism is weak or encounters an extremely strong stressor, symptoms may show up in the mental, emotional, or physical area as the vital force struggles to correct the disharmony. The latter point explains why homeopaths feel that suppressing symptoms is dangerous: It fights the body's physiological attempts to regain healthy balance.

Hahnemann felt that "mistunements" of this vital force underlie all physical, mental, and emotional symptoms that patients experience and that only applications of medicines that correctly act on the vital force can restore health. For him, the "mistunement" of the vital force as a unified whole was the disease needing treatment, and the symptoms merely provided the unique picture of how this was deranged. Consistent with these conceptualizations, recent research has suggested that cell walls have a nanomechanical motion at particular frequencies that generate audible, low-level sounds (Pelling et al. 2004). For example, cancer cells exhibit a noisy, disorganized motion (Pelling 2004). Moreover, individual cells also self-organize into communicating networks of cells, even the more primitive organisms such as yeast cells (Barabasi 2003).

At a clinical level, a recent study found significant correlations between classical homeopaths' ratings of fibromyalgia patients' vital force and scores on standardized conventional rating scales. The data, collected under double-blind conditions, included correlations between greater vital force ratings and less severe illness on observer-rated Clinical Global Impression scores (by both homeopaths and an independent conventional medical examiner), as well as lower patient-rated mental confusion and higher vigor on the Profile of Mood States questionnaire and greater positive states of mind on the Positive States of Mind scale (Bell et al. 2004c). Thus, historical notions of vital force may soon be incorporated into systematic empirical studies at the cellular and clinical levels of scale.

Not only do people embody a vital force, but also, as the visionary Hahnemann recognized, the remedy for each disorder has its own highly specific vibrational or spectral information energy (Oschman 2000; Rey 2003; Turin 1996) and applying the correct agent can strengthen a patient's vital force (Bailey 2002). In addition, materials science research has shown that different homeopathically prepared compounds discharge energy in highly specific ways (Elia and Niccoli 1999, 2004; Rey 2003; see also section titled "Objective Basic Science and Preclinical Evidence in Homeopathy," later in chapter). According to Bailey (2002),

> it is now assumed that homeopathic medicines work by resonance between the energy in the medicinal solution and the "body energy" of the patient. This accounts for the fact that generally one homeopathic remedy will have a profound healing effect on the patient, while the other hundreds of homeopathic remedies will usually have no effect. (p. 402)

As an analogy, when placing a tuning fork near a piano or guitar string, only the correct frequency (or a harmonic) evokes vibration (resonance). As noted above, scientific and technological advances can now facilitate rigorous examination of the resonance hypothesis in homeopathy (Oschman 2000).

Law of Minimum Dose

Hahnemann felt strongly that "the physician's highest and only calling is to make the sick healthy, to cure, as it is called. The highest ideal of cure is the rapid, gentle, and permanent restoration of health; that is, the lifting and annihilation of the disease in its entire extent in the shortest, most reliable, and least disadvantageous way, according to clearly realizable principles" (Hahnemann 1843/1996, p. 60 [Aphorisms 1 and 2]). Continually working to make his methods safer and more efficient, Hahnemann diluted some of his medicines because they were toxic in their crude form (the form used by his conventional contemporaries). He was surprised to find that the more diluted medicines worked more curatively for his patients; he also found he could make his medicines still more effective by vigorously shaking (*succussing*) them between dilutions. He proposed that the energy of the diluted medicine might be more subtle and affect the patient's vital force more efficiently and gently.

This dilution and shaking (*succussion* or *potentization*) process used to make remedies remains one of the features of homeopathy that conventional medical professionals find the most controversial (Jonas et al. 2003). During preparation, many commonly used homeopathic medicines are diluted past the point of Avogadro's number of molecules of material substance. On the health food store shelf, this would mean anything beyond 24X (1:10 serial dilution steps, followed by succussions, repeated 24 times) or 12C (1:100 serial dilution steps, followed by succussions, repeated 12 times). The *succussion* (shaking) process is done between dilution steps, and both processes are necessary for *potentization* (strengthening or bringing about the effectiveness) of the medicine. The higher the number, the more dilution and succussion steps have been done; it is thus called a higher "potency." Because professional homeopaths frequently use potencies of 200C and above, conventional physicians question what can be curative in the medicine. Homeopaths find in clinical treatment that these higher potencies (i.e., medicines whose effective properties have been brought out through more stepwise dilutions and succussions compared to those with less), when given to the correct patient with the correct kind of complaints, often produce more complete and lasting results than lower ones. This effect can be most pronounced in the treatment of patients with chronic emotional or mental symptoms, even though lower potencies such as 6X certainly have their place, especially in first aid and acute illness.

Also in contrast to the physicians of his day, Hahnemann recommended one medicine (*remedy*) at a time for the integrative pattern of the whole person at a dose corresponding exactly to the patient's need. This practice is one of the features differentiating classical (single-remedy) homeopathy from other sorts of homeopathy available today. Some homeopathic practitioners use remedy combinations (*complex homeopathy*) for specific symptoms or select remedies through electronic instrumentation, intuition, muscle testing, or other techniques (Jonas et al. 2003). Hahnemann did not practice any of these methods, although he updated his *Organon of the Medical Art* six times as his clinical experience grew. In that work, Hahnemann (1843/1996) decried the practice of mixing multiple therapeutic agents because of their uncertain effects and potential danger to patients. Psychiatry has had its own controversies about polypharmacy, especially in consultation-liaison (psychosomatic medicine) practices caring for patients with complex medication interactions and side effects. Still, it is rare today to find a psychiatric (or general medical) patient taking only one medicine. Even in conventional psychopharmacology, optimal dosing is an art that becomes more challenging with the increasing number of interactions a clinician must juggle.

Provings

To learn the properties of individual medicines, homeopaths conduct *provings* (Hahnemann coined the term *prüfung,* the German word for "test") according to strict protocols (Sherr 1994). This process is like a Phase I drug trial but with healthy rather than ill people taking an unknown substance and the clinician carefully recording every symptom (side effect) experienced. From the patterning of these symptoms, a *drug picture* is developed that can then guide homeopaths in using the now "proven" medicine (remedy) for healing sick patients. The collected information is categorized into each system affected and recorded into *repertories,* or books, that systematically list these symptoms along with the medicines known to cause or cure them. Although the well-known Greek physician Galen was the first to suggest using healthy people for such testing, Hahnemann was the first to rigorously conduct such testing (Carlston 2003). With the help of his family, friends, and about 50 of his physician colleagues, he proved approximately 100 substances during his lifetime. The proving of new medicines continues today because human need continues to evolve. Some question whether an historic repertory of symptoms accurately describes twenty-first-century human experience, so reproving of older remedies is performed as well. Most of the proven remedies are made from natural botanical, mineral, or animal substances; certain pharmaceuticals (such as haloperidol) and ubiquitous dietary items (such as Coca-Cola) have been homeopathically prepared and proven also. Other ways to learn about remedies include cured cases and toxicology; homeopaths access all these databases when studying their patients and corresponding remedy pictures. Software search engines such as ReferenceWorks, Encyclopedia Homeopathica, and ISIS help with this.

Totality of Symptoms

Selecting the appropriate remedy from the more than 3,000 now available can be difficult. To accomplish this, the homeopath must come to know the patient as deeply as possible through a lengthy interview that explores the patient's very being as much as his or her symptomatic complaints. A crucial principle of homeopathy is to recognize that a human is an integrated, whole entity rather than merely a sum of parts (Vithoulkas 1980). This being said, the world impinges on patients as a totality, but patients may show symptoms primarily in one central area—mental, emotional, or physical (center of gravity) (Vithoulkas 1980). The person's overall health and constitutional weaknesses determine where symptoms appear most prominently. Skeptics often assert that the in-depth interview process and the patient–provider alliance contribute more than the actual remedies to the favorable outcomes in homeopathy. This claim loses any relevance in considering self-care uses of homeopathy. For practitioner-provided care, the data are mixed in support for (Jacobs et al. 2005) or against (Bell et al. 2004a) the critics' hypothesis.

Hahnemann (1843/1996) did not view mental or emotional illness as distinct from physical illness, saying, "in all of the so-called somatic diseases as well, the mental and emotional frame of mind is always altered" (p. 196 [Aphorism 210]). However, he did hold that the emotional state is an extremely important guide to understanding the person's energetic imbalance: "The preeminent importance of the emotional state holds good to such an extent that the patient's emotional state often tips the scales in the selection of the homeopathic remedy" (p. 197 [Aphorism 211]). In addition, the remedies themselves affect mental and emotional states in specific, unique ways, so that matching a remedy to a patient is possible.

An appreciation of patient individuality becomes extremely important in understanding and treating chronic illnesses, illnesses that conventional medical practitioners find most challenging to treat. Two patients with identical DSM-IV-TR (American Psychiatric Association 2000) diagnoses, for example, may need different homeopathic remedies based on their unique individual characteristics. A depressed patient who cries easily, is openly emotional, clings to others, and wants consolation might benefit from the remedy *Pulsatilla* (windflower, a plant), but one who is more stoic and reserved in public, hates consolation, yet holds grudges and sobs uncontrollably when alone might need *Natrum muriaticum* (table salt, a mineral). Remembering that different patients with the same diagnosis of major depressive disorder may have very different responses to the same conventional antidepressant may help relate this idea to current psychiatric practice. Some may respond with symptom amelioration, some may experience no result at all, and a third group may respond with intolerable side effects. In addition, many psychiatric patients experience symptoms that do not fit into the DSM-IV-TR categories yet persist throughout treatment. Classical homeopathy at least provides some way to use these seemingly "eccentric" characteristics; in fact, some are strange and peculiar enough to lead right to the curative remedy.

Homeopaths have developed a hierarchy of levels of human functioning, based on the importance of the function to the expression of the individual as a human being. Engel (1977) also described a hierarchy of functional levels in his biopsychosocial model for conventional medicine and psychiatry. A homeopath can assess a patient's degree of health or illness by examining his or her mental/ spiritual, emotional, and physical levels as they impact the patient's ability to seek unconditional and continuous freedom from dysfunctional patterns (i.e., happiness) (Vithoulkas 1980). This happiness is more than a simple mood state; it evolves from the unselfish and creative expression of one's deepest purpose in life. Symptoms on any level (physical, emotional, or mental) limit a person's sense of well-being and ability to experience this form of happiness.

In this hierarchical model, psychiatrists might appreciate the homeopathic view that mental illness is the deepest type of illness that humans can experience, because it affects the expression of the person's very essence. Optimal mental functioning includes "clarity, rationality, coherence, logical sequence and creative service for the good of others as well as for the good of oneself" (Vithoulkas 1980, p. 27). Disturbances at the mental level may lead to dysfunction in the next-outer level, the emotional level, such as depression, anxiety, irritability, and anger. Also, according to Vithoulkas (1980), emotional health is "a state of being capable of freely feeling the full range of human emotions without being enslaved by them from moment to moment…The individual experiences an absolute dynamic calmness combined with love for self, others, and the environment" (pp. 31–32, 40). Feeling part of something larger than oneself is a necessity for good health. The still important, but mostly external, physical layer can reveal disturbances from the underlying two layers as well as be diseased itself. Conventional research has shown that a sense of meaning and purpose in life explains additional amounts of the variance in greater hope and lower levels of depression, even after controlling for baseline mood and personality traits (Mascaro and Rosen 2005).

Beyond these basic layers, the homeopath also needs to discern symptom intensity in each level. For example, even at the deepest mental level, absent-mindedness impairs the person less than delusional thinking and is a less pervasive symptom than complete confusion. Symptoms lie on a continuum of intensity. At the emotional level, irritability is a less severe symptom (and shows less systemic illness) than suicidal depression. Physical illnesses range in seriousness from organic brain disease (e.g., strokes) at the deepest level to lung and kidney disease near the middle to skin rash at the most superficial level. The homeopathic clinician can follow the historical process of symptom development and recession to see how a person's health is stabilizing or illness is progressing.

Laws of Cure

Closely related to the totality of symptoms idea is the concept that healing from illness proceeds in an organized, understandable fashion (Vithoulkas 1980). (The development of disease follows a similar process as well, but in the opposite direction.) Understanding this principle provides a way for the caregiver to assess the effectiveness of treatment, monitor a patient's clinical progress, and direct further interventions, no matter what type of therapy is used. Dr. Constantine Hering, father of homeopathy in the United States, is credited with developing these Laws of Cure. With considerable patient care experience, he noted the following:

- Symptoms resolve in reverse order of their appearance in time; healing progresses from the most recently developed condition to the oldest.
- Healing progresses from upper body parts to lower ones.
- The first symptoms to resolve are those involving deeper, more important organs and tissues, with symptoms in more superficial ones being resolved later. One might see a long-lasting skin rash while liver disease is healing, for example.

- Healing begins with the organs whose dysfunction is most life-threatening for immediate survival, then moves on to the less vital ones.

Holding these laws in mind enables physicians to see the vital force (i.e., the entire complex system that is the person) respond to therapeutic measures. For example, a clinician can suppress a patient's physical skin rash with steroids only to find that the patient develops asthma in the ensuing months, or it is possible for the clinician to successfully treat the asthma only to have the patient return showing more irritability and anxiety. By noting these hierarchies and continua and the direction of healing, the clinician can see that the symptoms' center of gravity has moved deeper, indicating deterioration of overall health even though the chief complaints are ameliorated. Another example might be treating panic disorder and depression with a homeopathic remedy and having those symptoms ameliorate while the patient develops allergic rhinitis. In this example, healing is occurring at the emotional level, but symptoms are appearing at the physical level, specifically in the nose. Although these latest symptoms are temporarily bothersome for the patient, healing is still proceeding in a positive direction, and interfering with the body's homeostatic wisdom would be countertherapeutic. If treatment is absolutely required during this temporary period, using nonsuppressive therapies that support the body's process would be more helpful to the patient's overall health. The Laws of Cure are compatible with principles of nonlinear dynamical self-organization in complex living systems described in the complexity-science literature (Bellavite 2003).

CLINICAL USE AND SAFETY OF HOMEOPATHY

Safety of Homeopathic Remedies

Unlike botanical medicines and nutritional supplements, homeopathic remedies are regulated by the U.S. Food and Drug Administration. To be sold in the United States, remedies must be proven and listed in the Homeopathic Pharmacopoeia of the United States (www.hpus.com). The dilution process used in their preparation renders them nontoxic, and they do not interact with conventional medications. However, some pharmaceuticals and dietary substances (e.g., steroids, antibiotics, coffee) may interfere with the activity of homeopathic medicine. Health food stores often carry popular homeopathic remedies in lower potencies (up to 30C), but more specialized homeopathic pharmacies and companies carry a wider supply at a full range of potencies. In contrast to the cost for psychotropic medications, homeopathic remedies are usually around $10 for an entire course of treatment. Initial results from observational studies conducted in Belgium (Van Wassenhoven and Ives 2004) and Israel (Frenkel and Hermoni 2002) suggest the potential for marked health care cost savings through wider use of homeopathic remedies.

Patients can be treated with homeopathic medicines while still taking conventional pharmaceuticals, although such combined usage can present complications. The pharmaceuticals may be gradually tapered as a patient makes clinical progress and with the concurrence of the patient's other physicians. Not only might the patient's psychiatric and other symptoms remit, but the patient's progress in psychotherapy and human development itself might increase also (Bailey 2002).

Practitioner Licensure and Training

With practitioners of many diverse backgrounds, homeopathic training and certification in the United States is a politically "hot" issue. Some, such as M.D.s and D.O.s, are licensed in all states and can use homeopathy within existing scopes of practice; Arizona, Nevada, and Connecticut even have designated homeopathic medical boards and licensure. Other licenses under which people practice homeopathy include acupuncture, naturopathic medicine, chiropractic, and nurse practitioner (Carlston 2003), but laws concerning the scope of practice differ among states. In addition, there are many highly skilled but unlicensed professional homeopaths whose practices are in legal "gray zones," depending on state precedent.

There are 35–40 comprehensive homeopathic training programs in the United States (Rowe 2004), which vary in length and intensity, depending on the population targeted. Most are classroom based, some include clinical training, and others rely on distance learning. Naturopathic medical schools also offer some homeopathic training, usually consisting of fewer hours than dedicated homeopathic programs. The Council on Homeopathic Education assesses and accredits homeopathic educational programs, and there are several certification bodies that review the training of individual homeopaths. These bodies are currently determining how best to work together, but the differing backgrounds create divergent viewpoints about this. For example, some feel homeopathy ought to be a branch or specialty of medicine, but unlicensed practitioners generally do not support this view. Some skilled homeopaths have certification in classical homeopathy (designated by the initials "CCH" after their names), but many have not chosen to take this examination, which is not a requirement for homeopathic practice. With these currently unresolved issues, a prospective patient may be able to develop a fairer view of a specific practitioner's qualifications by asking the individual homeopath about his or her training, experience, and philosophy than is indicated by the practitioner's professional designations alone. Referral resources for homeopathic practitioners include the National Center for Homeopathy (www.homeopathic.org), the American Institute of Homeopathy (www.homeopathyusa.org), the Homeopathic Academy of Naturopathic Physicians (www.hanp.net), and the North American Society of Homeopaths (www.homeopathy.org).

CURRENT DEVELOPMENTS IN HOMEOPATHY

Hahnemann continued refining homeopathy throughout his years of practice, updating his Organon of the Medical Art six times before his death in 1843. In this same spirit of inquiry and while searching for more consistent ways to help patients, homeopathy has continued to evolve. Current controversy in the field involves methods of interviewing patients, analyzing cases, and selecting remedies. For example, the Dutch homeopath Dr. Jan Scholten has made great strides in clinically applying mineral remedies through his understanding of the periodic table (Scholten 1996), but some claim his findings are too theoretical for practical use. Drs. Rajan Sankaran (1997, 2000, 2002) and Jayesh Shah and others at the Bombay School have furthered homeopathic prescribing by extensively examining patient sensations and linking these to substances from the natural world. When interviewing a patient, Drs. Sankaran and Shah seek a "non-human-specific" sensation that can reliably guide them to the helpful remedy. Dissenting voices claim that these methods wander too far from Hahnemann's original practice. Dr. Divya Chhabra, also from India, has deepened her understanding of patient symptoms through using free association. Her notion of finding a "confluence point" where mental, emotional, and physical symptoms unite is unique within homeopathy; this might also be useful to other medical systems dealing with patients' psychosomatic symptoms. The contributions of George Vithoulkas, a leading contemporary Greek homeopath, have been invaluable in spreading homeopathic medicine throughout the world, yet he himself disputes the approaches of these other clinicians. All of these practitioners and many more continually open their clinics and offer seminars to those wishing to learn their methods.

One might note that the themes of pattern recognition and finding where the patient is most "stuck" recur over and over (Davidson 1994) and have particular application in psychiatric medicine. A recent systematic qualitative study of homeopathic practitioners confirmed the importance of classical homeopathic treatment in facilitating the release of a patient from being chronically "stuck" in dysfunctional life patterns (Bell 2003; Saine 1997). Despite existing controversies, all homeopaths seem to seek genuine healing for patients on all levels. Other whole systems of CAM (e.g., traditional Chinese medicine) also report these types of global and multidimensional changes in patients undergoing treatment for many different chronic conditions (Gould and MacPherson 2001; Paterson 2005; Verhoef et al. 2005).

Case Example

The following case example, taken from Messer (2003), illustrates the individualized approach of homeopathic medicine.

George was a 42-year-old interior designer who came to the clinic because of his lifelong bouts of depression. He remembered having these problems as far back as when he was age 7 years, but he did not seem to have had a particularly traumatic or stressful childhood. He had tried many things, including drugs, but nothing seemed to help much. Over the 2 years prior to his coming to the clinic, he had been undergoing counseling, which seemed to have helped a little bit. He felt a little better from exercise and often self-medicated with beer.

George's depression tended to start from some trigger in his daily life and then build slowly until it was unbearable. It often began when he made a small mistake at work, after which he would berate himself and thus begin a downward spiral. George also said that he was not really following his true passion, which was to make and record music. He felt too overwhelmed by responsibilities to give time to this. During the times when he was depressed, he felt ashamed of himself and humiliated that he could not make the depression go away. At such moments, he was unmotivated and did not want to play his guitar, go to work, or do anything. He reproached himself at these times and felt worthless and like a failure. He was sad and said he felt embarrassed because he should be a better person. He also reported feeling physically weak and found getting out of bed to be a real chore. He described a depressive episode as living "incarcerated in the cell of my own mind."

George also had trouble with anxiety. When the phone rang, he was afraid to answer it, not knowing who might be calling and worrying that somehow this call might lead to a confrontation he wanted to avoid. He was afraid to answer his door or have people over to his house. He had trouble with relationships since he was afraid of people getting to know him. He was ashamed of revealing his feelings and ordinarily would not talk much or allow himself to show emotion. He tried to pretend everything was okay, telling people "what I think they want to hear, a candy-coated version of the truth." He could get angry but in general did not lose his temper. For example, in a restaurant once, he observed a nearby patron being rude to the server. His felt his blood pressure and heart rate going up and he felt a lot of anger, but he did not do anything. He reported often feeling sad but kept himself from crying, although he said "the feeling is always there."

A review of his bodily symptoms revealed that George had some nasal congestion in the morning, but otherwise his physical health was unremarkable. A review of his general symptoms found that he had some trouble sleeping; he was a light sleeper and often might wake during the night. He liked spicy food and wanted to have some with every meal. He confirmed again that he easily felt guilty if he thought he had done something wrong; he was fearful of any confrontation and was sensitive to music. If reprimanded, he felt terribly embarrassed and would avoid any person involved in the incident and try to never deal with them again. He was sensitive to others' feelings when he saw someone being rude to them. The patient felt less well overall when he became too hot, even though he could tolerate being in the sun. These are important "general symptoms" in homeopathic constitutional states.

The remedy in this case needed to fit the patient's particular and unique form of depression. After other remedies were considered, George was given *Pulsatilla* because of the following unique and characteristic symptoms:

- Strong fear of conflict and confrontation (repertory rubrics were "mind, yielding disposition" and "mind, timidity")
- Tendency to self-criticism
- Sensitivity to music

George was given a 1M dose of *Pulsatilla*. He returned 1 month later for follow-up and reported feeling "really good." For a couple of days after taking the remedy, he had felt a bit "dreamy," as if he needed to sit down, and also "spacey." A few days after this he felt a bit anxious, nervous, and itchy all over. He also developed a strange taste in his mouth. At 1 week after his dose of *Pulsatilla*, he said that he started to "feel great" and that this feeling had continued since.

George denied any current feelings of anxiety or depression. He reported feeling more ambitious and was able to maintain a positive attitude. Little things did not seem to bother him. He was no longer irritable, and his energy level had improved. His sleep had improved only slightly, but he was feeling more rested on awakening. Because he seemed to be having a good response to the initial dose of the remedy, it was not repeated at this time.

At George's 2-month follow-up, he said that he continued to feel fine. He was recording more music and experiencing no depression. He said that this was the first enjoyable Thanksgiving he had ever had. He was doing so well that he and his counselor decided to stop therapy sessions because he no longer needed to discuss problems and they were only talking about his hobbies and so on. The counselor was still available if George needed him. Again, George seemed to still be responding to the first dose of *Pulsatilla*, so no new prescription was indicated. He continued to do well for 9 months following this, and his continued well-being was confirmed by telephone-based follow-up.

The treatment given to George differed substantially from what he would have received in a standard psychiatric clinic. He needed only one dose of his homeopathic remedy over the year he was seen, whereas if he was being treated with conventional medicine, he would have been given antidepressants, dosed daily, for many months. With George's having experienced sadness, anxiety, and depression since age 7 years, it is likely he would have been on long-term antidepressant maintenance.

If George had relapsed while being treated homeopathically, it is likely that the same remedy would have been repeated once and the response observed over time (weeks to months), as the symptom picture indicated. If the symptom picture had changed from that of *Pulsatilla*, a single dose of a different indicated remedy would have been given, in the manner described above. Leading homeopaths might consider him as having been "cured" of his mood disorder if he remained free of symptoms for at least 2 years after his last indicated remedy dose.

Information from the proving of *Pulsatilla* helped in selecting the remedy for this patient. George's picture was not the clinically stereotypical one for *Pulsatilla*, yet the original proving data prominently listed his symptoms of anger, anxiety, and reluctance to share his emotions. His rare presentation of symptoms showed the need to study remedies carefully and in detail rather than making a snap judgment based on external symptoms alone. Another patient with dysthymia and recurrent depression might or might not require *Pulsatilla*, depending on that person's unique biopsychosocial symptom pattern. In short, it is the full context of the clinical presentation of a given patient, not the specific conventional diagnosis, that guides the treatment plan.

As is common in homeopathic practice, the patient saw the practitioner far less frequently than he would have seen a psychotherapist. This observation raises a question as to the extent to which clinical interpersonal factors versus the effects of the remedies themselves can contribute to catalyzing a favorable change within a patient. If the homeopathic encounters are highly beneficial per se apart from the remedies, then further research should address what elements are particular to a homeopathic session that stimulate change in a more cost-effective manner (i.e., in fewer sessions) than does conventional psychotherapy.

HOMEOPATHIC RESEARCH: STATE OF THE SCIENCE

Clinical Studies

In the 200-year history of classical homeopathy, the collected clinical literature includes hundreds of positive case reports assembled for many different psychiatric and neuropsychiatric disorders in professional specialty journals (e.g., *Homeopathy* [formerly the *British Homeopathic Journal*]; *Homeopathy: The Journal of the Faculty of Homeopathy; Homeopathic Links: International Journal for Classical Homeopathy; Simillimum: The Journal of the Homeopathic Academy of Naturopathic Physicians; The American Homeopath; American Journal of Homeopathic Medicine; The Homeopath: Journal of the Society of Homeopaths;* and numerous non–English language sources), lay publications (e.g., *Homeopathy Today*), books (e.g., Herscu 1990; Lansky 2003; Reichenberg-Ullman 2000; Reichenberg-Ullman and Ullman 2000, 2002; Saine 1997; Ullman and Reichenberg-Ullman 1999), software programs with sophisticated search engines (e.g., ReferenceWorks; Encyclopedia Homeopathica [www.wholehealthnow.com/homeopathy_software/eh.html]), and online Web sites (e.g., www.lyghtforce.com/homeopathyonline; www.homeopathycured-cases.com). Disorders that homeopaths routinely treat with reportedly good clinical success include depression; acute grief reactions; anxiety, including social phobia and panic disorder; posttraumatic stress disorder; premenstrual dysphoric disorder; insomnia; somatoform spectrum disorders such as fibromyalgia; chronic fatigue syndrome; multiple chemical sensitivities; alcohol abuse; attention-deficit/hyperactivity disorder; autism; traumatic brain injury; epilepsy; stroke; dementia; chronic headache; and vertigo. Currently the systematic research data on homeopathy for each of these conditions are extremely limited. Table 9–1 summarizes the status of research in the field; citations refer to peer-reviewed papers relevant to a given disorder.

The state of the science is such that homeopathy has always lacked a critical mass of researchers worldwide; there is no network of homeopathic research training programs and an insufficient research funding base to attract new homeopathy investigators. Almost all contemporary homeopaths are clinicians with limited training in research methodology. The rigorous research and reporting standards articulated by mainstream medical researchers, such as CONSORT (Moher et al.

TABLE 9–1.   Evidence for use of homeopathy in psychiatric/neuropsychiatric disorders

Disorder or symptom treated	CAM treatment used	Supporting evidence	Rating of supporting evidence	Comments
Acute grief reactions	Classical homeopathy	Davidson and Gaylord 1995	2	Many case reports; no studies
Alcohol abuse	Classical homeopathy	Rogers 1997; A. Sukul et al. 1999	2	Many case reports; animal studies suggest capacity to reduce alcohol-induced sleep time
Attention-deficit/ hyperactivity disorder	Classical homeopathy	Frei and Thurneysen 2001; Frei et al. 2005; Jacobs et al. 2005; Lamont 1997	3	Many case reports and some popular books; one positive controlled study, one good observational study, one negative controlled pilot study
Autism	Classical homeopathy	Lansky 2003	2	Many case reports; no controlled studies
Chronic headache	Classical homeopathy	Walach et al. 1997, 2000	1	Many case reports; one negative controlled study

TABLE 9–1. Evidence for use of homeopathy in psychiatric/neuropsychiatric disorders *(continued)*

Disorder or symptom treated	CAM treatment used	Supporting evidence	Rating of supporting evidence	Comments
Dementia	Classical homeopathy	Caville 2002; Jonas et al. 2001; Marotta et al. 2002, 2003; McCarney et al. 2003	2	Some case reports; animal studies suggest possible benefit of isopathic treatment with glutamate
Depression	Classical homeopathy	Davidson 1994; Davidson et al. 1997	2	Many case reports; one small case series; large-magnitude placebo effects with drugs make small pilot studies less feasible
Epilepsy	Classical homeopathy	Tandon et al. 2002	2	Many case reports
Generalized anxiety	Classical homeopathy	Bonne et al. 2003	2	One negative controlled study, one positive large-scale observational study
Insomnia	Classical homeopathy	Ruiz and Torres 1997; Ruiz-Vega et al. 2002	2	Many case reports; some animal studies; no clinical studies

TABLE 9–1. Evidence for use of homeopathy in psychiatric/neuropsychiatric disorders *(continued)*

Disorder or symptom treated	CAM treatment used	Supporting evidence	Rating of supporting evidence	Comments
Panic disorder	Classical homeopathy	Davidson et al. 1997	2	Many case reports; one small case series
Posttraumatic stress disorder	Classical homeopathy	Coll 2002; Morrison 1993	2	Many case reports; no studies
Premenstrual dysphoric disorder	Classical homeopathy	Yakir et al. 2001	2–3	Many case reports; one small study
Social phobia	Classical homeopathy	Davidson and Gaylord 1995; Davidson et al. 1997	2	Many case reports; one small study
Somatoform spectrum disorders	Classical homeopathy	Bell et al. 2004a, 2004b, 2004c, 2004d; Fisher et al. 1989; Geraghty 2002; Weatherley-Jones et al. 2004	3–4	Many case reports; two positive controlled studies of fibromyalgia; one equivocal controlled study of chronic fatigue syndrome

TABLE 9–1. Evidence for use of homeopathy in psychiatric/neuropsychiatric disorders (*continued*)

Disorder or symptom treated	CAM treatment used	Supporting evidence	Rating of supporting evidence	Comments
Stroke	Classical homeopathy	Jonas et al. 1999	2	Some case reports; animal studies suggest possible benefit of isopathic treatment with glutamate (see dementia)
Traumatic brain injury	Classical homeopathy	Chapman 2002; Chapman et al. 1999	2–3	Many case reports; one positive controlled study
Vertigo	Combination homeopathy	Weiser et al. 1998	2	Many case reports; one positive controlled study

Note. CAM = complementary and alternative medicine. Rating key: 5 = established use of specified CAM modality supported by systematic review; 4 = established use of specified CAM modality supported by three or more controlled, double-blind, randomized trials; 3 = use of specified CAM modality supported by consistent findings from open trials; 2 = use of specified CAM modality supported by consistent anecdotal reports, but few or no studies; 1 = specified CAM modality is in common use to treat mental health problems but is not supported by anecdotal or research evidence.

2001), do not as yet have parallels in homeopathy (Bell 2003). Moreover, although double-blind research in homeopathy would seem to be comparatively straightforward, given the physical capability to blind observers and subjects to homeopathic remedies versus placebo, data and anecdotal observations indicate that many such randomized clinical trials are methodologically problematic (Bell 2003; Walach 2002, 2003; Walach and Jonas 2002). Concerns about homeopathic clinical trials include the failure to select remedies in the highly individualized manner standard with classical homeopathy (the most developed clinical system in the field), failure to provide flexibility to change remedy selection or dose in accordance with emerging changes in the symptom pattern, failure to provide flexibility in timing and duration of treatment (pretreatment before a symptom has developed and overtreatment once improvement has begun are common in the controlled clinical literature, but both courses are known to lead to worsening of the patient's condition in terms of homeopathic clinical principles).

Several homeopathic researchers have begun to call for a greater focus on observational data to generate a better basis for future study designs (Fisher 2001; Frei and Thurneysen 2001; Van Wassenhoven and Ives 2004; Walach 2003; Walach and Jonas 2002b; Walach et al. 2005). Although national and international consensus panels have emphasized the need to test homeopathy interventions in a manner that respects and incorporates actual clinical practice in a given field (Kron et al. 1998; Levin et al. 1997), trials of homeopathic medicine set up according to conventional rigorous randomized, controlled designs ignore fundamental homeopathic principles. Such trials rank well in meta-analytical reviews of homeopathy (Linde et al. 1999), but the criteria for rating study quality fail to include or to weight scores for the integrity of the clinical practice used and the patient-centered—as opposed to disease-centered—nature of the outcomes (Bell 2003).

Furthermore, homeopathy is one of a number of CAM modalities, including traditional Chinese medicine, Ayurveda, and naturopathy, that claim personwide effects during the course of treatment. Consequently, the assumptions implicit in conventional medical research design often lead to inappropriate or incomplete evaluation of outcomes (Bell et al. 2002b; Jonas 2005); that is, homeopathy purports to mobilize changes over time that gradually shift the center of gravity of the illness (the subsystem of greatest pathology at a given time) from mental to emotional to physical planes, with concurrent symptoms often changing in all planes. A patient with depression who begins to respond appropriately to homeopathy could exhibit a lessening of the mood disorder and increased energy early in treatment but experience an apparent reemergence of prior somatic conditions such as asthma or eczema. Other symptoms that the patient did not think to report in the intake interview may resolve during homeopathic treatment. A rating scale for depression used in a study of homeopathy has no capacity to detect the types of emergent changes in nondepressive symptomatology commonly reported with homeopathic treatment.

Continued homeopathic treatment reportedly leads to resolution of the somatic problems over many months as well as to the emergence of a greater resilience to life stressors over several years (Bell et al. 2003). However, most psychiatric clinical trials are short, lasting only 12–16 weeks, and leave inadequate time to document the reportedly multisystem, multidimensional changes claimed in homeopathy (Bell et al. 2003). In summary, outcome measures drawn from conventional trial designs are focused on the disease rather than the patient, making it possible to miss documenting the full picture of clinical effects during the course of homeopathic treatment in an otherwise well-designed study (Bell 2005).

Objective Basic Science and Preclinical Evidence in Homeopathy

Most skeptics of homeopathy acknowledge that many clinical studies in the field, whether randomized clinical trials or observational studies, report findings consistent with anecdotal claims (Goldstein and Glik 1998; Linde et al. 1997; Thompson and Reilly 2002; van Haselen 2000; Van Wassenhoven and Ives 2004). However, skeptics typically find homeopathy to be implausible as a valid biologically active intervention because of the basic nature of the remedies (Langman 1997; Vandenbroucke 1997; Vandenbroucke and de Craen 2001).

The skeptics' perspective is that homeopathy can only be a placebo (Shang et al. 2005). Recent objective psychophysiological approaches are beginning to test the placebo hypothesis for homeopathy. For example, new electroencephalographic (EEG) evidence from a double-blind, randomized study of classical homeopathy in the treatment of fibromyalgia shows that active remedy and placebo effects on relative EEG alpha magnitude diverge over time in treatment (Bell et al. 2004b). Prefrontal EEG cordance, a derivative of relative and absolute EEG that differentiates those who actively respond to an antidepressant drug from those who respond to a placebo (Cook and Leuchter 2001; Cook et al. 2002; Leuchter et al. 2002), also distinguishes those who respond exceptionally well to active individualized homeopathy from all other study participants (i.e., those taking clinically less effective homeopathic medicines and those taking placebo) (Bell et al. 2004d).

In basic science, the data on homeopathic remedies are mixed (Bellavite 2002). On the one hand, dilution beyond Avogadro's number, which is characteristic of homeopathic remedies at doses of 12C and higher (where 200C or 1,000C to 1M are commonly used in treating psychiatric disorders), can lead to a loss of conventional molecular biological activity. On the other hand, homeopathic remedies are not prepared using only dilution; rather, each dilution step is followed by vigorous shaking (succussion).

New scientific data suggest that it is the succussion that may lead to persistent changes in the solvent structure of homeopathically prepared agents. For example, in replicated studies, the addition of alkali to homeopathically prepared remedies has led to a measurable excess heat generation compared with plain solvent or plain dilutions without succussion (Elia and Niccoli 1999, 2004). The heat indicates possible disruption of order in the water solvent molecular network organization per se. In other work, homeopathically prepared remedies (e.g., sodium chloride, lithium chloride) have exhibited a characteristic thermoluminescence pattern under experimental conditions of freezing, radiation treatment, and slow rewarming (Rey 2003). The latter findings suggest unique hydrogen bonding patterns between the water molecules of the homeopathically prepared remedies. Taken together, the materials science researchers involved in such studies suggest that homeopathically prepared remedies show evidence of formation of water clusters, altered hydrogen-bonded networks of water molecules, and/or nano-bubbles formed as a consequence of the preparation method. These conclusions are consistent with current materials science research on the fundamental properties of water solutions, but are typically rejected by skeptics of homeopathy using Newtonian physics notions of the nature of water. Consistent with this newer research, one older study demonstrated that the "higher" potencies of certain homeopathic remedies (i.e., no source molecules remaining in the remedy solvent) could prolong haloperidol-induced catalepsy in animals for longer periods of time than could "lower" potencies of the same remedies (i.e., more source molecules potentially remaining in the remedy solvent) (N.C. Sukul et al. 1986).

Homeopathy may map best to concepts drawn from network and complex systems theory at the levels of both scale of the remedy and changes in the patient during treatment. At the level of the patient, a number of contemporary homeopathic researchers have noted the striking overlaps between homeopathic constructs and the modern science of complex adaptive systems and interactive networks (Bell et al. 2002a, 2004b; Bellavite 2003; Bellavite and Signorini 2002; Hyland 2003; Hyland and Lewith 2002; Milgrom 2002; Shepperd 1994; Torres 2002; Waldo and Torres 2003). In complex systems theory, a person is an intact, indivisible network of interactive, interrelated parts with a nonlinear dynamic pattern of behaviors. The whole system is more than the sum of its parts; that is, a person exhibits emergent behaviors/properties that are not predicted by understanding the properties of the lower-order parts in isolation such as lung, liver, heart, and brain (Engel 1977). The homeopathic concepts that 1) a single remedy treats the entire individual's pattern of mental, emotional, and physical symptoms; and 2) changes occur over time throughout the person, not just in the chief complaint, are consistent with an integrated network view of the human being (Barabasi 2003).

CONCLUSION

Overall, the basic and preclinical science evidence offers heuristically useful ways to conceptualize and perform appropriate, hypothesis-driven research in homeopathy. The challenge remains to follow up the promising preclinical and scientific data, the anecdotal clinical evidence, and initial systematic studies with higher-quality research (Jonas 2005; Jonas et al. 2003).

In summary, consumers have used and continue to use homeopathy worldwide in growing numbers for acute and chronic conditions. Some psychiatrists might feel repelled by the paradigm shift required to consider homeopathic concepts. Others might see some heuristic value in understanding the interest of a substantial subset of consumers in homeopathy as one of a number of CAM systems. Personality trait data suggest, for example, that individuals who score high in Openness are more likely to use Chinese medicine or homeopathy than are those with low levels of Openness (Honda and Jacobson 2005). In either event, patients are best served when their physicians know when their patients combine conventional and alternative approaches. The laws of healing and cure that the early homeopaths have articulated offer a valuable conceptual framework in which to consider the process of whole-person healing, regardless of modality. Inherently integrative and interdisciplinary in nature, the homeopathic perspective on health and disease is especially applicable to patients with complex medical and psychiatric symptoms. New discoveries and emerging research evidence from scientific disciplines outside conventional medicine with relevance to homeopathy promise the possibility of enlarging our understanding of human beings and of life itself (Hyland 2003; Hyland and Lewith 2002; Whitmont 1991).

REFERENCES

American Psychiatric Association: Diagnostic and Statistical Manual of Mental Disorders, 4th Edition, Text Revision. Washington, DC, American Psychiatric Association, 2000

Astin JA: Why patients use alternative medicine: results of a national study. JAMA 279:1548–1553, 1998

Bailey P: Homeopathy, in Handbook of Complementary and Alternative Therapies in Mental Health. Edited by Shannon S. San Diego, CA, Academic Press, 2002, pp 401–429

Bannerman R, Burton J, Wen Chieh C: Traditional Medicine and Health Care Coverage. Geneva, World Health Organization, 1983

Barabasi AL: Linked: How Everything Is Connected to Everything Else and What It Means for Business, Science, and Everyday Life. Cambridge, MA, Plume, 2003

Bell IR: Evidence-based homeopathy: empirical questions and methodological considerations for homeopathic clinical research. American Journal of Homeopathic Medicine 96:17–31, 2003

Bell IR: All evidence is equal, but some evidence is more equal than others: can logic prevail over emotion in the homeopathy debate? J Altern Complement Med 11:763–769, 2005

Bell IR, Baldwin CM, Schwartz GE: Translating a nonlinear systems theory model for homeopathy into empirical tests. Altern Ther Health Med 8:58–66, 2002a

Bell IR, Caspi O, Schwartz GE, et al: Integrative medicine and systemic outcomes research: issues in the emergence of a new model for primary health care. Arch Intern Med 162:133–140, 2002b

Bell IR, Koithan M, Gorman MM, et al: Homeopathic practitioner views of changes in patients undergoing constitutional treatment for chronic disease. J Altern Complement Med 9:39–50, 2003

Bell IR, Lewis DAI, Brooks AJ, et al: Improved clinical status in fibromyalgia patients treated with individualized homeopathic remedies versus placebo. Rheumatology 43:577–582, 2004a

Bell IR, Lewis DAI, Lewis SE, et al: EEG alpha sensitization in individualized homeopathic treatment of fibromyalgia. Int J Neurosci 114:1195–1220, 2004b

Bell IR, Lewis DAI, Lewis SE, et al: Strength of vital force in classical homeopathy: bio-psycho-social-spiritual correlates in a complex systems context. J Altern Complement Med 10:123–131, 2004c

Bell IR, Lewis DAI, Schwartz GE, et al: Electroencephalographic cordance patterns distinguish exceptional clinical responders with fibromyalgia to individualized homeopathic medicines. J Altern Complement Med 10:285–299, 2004d

Bellavite P: Complexity science and homeopathy: a synthetic overview. Homeopathy 92:203–212, 2003

Bellavite P, Signorini A: The Emerging Science of Homeopathy: Complexity, Biodynamics, and Nanopharmacology. Berkeley, CA, North Atlantic Books, 2002, p 408

Bonne O, Shemer Y, Gorali Y, et al: A randomized, double-blind, placebo-controlled study of classical homeopathy in generalized anxiety disorder. J Clin Psychiatry 64:282–287, 2003

Calabrese EJ: Toxicological awakenings: the rebirth of hormesis as a central pillar of toxicology. Toxicol Appl Pharmacol 204:1–8, 2005

Calabrese EJ, Baldwin LA: Hormesis: a generalizable and unifying hypothesis. Crit Rev Toxicol 31:353–424, 2001

Carlston M: Classical Homeopathy (Medical Guides to Complementary and Alternative Medicine Series). Series edited by Micozzi M. Philadelphia, PA, Churchill Livingstone, 2003

Caville P: Homeopathy in dementia and agitation. Homeopathy 91:109–112, 2002

Chapman E: Placebo reaction versus homeopathic effect: how to distinguish the two. American Journal of Homeopathic Medicine 95:157–163, 2002

Chapman EH, Weintraub RJ, Milburn MA, et al: Homeopathic treatment of mild traumatic brain injury: a randomized, double-blind, placebo-controlled clinical trial. J Head Trauma Rehabil 14:521–542, 1999

Coll L: Homeopathy in survivors of childhood sexual abuse. Homeopathy 91:3–9, 2002

Cook IA, Leuchter AF: Prefrontal changes and treatment response prediction in depression. Semin Clin Neuropsychiatry 6:113–120, 2001

Cook IA, Leuchter AF, Morgan M, et al: Early changes in prefrontal activity characterize clinical responders to antidepressants. Neuropsychopharmacology 27:120–131, 2002

Davidson J: Psychiatry and homeopathy: basis for a dialogue. Br Homeopath J 83:78–83, 1994

Davidson J, Gaylord S: Meeting of minds in psychiatry and homeopathy: an example in social phobia. Altern Ther Health Med 1:36–43, 1995

Davidson JR, Morrison RM, Shore J, et al: Homeopathic treatment of depression and anxiety. Altern Ther Health Med 3:46–49, 1997

Druss B, Rosenheck R: Use of practitioner-based complementary therapies by persons reporting mental conditions in the United States. Arch Gen Psychiatry 57:708–714, 2000

Eisenberg DM, Davis RB, Ettner SL, et al: Trends in alternative medicine use in the US, 1990–1997: results of a follow-up national survey. JAMA 280:1569–1575, 1998

Elia V, Niccoli M: Thermodynamics of extremely diluted aqueous solutions. Ann N Y Acad Sci 879:241–248, 1999

Elia V, Niccoli M: New physico-chemical properties of extremely diluted aqueous solutions. Journal of Thermal Analysis and Calorimetry 75:815–836, 2004

Engel GL: The need for a new medical model: a challenge for biomedicine. Science 196:129–136, 1977

Fisher P: Research for whom? Br Homoeopath J 90:178–179, 2001

Fisher P, Greenwood A, Huskisson EC, et al: Effect of homeopathic treatment on fibrositis (primary fibromyalgia). BMJ 299:365–366, 1989

Frei H, Thurneysen A: Treatment for hyperactive children: homeopathy and methylphenidate compared in a family setting. Br Homoeopath J 90:183–188, 2001

Frei H, Everts R, von Ammon K, et al: Homeopathic treatment of children with attention deficit hyperactivity disorder: a randomised, double blind, placebo-controlled crossover trial. Eur J Pediatr 164:758–767, 2005

Frenkel M, Hermoni D: Effects of homeopathic intervention on medication consumption in atopic and allergic disorders. Altern Ther Health Med 8:76–79, 2002

Geraghty J: Homeopathic treatment of chronic fatigue syndrome: three case studies using Jan Scholten's methodology. Homeopathy 91:99–105, 2002

Goldstein MS, Glik D: Use of and satisfaction with homeopathy in a patient population. Altern Ther Health Med 4:60–65, 1998

Gould A, MacPherson H: Patient perspectives on outcomes after treatment with acupuncture. J Altern Complement Med 7:261–268, 2001

Hahnemann S: Organon of the Medical Art (1843), 6th Edition. Edited by O'Reilly WB, translated by Decker S. Redmond, WA, Birdcage Books, 1996

Herscu P: Homeopathic Treatment of Children: Pediatric Constitutional Types. Berkeley, CA, North Atlantic Books, 1990

Honda K, Jacobson JS: Use of complementary and alternative medicine among United States adults: the influences of personality, coping strategies, and social support. Prev Med 40:46–53, 2005

Hyland M: Extended network generalized entanglement theory: therapeutic mechanisms, empirical predictions, and investigations. J Altern Complement Med 9:919–936, 2003

Hyland ME, Lewith GT: Oscillatory effects in a homeopathic clinical trial: an explanation using complexity theory, and implications for clinical practice. Homeopathy 91:145–149, 2002

Jacobs J, Williams AL, Girard C, et al: Homeopathy for attention-deficit/hyperactivity disorder: a pilot randomized controlled trial. J Altern Complement Med 11:799–806, 2005

Jonas WB: Building an evidence house: challenges and solutions to research in complementary and alternative medicine. Forsch Komplementarmed Klass Naturheilkd 12:159–167, 2005

Jonas W, Lin Y, Williams A, et al: Treatment of experimental stroke with low-dose glutamate and homeopathic *Arnica montana*. Perfusion 12:452–462, 1999

Jonas W, Lin Y, Tortella F: Neuroprotection from glutamate toxicity with ultra-low dose glutamate. NeuroReport 12:335–339, 2001

Jonas WB, Kaptchuk TJ, Linde K: A critical overview of homeopathy. Ann Intern Med 138:393–399, 2003

Kessler RC, Davis RB, Foster DF: Long-term trends in the use of complementary and alternative medical therapies in the United States. Ann Intern Med 135:262–268, 2001a

Kessler RC, Soukup J, Davis R: The use of complementary and alternative therapies to treat anxiety and depression in the United States. Am J Psychiatry 158:289–294, 2001b

Kornfeld D: Consultation-liaison psychiatry: contributions to medical practice. Am J Psychiatry 159:1964–1972, 2002

Kron M, English JM, Gaus W: Guidelines on methodology of clinical research in homeopathy, in Homeopathy: A Critical Appraisal. Edited by Ernst E, Hahn EG. Oxford, Butterworth-Heinemann, 1998, pp 9–47

Lamont J: Homeopathic treatment of attention deficit hyperactivity disorder: a controlled study. Br Homoeopath J 86:196–200, 1997

Langman MJS: Homeopathy trials: reason for good ones but are they warranted? Lancet 350:825, 1997

Lansky AL: Impossible Cure: The Promise of Homeopathy. Portola Valley, CA, RL Ranch Press, 2003

Leuchter AF, Cook IA, Witte EA, et al: Changes in brain function of depressed subjects during treatment with placebo. Am J Psychiatry 159:122–129, 2002

Levin JS, Glass TA, Kushi LH, et al: Quantitative methods in research on complementary and alternative medicine: a methodological manifesto. NIH Office of Alternative Medicine. Med Care 35:1079–1094, 1997

Linde K, Clausius N, Ramirez G, et al: Are the clinical effects of homeopathy placebo effects? a meta-analysis of placebo-controlled trials. Lancet 350:834–843, 1997

Linde K, Scholz M, Ramirez G, et al: Impact of study quality on outcome in placebo-controlled trials of homeopathy. J Clin Epidemiol 52:631–636, 1999

Lipsitt D: Consultation-liaison psychiatry and psychosomatic medicine: the company they keep. Psychosom Med 63:896–909, 2001

Marotta D, Marini A, Banaudha K, et al: Nonlinear effects of cycloheximide in glutamate-treated cultured rat cerebellar neurons. Neurotoxicology 23:307–312, 2002

Marotta D, Marini A, Banaudha K, et al: Nonlinear effects of glutamate and KCl on glutamate toxicity in cultured rat cerebellar neurons. Int J Neurosci 113:45–56, 2003

Mascaro N, Rosen DH: Existential meaning's role in the enhancement of hope and prevention of depressive symptoms. J Pers 73:985–1013, 2005

McCarney R, Warner J, Fisher P, et al: Homeopathy for dementia. Cochrane Database Syst Rev (1):CD003803, 2003

Menninger C: Some reflections relative to the symptomatology and materia medica of typhoid fever. Transactions of the American Institute of Homoeopathy 1897, p 430

Merrell WC, Shalts E: Homeopathy. Med Clin North Am 86:47–62, 2002

Messer S: "I just don't feel happy...": a case of life-long depression. Homeopathy Today 23:26–29, 2003

Milgrom LR: Vitalism, complexity, and the concept of spin. Homeopathy 91:26–31, 2002

Moher D, Schulz KF, Altman D, et al: The CONSORT statement: revised recommendations for improving the quality of reports of parallel-group randomized trials. JAMA 285:1987–1991, 2001

Morrison R: Materia medica of post-traumatic stress disorder. J Am Inst Homeopath 86:110–118, 1993

Oschman JL: Energy Medicine: The Scientific Basis. Edinburgh, Churchill Livingstone, 2000

Paterson C, Dieppe P: Characteristic and incidental (placebo) effects in complex interventions such as acupuncture. BMJ 330:1202–1205, 2005

Pelling AE: The dark side of the cell: the singing cell. 2004. Available at: http://users.design.ucla.edu/~aniemetz/darksideofcell/bg.html

Pelling AE, Sehati S, Gralla EB, et al: Local nanomechanical motion of the cell wall of *Saccharomyces cerevisiae*. Science 305:1147–1150, 2004

Reichenberg-Ullman J: Whole Woman Homeopathy: The Comprehensive Guide to Treating PMS, Menopause, Cystitis, and Other Problems Naturally and Effectively. Rocklin, CA, Prima Lifestyles, 2000

Reichenberg-Ullman J, Ullman R: Ritalin-Free Kids: Safe and Effective Homeopathic Medicine for ADHD and Other Behavioral and Learning Problems. Rocklin, CA, Prima Lifestyles, 2000

Reichenberg-Ullman J, Ullman R: Prozac-Free. Berkeley, CA, North Atlantic Books, 2002

Rey L: Thermoluminescence of ultra-high dilutions of lithium chloride and sodium chloride. Physica A 323:67–74, 2003. Available at: www.vhan.nl/documents/Rey.thermoluminescence.pdf

Riley D, Fischer M, Singh B, et al: Homeopathy and conventional medicine: an outcomes study comparing effectiveness in a primary care setting. J Altern Complement Med 7:149–159, 2001

Rogers J: Homoeopathy and the treatment of alcohol-related problems. Complement Ther Nurs Midwifery 3:21–28, 1997

Rowe T: Choosing a Career in Homeopathic Medicine. Phoenix, AZ, Desert Institute Publishing, 2004

Rozman KK, Doull J: Scientific foundations of hormesis, 2: maturation, strengths, limitations, and possible applications in toxicology, pharmacology, and epidemiology. Crit Rev Toxicol 33:451–462, 2003

Ruiz G, Torres JL: Homeopathic effect on the sleep pattern of rats. Br Homoeopath J 86:201–206, 1997

Ruiz-Vega G, Perez-Ordaz L, Leon-Hueramo O, et al: Comparative effect of *Coffea cruda* potencies on rats. Homeopathy 91:80–84, 2002

Saine A: Psychiatric Patients: Back to the Roots. Steps in Taking Materia Medica Cases. Eindhoven, Netherlands, Lutra Services, 1997

Sankaran R: The Soul of Remedies. Bombay, India, Homeopathic Medical, 1997

Sankaran R: The System of Homeopathy. Mumbai, India, Homeopathic Medical, 2000

Sankaran R: An Insight Into Plants, Vols I & II. Mumbai, India, Homeopathic Medical, 2002

Scholten J: Homeopathy and the Elements. Utrecht, Netherlands, Stichting Alonnissos, 1996

Shalts E: Homeopathy, in Integrative Medicine: Principles for Practice. Edited by Kligler B, Lee R. New York, McGraw-Hill, 2004, pp 255–270

Shang A, Huwiler-Muntener K, Nartey L, et al: Are the clinical effects of homoeopathy placebo effects? comparative study of placebo-controlled trials of homoeopathy and allopathy. Lancet 66:726–732, 2005

Shepperd J: Chaos theory: implications for homeopathy. Journal of the American Institute of Homeopathy 87:22, 1994

Sherr J: The Dynamics and Methodology of Homeopathic Provings, 2nd Edition. Malvern, UK, Dynamis Books, 1994

Spence D, Thompson EA, Barron SJ: Homeopathic treatment for chronic disease: a 6-year university-hospital outpatient observational study. J Altern Complement Med 11:793–798, 2005

Stone J, Colyer M, Feltower S: "Psychosomatic": a systematic review of its meaning in newspaper articles. Psychosomatics 45:287–290, 2004

Sukul A, Sinhabau SP, Sukul NC: Reduction of alcohol induced sleep time in albino mice by potentized *Nux vomica* prepared with 90% ethanol. Br Homoeopath J 88:58–61, 1999

Sukul NC, Bala SK, Bhattacharyya B: Prolonged cataleptogenic effects of potentized homoeopathic drugs. Psychopharmacology 89:338–339, 1986

Tandon M, Prabhakar S, Prandhi P: Pattern of use of complementary/alternative medicine (CAM) in epileptic patients in a tertiary care hospital in India. Pharmacoepidemiol Drug Saf 11:457–463, 2002

Thompson EA, Reilly D: The homeopathic approach to symptom control in the cancer patient: a prospective observational study. Palliat Med 16:227–233, 2002

Torres JL: Homeopathic effect: a network perspective. Homeopathy 91:89–94, 2002

Turin L: A spectroscopic mechanism for primary olfactory reception. Chem Senses 21:773–791, 1996

Ullman D: Homeopathic Family Medicine: Integrating the Science and Art of Natural Health Care. Berkeley, CA, Homeopathic Educational Services, 2002

Ullman R, Reichenberg-Ullman J: Rage Free Kids. Rocklin, CA, Prima Lifestyles, 1999

Unutzer J, Klap R, Sturm R: Mental disorders and the use of alternative medicine: results from a national survey. Am J Psychiatry 157:1851–1857, 2000

Vandenbroucke JP: Homeopathy trials: going nowhere. Lancet 350:824, 1997

Vandenbroucke JP, de Craen AJ: Alternative medicine: a "mirror image" for scientific reasoning in conventional medicine. Ann Intern Med 135:507–513, 2001

van Haselen R: The economic evaluation of complementary medicine: a staged approach at the Royal London Homeopathic Hospital. Br Homoeopath J 89 (suppl 1):S23–S26, 2000

Van Wassenhoven M, Ives G: An observational study of patients receiving homeopathic treatment. Homeopathy 93:3–11, 2004

Verhoef MJ, Lewith G, Ritenbaugh C, et al: Complementary and alternative medicine whole systems research: beyond identification of inadequacies of the RCT. Complement Ther Med 13:206–212, 2005

Vithoulkas G: The Science of Homeopathy. New York, Grove Weidenfeld, 1980

Walach H: What happens in homeopathic remedy provings? results from a double-blind crossover study of belladonna 30CH and an analysis by grade of membership (GoM), in Future Directions and Current Issues of Research in Homeopathy. Edited by Chez RA. Freiburg, Germany, Samueli Institute, 2002, pp 110–133

Walach H: Entanglement model of homeopathy as an example of generalised entanglement predicted by weak quantum theory. Forsch Komplementarmed Klass Naturheilkd 10:192–200, 2003

Walach H, Jonas WB: Homeopathy, in Clinical Research in Complementary Therapies. Edited by Lewith G, Jonas WB, Walach H. Edinburgh, Churchill Livingstone, 2002, pp 229–246

Walach H, Haeusler W, Lowes T, et al: Classical homeopathic treatment of chronic headaches. Cephalalgia 17:101, 119–126, 1997

Walach H, Lowes T, Mussbach D, et al: The long-term effects of homeopathic treatment of chronic headaches: 1-year follow-up. Cephalalgia 20:835–837, 2000

Walach H, Jonas WB, Ives J, et al: Research on homeopathy: state of the art. J Altern Complement Med 11:813–829, 2005

Waldo R, Torres JL: Mutual information and the homeopathic effect. Homeopathy 92:30–34, 2003

Weatherley-Jones E, Nicholl JP, Thomas KJ, et al: A randomised, controlled triple-blind trial of the efficacy of homeopathic treatment for chronic fatigue syndrome. J Psychosom Res 56:189–197, 2004

Weiser M, Strosser W, Klein P: Homeopathic vs. conventional treatment of vertigo: a randomized double-blind controlled clinical study. Arch Otolaryngol Head Neck Surg 124:879–885, 1998

Whitmont EC: Psyche and Substance: Essays on Homeopathy in Light of Jungian Psychology. Berkeley, CA, North Atlantic Books, 1991

Winston J: The Faces of Homeopathy: An Illustrated History of the First 200 Years. Tawa, New Zealand, Great Auk Publishing, 1999

Witt C, Keil T, Selim D, et al: Outcome and costs of homoeopathic and conventional treatment strategies: a comparative cohort study in patients with chronic disorders. Complement Ther Med 13:79–86, 2005a

Witt CM, Luedtke R, Baur R, et al: Homeopathic medical practice: long-term results of a cohort study with 3981 patients. BMC Public Health 5:115, 2005b

Yakir M, Kreitler S, Brzezinski A, et al: Effects of homeopathic treatment in women with premenstrual syndrome: a pilot study. Br Homoeopath J 90:148–153, 2001

10

Ayurvedic Treatments

Sudha Prathikanti, M.D.

Ayurveda (pronounced "ah´ yoor vay da") is the indigenous health and healing system of India. Most scholars regard Ayurveda as the oldest extant medical tradition in the world, with Ayurvedic remedies appearing in the *Rig Veda* than 6,000 years ago. The word *Ayurveda* is derived from two Sanskrit roots: *ayu,* meaning "life" or "living," and *veda,* meaning "knowledge." Thus, Ayurveda is the "knowledge of living" and is concerned with maximizing health, vitality, and longevity through wise lifestyle choices. Ayurveda offers treatment for thousands of ailments, but its primary emphasis is on preventing illness and optimizing health through careful attention to one's nutrition, activity, circadian rhythms, seasonal and environmental influences, psychological attitudes, and spiritual practices. Ayurveda is holistic in its orientation, defining life as an inseparable union of body, mind, and spirit; an effective physician is viewed as one who attends to this integral whole:

> Life is an inextricable joining of body, mind and spirit. The three—body, mind and spirit—are like a tripod: the world rests on their combination; in them all life abides. This is the subject matter of Ayurveda. (Charaka 1949, VI 1.42, VI 1.46–47)
>
> A physician who cannot enter the innermost soul of the patient with the bright lamp of his or her own knowledge cannot successfully treat any disease. The physician should first study all factors, including environmental factors, that influence a patient's illness and then prescribe treatment. (Charaka 1949, III 4.14)

HISTORY OF AYURVEDA

In the 1920s, archeological discovery of the vast Harappan cities of the Indus-Saraswati Valley established India as one of first cradles of civilization, contemporaneous with early Egypt and Mesopotamia (S. Gupta 1996; Possehl 1982;

Rao 1991). The indigenous culture of ancient India is called Vedic culture and is at least 6,000 years old, arising in the Harappan period or earlier (Danino and Sujata 1996; Feuerstein et al. 1995; Lal 1997; Rajaram and Frawley 1995; B. Singh 1995; Talageri 2000). It is remarkable that many Vedic traditions (e.g., Ayurveda, yoga) have been preserved in India through six millennia into the modern era.

Given its antiquity, Ayurveda influenced the medical systems of many early cultures outside the subcontinent of India. There is evidence of extensive sea travel from India to Mesopotamia as far back as 2500 B.C.E. (S. Gupta 1996; Rao 1991), with Indian sea traders bringing with them many precious commodities, including Ayurvedic herbs. During the first millennium B.C.E., India established diplomatic embassies in Egypt, Greece, and the Roman Empire (Harle 1992; Singhal 1969); core concepts from Vedic medicine, science, and mathematics played a key role in the technological advances of these civilizations (Filliozat 1970; Halbfass 1988; Ifrah 2000; Kak 1999, 2005b; Rawlinson 1975; Subbarayappa 1970). Ayurveda was taught at famous Indian universities such as Takshashila (founded circa 700 B.C.E.), where foreign students came from great distances to study alongside their Indian counterparts (Keay 2000; Mookerji 1947). During a brief military excursion into India in 326 B.C.E., Alexander the Great was much impressed by the Indian system of medicine and added several Ayurvedic physicians to his retinue (Jaggi 1981; Svoboda 1992). Starting in 300 B.C.E., Indian monks began to spread Buddhist teachings to China, Tibet, Japan, and Southeast Asia; these monks carried Ayurvedic texts, which had a profound and lasting effect on Chinese medicine and the healing traditions of many other Asian cultures (Jaggi 1981; Mookerji 1947; Svoboda and Lade 1995). In the ancient world, important Ayurvedic works were translated from Sanskrit into Greek, Latin, Persian, Arabic, Chinese, and Pali (Jee 1895/1993; Lele 1986).

After a golden age of science and art that lasted more than a millennium, India was beset by a series of foreign invasions beginning around 1200 C.E. Invaders destroyed many libraries and repositories of traditional Ayurvedic knowledge and enforced their own systems of medicine (Ghosh 2001; Svoboda and Lade 1995). Major Ayurvedic compendiums such as the *Charaka Samhita* and the *Sushruta Samhita* survived only because they had been memorized, transcribed, or translated so widely. More esoteric Ayurvedic texts were lost forever. During the British colonial occupation of India in the nineteenth and early twentieth centuries, the practice of Ayurveda suffered further; the British outlawed Ayurvedic education and shut down Ayurvedic schools in an effort to promulgate Western medicine (Vaidya et al. 2002). Even during this period of great suppression, Ayurveda continued to enrich the Western world when the millennia-old surgical procedures of the *Sushruta Samhita* were translated into European languages and formed the basis for the allopathic specialty of reconstructive plastic surgery (Hauben 1984; McDowell 1977; Rana and Arora 2002).

Despite serious historical setbacks, Ayurveda survives to this day in India because its essential teachings were transmitted via oral tradition from generation to generation of Ayurvedic healers. After winning independence from Britain in 1947, India began to revitalize the teaching of Ayurveda in major universities and colleges across the subcontinent (Jaggi 1981; Khor and Lin 2001). India's efforts have been encouraged and strengthened by the World Health Organization, which recognizes that indigenous medicine is the primary form of health care for most of the global population (World Health Organization 2002). In the United States and other Western countries, there recently has been burgeoning interest in the use of Ayurveda as a complementary and alternative medicine; this, too, has contributed to the renewal of Ayurvedic studies.

TRADITIONAL AYURVEDIC TRAINING

The training of Ayurvedic physicians in ancient times has been well recorded (Ghosh 2001; Jaggi 1981; Kak 2005a; Mookerji 1947). Students aspiring to learn Ayurveda were first required to complete 12 years of basic education in Sanskrit poetry and literature, mathematics, logic, grammar, and the Vedas. Next, admission to a center of Ayurvedic learning, such as Takshashila or Nalanda, had to be secured by passing a competitive entrance exam and obtaining the approval of an erudite selection committee that scrutinized the personal qualities of the candidate. Once admitted, students underwent a rigorous 7-year curriculum involving didactic and clinical components. Three major redactions of Ayurvedic knowledge were memorized and learned in their entirety: the *Charaka Samhita* (compiled circa 1000 B.C.E.), the *Sushruta Samhita* (compiled circa 1000 B.C.E.), and the *Ashtanga Hridayam* (compiled 500 C.E.). Students became proficient in eight branches of Ayurvedic medicine, learning the relevant anatomy, physiology, pathology, and therapeutics within each branch:

1. Internal medicine (*Kaya Chikitsa*)
2. Obstetrics and pediatrics (*Bala Chikitsa*)
3. Psychiatry (*Graha Chikitsa*)
4. Ophthalmology and otorhinolaryngology (*Shalakya Chikitsa*)
5. Surgery (*Shalya Chikitsa*)
6. Toxicology (*Agada Tantra*)
7. Longevity and rejuvenation (*Rasayana*)
8. Sexuality and fertility (*Vajikarana*)

Students of Ayurveda were taught a great reverence for nature and its healing substances. They mastered the preparation of hundreds of herbal and mineral medicines, in the process learning about horticulture, metallurgy, distillation, the manufacture of sugars, analysis and separation of minerals, chelation of metals, and the production of alkalis. They also became adept in many surgeries, including rhinoplasty, skin grafting, bone setting, cesarean section, and cataract removal. Surgical interventions were reserved for clinical scenarios in which other therapies were not beneficial. Special attention was given to the art of interacting with patients in a compassionate and skillful manner. At the end of the 7-year training period, students had to pass a set of rigorous examinations to receive official authorization to practice medicine. In a formal graduation ceremony, the new physicians pledged to uphold a strict code of ethical conduct and continue to enrich their knowledge base through a process of lifelong learning.

PRINCIPAL CONCEPTS OF AYURVEDA

Five Elements and Three Doshas

In the Ayurvedic worldview, all aspects of the universe, including human beings, are a manifestation of *pancha maha bhuta* or five great elements: space, air, fire, water, and earth. *Bhuta* is often translated from Sanskrit as "element," but in this context, an element is not a concrete substance; rather, each great element may be viewed as a creative energy with its own special attributes. For example, the creative element of space has the attribute of expansiveness; air, the attributes of lightness and mobility; fire, the attributes of heat and luminosity; water, the attribute of moistness; and earth, the attribute of solidity. The manifestation of these five great elements in countless permutations and combinations gives rise to the cosmos.

The grossest expression of the five great elements is in physical matter, including structures of the human body. For example, the element of space manifests as all body cavities and the interstices between cells. Air is present as all gaseous substances of the body, whereas fire manifests as stomach acid and digestive enzymes. Water predominates in blood, saliva, and sweat, and earth predominates in the solid structures of the bones and teeth.

The five great elements are also manifested in more subtle, dynamic forms called *doshas,* or bioenergetic principles. Each dosha is a combination of two great elements (Figure 10–1) and possesses the attributes of its component elements. There are three doshas in all: *Vata, Pitta,* and *Kapha.* All of the physiological functions and bioenergetic processes collectively called life—from respiration and metabolism to feeling and thinking—are governed by Vata, Pitta, and Kapha.

Each dosha has specific expression at the somatic and mental levels. Vata is a combination of space and air, manifesting as the bioenergetic principle of expansion and movement within any living organism. At the somatic level, the inhalation of the lungs, the beating of the heart, and the contraction of skeletal muscle are all manifestations of Vata. At the mental level, the anxious wandering of the mind and creative flights of fancy are also an expression of Vata's energy

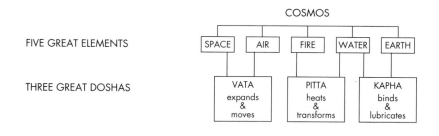

FIGURE 10–1.　The five great elements join in pairs to form the three great doshas.

of movement. Pitta is a combination of fire with a minute amount of water and manifests in living organisms as the bioenergetic principle of heating or transformation. At the somatic level, thermogenesis, digestion, and metabolism are all manifestations of Pitta. At the mental level, brightness of mind and flares of anger are also expressions of Pitta's fiery bioenergetic force. Kapha is formed from earth and water and is the bioenergetic principle of binding and lubricating. At the somatic level, Kapha governs the joining of cells to create muscle, fat, and body mass and controls the secretion of body fluids. At the mental level, the binding force of Kapha is expressed in emotional attachment and the power of memory. Thus, all living creatures embody the five great elements, not only in their physical structures but also in the doshas that govern somatopsychic functioning; the body and mind are simply gross versus subtle manifestations of the same five elements, obviating any duality.

Unique Constitution

All three doshas—Vata, Pitta, and Kapha—are necessary for life. However, at birth, each human being is endowed with a unique proportion of each dosha. This unique balance of Vata, Pitta, and Kapha is called the individual's *constitution*. The constitution influences somatopsychic functioning in specific ways, giving rise to individual strengths and vulnerabilities. In Figure 10–2, the three broad constitutional types (Vata-dominant, Pitta-dominant, and Kapha-dominant) are outlined to help illustrate the specific influence of each dosha on the body–mind complex.

It should be noted that discussion of a particular constitutional "type" is merely a heuristic device. In Ayurveda, no two individuals will have exactly the same constitution. Each person is a unique admixture of Vata, Pitta, and Kapha, possessing a tri-dosha constitution shared by no one else. The *Textbook of Ayurveda* (Lad 2002) discusses tri-dosha theory in much greater depth.

AYURVEDA: CONSTITUTIONAL TYPES

VATA	PITTA	KAPHA
AIR + SPACE	FIRE + WATER	WATER + EARTH
Lean, bony build	Medium build	Large, hefty build
Rapid walk & talk	Forceful walk & talk	Slow walk & talk
Erratic appetite & stamina	Strong appetite & stamina	Steady appetite & stamina
Sensitive to wind & cold	Sensitive to heat	Sensitive to fog & cold
Quick, flexible mind	Sharp, penetrating mind	Deliberate, steady mind
Learns quickly, forgets quickly	Learns intensely, retains well	Learns slowly, retains well
Enthusiastic, open to change	Strong-willed, likes to lead	Complacent, forgiving
Easily anxious, unsettled	Easily irritable, competitive	Easily depressed, clingy
Responds well to:	Responds well to:	Responds well to:
Regular, long sleep	Moderate sleep	Less sleep
Frequent meals: warm & rich	Regular meals: cool & sweet	Fewer meals: light & spicy
Warm, moist climate	Cool climate	Warm, dry climate

FIGURE 10–2. Three constitutional types, each with characteristic body–mind attributes.

Health and Illness

From an Ayurvedic perspective, one is healthy and has optimal somatopsychic functioning when all three doshas are "in balance"—that is, when the three doshas remain in the unique proportions characteristic of one's constitution. The three doshas in constitutional balance are said to confer enormous immunity, resilience, and recuperative energy. An individual who maintains tri-dosha balance has the intrinsic capacity to metabolize and heal from a great deal of physical and emotional stress. Throughout life, however, any number of factors—internal and external—can disturb one's tri-dosha balance. With a sustained imbalance of the three doshas, there is impaired capacity to meet biological and psychological challenges, and illness eventually ensues. Thus, health is a dynamic process that relies on each person's sustaining the doshas in the optimal proportions comprising his or her constitution. Health is sustained tri-dosha balance, whereas illness is sustained tri-dosha imbalance.

In Ayurveda, lifestyle has a profound effect on tri-dosha balance. As described earlier, every aspect of the universe is simply a combination or permutation of the five great elements. Thus, the foods eaten, music heard, colors seen, and mental and physical activities undertaken each contribute specific amounts of space, air, fire, water, and earth to one's body–mind complex. Poor choices in diet, activity, and environmental stimuli lead to a relative excess or deficit of specific elements, so that Vata, Pitta, and Kapha do not remain in constitutional balance. For example, eating spicier food than one can tolerate on a constitutional level leads to a relative excess of the fire element. Pitta subsequently becomes elevated and an illness of excess "heat," such as gastritis, may develop. The Ayurvedic model is keenly attuned to variations in individual constitutions; lifestyle choices that are harmful for one person might be tolerable or even beneficial to another. Therefore, very spicy foods may be perfectly healthy for one individual but may lead to gastritis in another. The key to health and well-being is to make lifestyle choices in harmony with one's unique tri-dosha constitution.

CLINICAL ASSESSMENT IN AYURVEDA

Tasks of the Physician

During a clinical evaluation, the Ayurvedic physician first ascertains the specific tri-dosha constitution (*prakriti*) of the patient and then identifies the presence and magnitude of any current dosha imbalance (*vikriti*). The goal of the physician is to restore or optimize the tri-dosha balance unique to each person, thereby helping to restore or optimize health and well-being. A person may consult an Ayurvedic physician not only to alleviate distress but also to clarify which lifestyle choices are the most health promoting for his or her unique constitution.

Ascertaining Constitution

To ascertain the specific tri-dosha constitution of a patient, the Ayurvedic physician begins with a detailed enquiry about the patient's somatopsychic functioning during good health, when the three doshas are understood to be in constitutional balance. The patient describes healthy baseline sleep and activity patterns, dietary preferences, bowel habits, climate tolerance, personality, cognitive style, and emotional strengths and vulnerabilities. Based on the patient's description, the physician determines the relative strength of Vata, Pitta, and Kapha in each domain of functioning. After the interview, the Ayurvedic physician conducts a classic eight-point physical examination of the patient, noting the pulse; condition of urine and stools; appearance of the tongue, eyes, and skin; quality of speech; and general appearance. Again, the relative strength of Vata, Pitta, and Kapha in the patient's constitution is determined through characteristic findings on examination. Throughout the interview and examination, the physician carefully checks with the patient as to whether any current body–mind attributes are significantly different from a healthy baseline. If so, body–mind attributes during good health are used to ascertain the patient's unique tri-dosha constitution.

Identifying Dosha Imbalance

If the patient reports a troubling new symptom or states that some aspect of current functioning has declined from a healthy baseline, this reflects a disturbance in tri-dosha balance. Based on the pattern of change in somatopsychic functioning, the Ayurvedic physician identifies which dosha or doshas are most perturbed at the time. For example, an individual who complains of anxiety, weight loss, and cold sensitivity suffers from Vata elevation, whereas an individual with irritability, dyspepsia, and hot flashes suffers from Pitta elevation. In the Ayurvedic model, individuals are most likely to develop symptoms that represent an elevation of their dominant dosha. If more than one dosha is disturbed, considerable skill may be required on the physician's part to interpret the ensuing pattern of symptoms.

Restoring Dosha Balance

The goal of Ayurvedic treatment is to restore tri-dosha balance, thereby restoring the individual's capacity for self-healing. Each therapeutic technique introduces the appropriate combination of the five great elements to rebalance Vata, Pitta, and Kapha in the suffering person. For example, if clinical assessment shows that Vata is elevated and Kapha is diminished, then therapeutic interventions must reduce air and space elements to pacify Vata but increase water and earth elements to strengthen Kapha.

Because every aspect of the universe is comprised of one or more of the five great elements, anything in the universe theoretically may serve as a treatment—when used in the right context. Thus, Ayurvedic treatment methods are broad-ranging and include dietary changes, herbal medicine, oil massage, aromatherapy, sound therapy, color therapy, yoga postures, breathing exercises, and meditation practices. A skilled Ayurvedic physician prescribes the specific foods, herbs, yoga postures, and other interventions that offer the correct balance of great elements to pacify an aggravated dosha or strengthen a depleted dosha. According to the *Charaka Samhita,* "there in nothing in this creation which cannot be used as medicine," as long as the physician understands its appropriate application. This Ayurvedic concept is illustrated in a story from the life of Jivaka, the personal physician to Buddha in the sixth century B.C.E.:

> Many are the stories of Jivaka's amazing cures, and his studentship at Takshashila was apparently no less amazing. After 7 full years of [Ayurvedic] studies there, his guru handed him a spade and sent him out for his final examination: to search within a radius of several miles for any plant bereft of all medicinal value. Jivaka passed his exam when he returned unable to find any such substance. (Svoboda 1992, p. 2)

AYURVEDIC PSYCHIATRY (GRAHA CHIKITSA)

Ayurveda views the mind (*manas*) as being created and sustained by the same five great elements as the body (*shareera*). However, in the mind, the generative potential of the great elements is not manifested as tangible body tissues but as subtle "structures" of consciousness, such as ego (*ahankara*), will (*ittcha*), and intellect (*buddhi*). Vata, Pitta, and Kapha, the bioenergetic principles derived from the great elements, govern not only different somatic functions but also different mental functions. Vata, the bioenergetic principle of movement and expansion, enables the mind to be mobile, perceptive, and expressive. Pitta, the bioenergetic principle of heating and transformation, allows the mind to properly "digest" sensory input and formulate correct responses. Kapha, the bioenergetic principle of binding and stabilizing, allows the mind to have equipoise and long-term memory. In concert, the three doshas create unique patterns of perceiving, thinking, feeling, remembering, and reacting that comprise an individual's personality and temperament.

When Vata, Pitta, and Kapha are in balance, harmony prevails at the psychological and physical levels. Sustained imbalance of any dosha tends to precipitate illness, which may be classified broadly as follows: 1) illness with predominance of somatic disturbance, 2) illness with predominance of psychological disturbance, or 3) illness with significant somatic and psychological disturbance. The tendencies toward a specific dosha imbalance and toward developing illness with significant psychological features are both influenced by the person's unique constitution as well as his or her lifestyle and environment.

In ancient Ayurvedic nosology, insanity (*unmada*) is classified as an illness with significant somatic and psychological disturbance. According to the *Charaka Samhita,* unmada is characterized by abnormalities in behavior, speech, cognition, affect, and body habitus:

> [A person with unmada] shows confusion of the intellect, extreme fickleness of mind, agitation of the eyes, unsteadiness, incoherence of speech, mental vacuity...and is unable to know pleasure from pain, and right behavior or duty. Deprived of memory, understanding or his wits, he keeps his mind wavering restlessly...and [may be] wasted in his body. (*Charaka Samhita,* quoted in Haldipur 1984, p. 336)

Moreover, the nature of psychological and somatic symptoms associated with unmada varies according to whether the afflicted individual is of Vata, Pitta, or Kapha predominance:

> [A Vata-type unmada is marked by] laughing, smiling, dancing, singing, speaking, bodily movements and weeping—all of which are out of place—and leanness of the body and reddish complexion. [A Pitta-type unmada is marked by] impatience, fury, nudity, wrathful abuse of others, running away, heat of body, rage, desire for cool food and drink, and a yellow complexion. [A Kapha-type unmada is marked by] excessive sleep, silence, little disposition for movement, dribbling of saliva or nasal discharge, disinclination for food, love of solitude, and pallor. (*Charaka Samhita,* quoted in Haldipur 1984, p. 337)

In general, Vata imbalance with extreme psychological disturbance may result in paranoia, hallucinations, or manic features. Pitta imbalance with extreme psychological disturbance tends to be associated with aggression, violence, or antisocial behavior. Finally, Kapha imbalance with extreme psychological disturbance involves apathy, abulia, social withdrawal, or mutism.

From the various ancient descriptions of unmada, it seems this Ayurvedic diagnosis may have encompassed a wide range of modern psychotic presentations, including bipolar mania, schizophrenia, depression with psychosis, or delirium with psychosis. A one-to-one correspondence between Ayurvedic and DSM-IV-TR (American Psychiatric Association 2000) diagnoses is unlikely. Still, in perusing the ancient texts, there is a clear concordance between many Ayurvedic syndromes and modern categories of psychiatric illness. For example, Ayurvedic signs and symptoms for *cittavasada* (depression), *cittodvega* (anxiety disorder), *atattvabhinivesa* (obsession), *apatantraka* (hysteria/conversion disorder), *gagodvega* (hypochondriasis), and *madatyaya* (alcoholism) quickly strike chords of recognition in the modern physician. According to the *Charaka Samhita,* all of these disorders involve varying dysfunction of eight essential aspects of mind: emotion, reasoning, orientation, learning/memory, attachment, habit, psychomotor function, and behavior.

Neurological disorders such as delirium, epilepsy, neurasthenia, Parkinson's disease, vertigo, coma, and mental retardation are also considered part of Graha Chikitsa. As early as thousands of years ago, Ayurvedic physicians seemed to appreciate the fundamental connection between neurology and psychiatry and the fallacy of separating "organic" from "functional" disorders. Ayurveda recognizes that for some neuropsychiatric conditions, dosha disturbance may begin at the mental level but become manifest more at the somatic level (conversion disorder); at other times, dosha disturbance may begin at the somatic level but become manifest more at the mental level, altering consciousness (neurological disorders). However, for the Ayurvedic physician, the diagnostic focus is not on deciding whether the patient's condition is somatically based or "all in the head"; rather, the focus is on identifying which dosha or set of doshas is disturbed in the patient as evidenced by the overall pattern of somatic and psychological symptoms. Treatment then involves correcting the specific dosha imbalance through appropriate physical, psychological, and spiritual remedies. According to the *Charaka Samhita,* "The number of diseases is uncountable, but the number of doshas is definitely three" (Charaka 1949, III 6.5). Thus, Charaka contended that an astute Ayurvedic physician should feel no reluctance in treating a novel disorder previously undescribed in medical texts; each symptom of the disorder can ultimately be identified and treated in terms of a specific dosha imbalance. (For a more in-depth discussion of psychopathology and its treatment within Ayurveda, readers are referred to S.P. Gupta [1977].)

Ayurvedic treatment of any illness, including neuropsychiatric illness, is encapsulated in Charaka's famous adage: "purify, pacify, and remove the cause of disease" (Charaka 1949, I 1.3). The first therapeutic step is to purify the body–mind complex through cleansing procedures (*panchakarma*) intended to remove gross and subtle toxins that accumulate with dosha imbalance; the longer the dosha imbalance has been in place, the more rigorous should be the purification process. Next, pacification of dosha imbalance is undertaken: this may involve nutritional therapy, yoga postures, herbal medicine, and a number of lifestyle changes designed to soothe an aggravated dosha and strengthen a depleted dosha. Finally, the cause of illness is removed. In Ayurveda, illness may be caused by external factors such as pathogens, trauma, and poor lifestyle choices, as well as by internal factors such as maladaptive cognitions and affects; these etiological factors must be removed whenever possible to prevent a recurrence of illness. However, an even deeper etiological factor must also be addressed: In Ayurveda, the ultimate source of all illness and suffering is one's fundamental alienation from the cosmic consciousness (*Atman*) that is said to underlie the entirety of the manifest universe. Thus, psychospiritual intervention through a variety of meditative and metaphysical practices is considered to be an integral aspect of the Ayurvedic physician's healing art (Frawley 1997).

Psychospiritual practices are said to strengthen qualities of *sattva* within the mind while attenuating qualities of *rajas* and *tamas*. In brief, *sattva* is the primal force of goodness, compassion, luminous understanding, and peace; the more one develops sattvic qualities, the more easily one may remove the ultimate source of suffering. *Rajas* is the primal force of passion, dynamism, and turbulence; rajasic qualities of mind facilitate worldly accomplishments, egotistical pursuits, and the quest for power and pleasure. *Tamas* is the primal force of dullness, inertia, and ignorance; tamasic qualities of mind lead to stagnation, insensitivity, disintegration, and decay. Sattva brings one closer to the direct apprehension of cosmic consciousness, whereas rajas and tamas exacerbate one's (mis)-perception of separation from cosmic consciousness.

RESEARCH ISSUES IN AYURVEDA

Challenges in Conducting Ayurvedic Research

Modern researchers confront several perplexing issues when evaluating Ayurvedic therapies through the scientific standard of the randomized, double-blind, placebo-controlled clinical trial. First, the concept of randomly assigning the same treatment to all members of a given study group is entirely counter to traditional Ayurvedic practice. Ayurveda emphasizes the unique constitution of each person and therefore insists on a highly individualized treatment regimen for each patient. Second, double-blind placebo or sham interventions may be impossible to construct for many behavioral therapies in Ayurveda, such as those involving massage, yoga, or cleansing procedures such as enemas. Third, most scientific trials attempt to isolate the effects of one specific intervention on the final clinical outcome. However, it is rare in Ayurveda to use only one remedy in treating a patient's illness. It is more common for a variety of treatments to be used in concert to restore tri-dosha balance; these treatments are believed to act synergistically at multiple levels—somatic, psychological, and spiritual—to pacify an aggravated dosha or strengthen a depleted dosha.

Source and Quality of Ayurvedic Research

In India, the government's Central Council for Research in Ayurveda and Siddha is comprised of 30 regional institutes across the country; collectively, these institutes have produced much of the scientific database on Ayurvedic therapies over the past 50 years. Premier Indian academic centers such as the All India Institute of Medical Sciences have also been important sources of Ayurveda research. In the United States and other Western countries, Ayurvedic treatment modalities have been studied at major universities with increasing frequency over the past three decades. The Maharishi International University and its affiliates have produced many high-quality clinical trials related to Ayurvedic therapies; however, some scholars contend that because the Maharishi organizations may derive financial benefit from research promoting Maharishi Ayurvedic therapies, findings from their research should be interpreted with caution until replicated by independent trials.

Most Ayurvedic studies from India are inaccessible for review outside the subcontinent, as they may be absent from international medical databases, unavailable online, or written in a regional Indian language. Among accessible English-language studies of Ayurvedic therapies from all countries, significant methodological shortcomings exist. Randomized, controlled trials are few in number, especially when nonherbal therapies are being investigated. Studies often have an extremely small number of subjects and thereby lack the power to detect even a large effect size or make meaningful generalizations about the efficacy of a particular therapy in a larger population. Studies of nonherbal Ayurvedic therapies may include significant co-interventions, making it difficult to conclude that beneficial outcomes are attributable to a specific Ayurvedic therapy alone. Despite these limitations, Bodeker (2001) observed that the pool of results from preliminary Ayurvedic research "is consistent with the clinical expectations of Ayurvedic practitioners and constitutes a first round of data that can provide the basis for more rigorous clinical trials" (p. 390).

RESEARCH ON AYURVEDIC HERBAL THERAPIES

The Ayurvedic pharmacopoeia contains several thousand medicinal plants that may be used singly or in complex multiherb formulas. Among Ayurvedic therapies, herbs have the largest evidence base because they are the most easily studied intervention using conventional research protocols. Highly purified subcomponents of herbs (the hypothesized active ingredients) are typically used in studies, even though the whole plant extract may be used in traditional Ayurvedic therapy. The study of isolated portions of the herb may not always yield accurate data about the efficacy and safety of the herb's use in a traditional context.

Ayurvedic Herbs for Psychiatric Conditions

In classical Ayurveda texts, two groups of herbs—the *medhya* and the *vajikarana* herbs—comprise the most common botanical remedies for neuropsychiatric ailments. According to tradition, medhya herbs provide special nourishment to neuronal tissue and are thus used to enhance memory, cognition, and the ability to cope with psychological disturbance. Medhya herbs include *brahmi* (*Bacopa monnieri*), *mandukaparni* (*Centella asiatica*), *shankapushpi* (*Convolvulus pluricaulis*), *ashwagandha* (*Withania somnifera*), *sarpagandha* (*Rauwolfia serpentina*), *jatamansi* (*Nardostachys jatamansi*), and *vacha* (*Acorus calamus*). The vajikarana herbs are said to enhance libido, vigor, and zest for life; these herbs are traditionally used as aphrodisiacs and antidepressants. The vajikarana herb most commonly used in psychiatric conditions is *kapikacchu* (*Mucuna pruriens*). Although medhya and vajikarana herbs may be used singly, they are more often administered in poly-herb formulas called *rasayanas*. Rasayanas may consist of only a few herbs or may include complex combinations of several hundred herbs and minerals.

Table 10–1 lists psychiatric indications for some Ayurvedic herbs, along with the supporting scientific evidence for their use. Because many Ayurvedic studies from India could not be accessed for this review, the rating of evidence in these tables may not reflect the complete database. Among the herbs listed, *unmada gaja kesari, smriti sagar rasa,* and *yogabalacurna* are traditional medhya rasayanas; *Brahmyadiyoga* is a modified rasayana containing *Centella, Rauwolfia,* and *Acorus* among its herbal ingredients. Included in Table 10–1 are a few proprietary poly-herbal formulas. Geriforte is comprised largely of *chyavanprash,* a traditional Ayurvedic rasayana containing many medhya herbs. Similarly, Mentat, Memorin, and the Maharishi Amrit Kalash all contain medhya herbs as primary ingredients, with *Bacopa monnieri* being the predominant ingredient in Mentat.

Depressive Disorders

To date, Indian case reports, open trials, and a few placebo-controlled, single-blind trials suggest that Ayurvedic herbs may have a role in the treatment of depressive disorders. Nearly all these trials described subjects as having "depressive neurosis" or "mild-to-moderate depressive illness" according to ICD-9 diagnostic criteria (World Health Organization 1975); these subjects most likely would meet DSM-IV-TR criteria for dysthymia rather than major depressive disorder. Limitations to the clinical investigations examined in this review included small sample sizes, incomplete descriptions of eligibility criteria, and inadequate mention of instruments for measuring clinical improvement; among studies that used a placebo control, it was often unclear whether or how subjects were randomized into the different intervention groups.

With these caveats in mind, *Withania somnifera, Mucuna pruriens, Acorus calamus, Convolvulus pluricaulis,* and *Celastrus panniculatus* all have shown positive re-

TABLE 10–1. Ayurvedic herbs with potential benefit in the treatment of psychiatric conditions

Psychiatric indication	Herbs and polyherb formulas	Supporting evidence	Evidence rating	Comments
Depressive disorders	*Withania somnifera, Mucuna pruriens*	R.K. Tripathi and Singh 1983; Koirala 1992	3	Herbs used together for depressive neurosis
	Convolvulus pluricaulis	Kushwaha and Sharma 1992	3	Depressive neurosis
	Yogabalacurna[a]	S.K. Gupta and Singh 2002	3	Depressive disorder
	Geriforte[a]	Damle and Gore 1982; De Sousa et al. 1989; Malhotra 1986	3	Most promising in dysthymia
	Mentat[a]	K.P. Sharma et al. 1993	3	Depressive neurosis
Bipolar disorder	*Rauwolfia serpentina*	Bacher and Lewis 1979; Berlant 1986	3	May be useful in refractory mania
Schizophrenia and psychosis	*Rauwolfia serpentina*[b]	Christison et al. 1991[c]; Kline 1954; Lopez–Munoz 2004; Sen 1931	1	Used in schizophrenia; crude plant extract has few side effects compared with reserpine

TABLE 10–1. Ayurvedic herbs with potential benefit in the treatment of psychiatric conditions *(continued)*

Psychiatric indication	Herbs and polyherb formulas	Supporting evidence	Evidence rating	Comments
Schizophrenia and psychosis *(continued)*	Brahmyadiyoga[a,b]	Mahal et al. 1976[c]; Ramu 1983; Ramu et al. 1999[c]	2	Used in schizophrenia; crude *Rauwolfia* extract plus five other herbs
	Smriti sagar rasa[a]	J.S. Tripathi and Singh 1994	3	Residual schizophrenia
	Unmada gaja kesari[a]	Choudhuri 2001	3	Residual schizophrenia
	Menat[a]	Das and De Sousa 1989	3	Negative symptoms of schizophrenia
Anxiety disorders	*Bacopa monnieri*[b]	R. H. Singh and Singh 1980	3	Anxiety neurosis
		Stough et al. 2001[c]	3	Healthy subjects
	Centella asiatica[b]	R. H. Singh et al. 1981	3	Anxiety neurosis
		Kaushik and Singh 1982	3	Used with *Convolvulus*
		Bradwejn et al. 2000[c]	3	Healthy subjects
	Convolvulus pluricaulis	Kaushik and Singh 1982; R. H. Singh and Mehta 1977	3	Used with *Centella*
	Withania somnifera	Malviya 1976	3	Anxiety neurosis

TABLE 10–1. Ayurvedic herbs with potential benefit in the treatment of psychiatric conditions *(continued)*

Psychiatric indication	Herbs and polyherb formulas	Supporting evidence	Evidence rating	Comments
Anxiety disorders *(continued)*	Geriforte[a,b]	Boral et al. 1989; Chakraborty 1983	2	Anxiety neurosis
		Shah et al. 1990	2	Generalized anxiety
		Shah et al. 1993[c]	2	Anxiety/depression
	Mentat[a,b]	Agrawal et al. 1991[c]	3	Healthy subjects
Cognitive dysfunction (diverse etiology)	Bacopa monnieri[b]	Agrawal et al. 1993	3	Mental retardation
		Negi et al. 2000[c]; Srivastava et al. 2002[c]	2	Attention–deficit/ hyperactivity disorder
		H. Singh et al. 2004[c]; Srivastava et al. 2003[c]	2	Age-associated memory impairment
	Centella asiatica[b]	Appa Rao et al. 1973, 1977[c]	2	Mental retardation
	Mentat[a,b]	D'Souza and Chavda 1991[c]; Kalra et al. 2002[c]; R.B. Patel and Pereira 1991[c]	1	Attention–deficit/ hyperactivity disorder

TABLE 10–1. Ayurvedic herbs with potential benefit in the treatment of psychiatric conditions *(continued)*

Psychiatric indication	Herbs and polyherb formulas	Supporting evidence	Evidence rating	Comments
Cognitive dysfunction (diverse etiology) *(continued)*		Dave et al. 1993[c]; Dixit et al. 1992; Trivedi 1999	2	Mental retardation
		Upadhyay et al. 2002[c]	3	Learning disability
	Memorin[a,b]	Andrade et al. 1998[c]	3	Age-associated memory impairment
Cognitive enhancement	*Bacopa monnieri*[b]	Abhang 1993[c]; R. Sharma et al. 1987	2	Healthy children
		Roodenrys et al. 2002[c]; Stough et al. 2001[c]	2	Healthy adults
	Centella asiatica[b]	Kuppurajan et al. 1978[c]	3	Healthy children
	Withania somnifera[b]	Karnick 1991[c]	3	Healthy adults
	Six-herb formula[a,b]	Kaur et al. 1998[c]	3	Healthy children
	Maharishi Amrit Kalash[a,b]	Gelderloos et al. 1990[c]	3	Healthy elderly individuals
	Mentat[a,b]	Koti 1991[c]	2	Healthy children
		Agrawal et al. 1991[c]	2	Healthy adults

TABLE 10–1. Ayurvedic herbs with potential benefit in the treatment of psychiatric conditions *(continued)*

Psychiatric indication	Herbs and polyherb formulas	Supporting evidence	Evidence rating	Comments
Substance abuse	Geriforte[a]	R. H. Singh and Sinha 1979	3	Healthy elderly individuals
	Mentat[a]	Trivedi 1999	3	Alcoholism
Insomnia	*Valeriana jatamansi*[b]	Donath et al. 2000[c]; Leathwood and Chauffard 1985[c]; Leathwood et al. 1982[c]; Trevena 2004[c]; Ziegler et al. 2002[c]	1	Used a *Valerian* species closely related to *Valeriana jatamansi*
	Nardostachys jatamansi, Rauwolfia serpentina, Tinospora cordifolia	Rani and Naidu 1998	3	All three herbs used in combination

[a]Polyherb formulas, listed by traditional Sanskrit names or proprietary names, as appropriate.
[b]Herbs tested in randomized controlled trials.
[c]Randomized controlled trials.

sults in preliminary clinical trials with depressed subjects (S.K. Gupta and Singh 2002; Koirala 1992; Kushwaha and Sharma 1992; R.K. Tripathi and Singh 1983). Mentat and Geriforte, two proprietary mixtures of indigenous *medhya* herbs, have also demonstrated some antidepressant efficacy (Damle and Gore 1982; De Sousa et al. 1989; Malhotra 1986; K.P. Sharma et al. 1993). Generally, Ayurvedic herbs for depression are used in dyads, triads, or polyherb formulas rather than singly. For example, in one open study of 50 subjects with "depressive neurosis," *Withania* was given in the morning and *Mucuna* was given at bedtime; after 8 weeks, the investigators reported significant reductions in depressive symptoms as measured by the Hamilton Rating Scale for Depression (R.K. Tripathi and Singh 1983). However, at least one single-blind, placebo-controlled study of 20 subjects reported the efficacy of *Convolvulus* as an isolated herbal remedy for "mild-to-moderate depressive illness" (Kushwaha and Sharma 1992). In trying to gauge which depressed subjects may be best suited for treatment with Ayurvedic herbs, a single-blind, placebo-controlled trial compared the antidepressant effect of a polyherb formula in 134 subjects with different ICD-9 subtypes of depression; the investigators concluded that the herbal formula was significantly better than placebo in treating depressive disorders of "neurotic origin" (dysthymia) but not in treating more severe depressive disorders (Malhotra 1986). None of the clinical trials noted significant side effects for the herbal remedy being studied. Koirala (1992) did note that there were some data to suggest that serotonin autoreceptors may be sensitized with *Withania* and *Convolvulus*.

Bipolar Disorder

Case reports and series have suggested that reserpine, an alkaloid derivative of *Rauwolfia serpentina,* may represent an underutilized therapy in the management of bipolar disorder, particularly in manic episodes refractory to lithium and typical antipsychotics (Berlant 1986; Telner et al. 1986). Lithium plus reserpine may allow bipolar patients to achieve better clinical functioning than lithium plus conventional antipsychotics, and adjunctive reserpine therapy may allow patients to decrease their use of lithium (Bacher and Lewis 1979). These reports are consistent with the indigenous use of *Rauwolfia* to manage Vata-type unmada, which closely resembles current-day descriptions of mania.

Schizophrenia and Psychosis

For millennia, the root of *Rauwolfia serpentina* has had many medicinal uses in Ayurveda, including the calming of psychotically disturbed individuals. Indeed, in northern India, *Rauwolfia* is sometimes called *pagal-ki-dawa,* or "insane people's medicine." In 1931, Gananath Sen and Kartick Chandra Bose published the first scientific description of *Rauwolfia* as a potent antipsychotic tranquilizer (Sen and Bose 1931). They reported in *Indian Medicine World* that doses of 20 to 30 grains of [*Rauwolfia*] powder twice daily produce not only a hypnotic effect but also a reduction of blood pressure and violent symptoms. Within a week usually the patient's senses are restored, though he may [still] show some mental aberrations. Usually the treatment has to be continued for 4 to 6 weeks (sometimes more), the doses being reduced gradually. (Sen and Bose, as quoted in S.P.K. Gupta 2002, p. 2)

After a *New York Times* article in 1953 reported on the herbal treatment of mental illness in India, Nathan Kline investigated the psychotropic effects of *Rauwolfia* in a series of New York patients, publishing the first Western account of *Rauwolfia*'s antipsychotic efficacy (Kline 1954). Subsequently, clinical studies by a number of European and American researchers firmly established reserpine, an alkaloid extract of *Rauwolfia*, as one of the first pharmacological remedies for the allopathic diagnosis of schizophrenia (Lopez-Munoz et al. 2004).

Beyond its clinical use as an antipsychotic medicine, reserpine played another revolutionary role in psychiatry: observations of reserpine's tendency to cause depression, coupled with its measurable depletion of brain norepinephrine and serotonin, ushered in the "monoamine hypothesis" of depression, providing the first crucial links between the psychobiology of mental illness and potential pharmacotherapies. Reserpine was later supplanted by newer antipsychotic medicines, in part because of a side-effect profile that seemed to include extrapyramidal symptoms, nightmares, and depression. Yet 40 years after its "discovery" in the West, reserpine continued to be acknowledged as an important treatment option for schizophrenic patients unresponsive to other antipsychotics (Christison et al. 1991).

Several early papers in the Western psychiatric literature reported that the total alkaloid preparation of *Rauwolfia* appeared to be free of the side effects seen with the isolated reserpine alkaloid (Colabawalla 1958; Torsegno and Zucchi 1955). These reports were consistent with the benign side-effect profile of traditional Ayurvedic medicines using the crude plant extract of *Rauwolfia*. Therefore, Indian researchers decided to design a polyherb formula for schizophrenia that was modeled after traditional rasayanas containing crude plant extracts of *Rauwolfia*. The result was Brahmyadiyoga, a preparation of six Ayurvedic herbs that includes crude plant extracts of *Rauwolfia serpentina, Centella asiatica, Acorus calamus, Saussurea lappa, Valeriana wallichii,* and *Nardostachys jatamansi*. In true Ayurvedic tradition, investigators stated that the polyherb formula was intended to offer multiple neuropsychiatric benefits, including anticonvulsant, sedative-hypnotic, nootropic, and antipsychotic effects.

The antipsychotic effects of Brahmyadiyoga were subsequently demonstrated in a small open trial with 14 subjects with chronic schizophrenia (Ramu et al. 1983) and in two larger double-blind, placebo-controlled studies (Mahal et al. 1976; Ramu et al. 1999). In the study by Mahal et al. (1976), 136 subjects with acute exacerbation of schizophrenia were randomized to one of four intervention groups: Brahmyadiyoga, chlorpromazine, *Valeriana wallichii,* or placebo. At the end of 2 months, treatment effectiveness was measured using the Brief Psychiatric Rating Scale; the Brahmyadiyoga and chlorpromazine groups both showed significantly more clinical improvement than the *Valeriana* or placebo groups. The improvement shown by the Brahmyadiyoga group appeared comparable with that of the chlorpromazine group, but the former subjects had virtually no side effects. In the study by Ramu et al. (1999), 78 subjects with chronic schizophrenia were randomized to one of three intervention groups: Brahmyadiyoga, chlorpromazine, or placebo. Clinical outcomes were measured by scores on the Brief Psychiatric Rating Scale and the Fergus Falls Behavior Rating Scale. Both the chlorpromazine and Brahmyadiyoga groups showed significant clinical improvement over placebo, with the chlorpromazine group also showing a small but statistically significant improvement over the Brahmyadiyoga group. Subjects in the Brahmyadiyoga group had virtually no side effects compared with those in the chlorpromazine group. Based on these two well-designed studies, Brahmyadiyoga clearly has significant antipsychotic activity and is extremely well tolerated; it may be slightly less effective than a typical antipsychotic in treating schizophrenia. Ramu et al. (1999) suggest that Brahmyadiyoga may serve as an adjuvant to modern antipsychotics; blood pressure and liver function should be periodically assessed as a precaution.

The marked difference in the side-effect profiles of reserpine and the crude *Rauwolfia* extract in Brahmyadiyoga was evaluated through receptor-binding studies (Cott and Misra 1999). In contrast to reserpine, the crude *Rauwolfia* extract revealed a surprising affinity for GABAergic (γ-aminobutyric acid) and α_2-adrenergic receptors in addition to dopaminergic receptors. Previous studies have suggested that augmentation of typical antipsychotics with agents having GABAergic and α_2-adrenergic activity may improve clinical outcomes in schizophrenia (Frederiksen 1975; Litman et al. 1993). Thus, the antipsychotic efficacy and benign side-effect profile of crude *Rauwolfia* may be related to a biological mechanism of action very different from that of the isolated reserpine alkaloid.

In open trials, other Ayurvedic polyherb formulas have shown promise in the treatment of schizophrenia. *Smriti sagar rasa* and *unmada gaja kesari* are two complex polyherb-mineral rasayanas with reported efficacy in improving the negative symptoms of residual-phase schizophrenia (Choudhuri 2001; J.S. Tripathi and Singh 1994). Another Ayurvedic formula containing several medhya herbs such as *Acorus, Withania,* and *Bacopa* appeared to be effective and well tolerated in 10 subjects with psychosis (Dash et al. 1983). Mentat, a proprietary polyherb formula with *Bacopa* as its primary ingredient, improved negative symptoms in 20 subjects with chronic undifferentiated schizophrenia who underwent 8 weeks of treatment (Das and De Sousa 1989).

Anxiety Disorders

Nearly all the Indian clinical studies mentioned in this section involved subjects diagnosed with ICD-9 "anxiety neurosis." These subjects most likely would be diagnosed with anxiety disorder not otherwise specified under current DSM-IV-TR diagnostic criteria. Most of the studies had relatively small sample sizes. Studies conducted before 1990 tended to use psychometric instruments unfamiliar to Western researchers, whereas studies conducted after 1990 adopted standard Western instruments such as the Hamilton Anxiety Scale.

The medhya herb *Bacopa monnieri* has a long history of traditional use in many neuropsychiatric ailments, including anxiety. In an early open clinical trial (R.H. Singh and Singh 1980), subjects with anxiety neurosis showed marked reduction in anxiety after 2–4 weeks of treatment with *Bacopa*. More than two decades later, Australian researchers conducted a randomized, double-blind, placebo-controlled trial of *Bacopa* in healthy volunteers (Stough et al. 2001). The researchers reported that 12 weeks of *Bacopa* administration resulted in significantly reduced anxiety.

Other medhya herbs have been studied for their efficacy in treating anxiety. Open trials support the use of *Centella asiatica* in the treatment of anxiety neurosis (Kaushik and Singh 1982; R.H. Singh et al. 1981). In a recent double-blind, placebo-controlled study with healthy subjects, *Centella* was found to significantly reduce acoustic startle response measured 30 and 60 minutes after administration of a one-time dose (Bradwejn et al. 2000); because a hyperstartle response is characteristic of many patients with anxiety disorders, this study invited further investigation of *Centella* as an anxiolytic agent. Open trials also indicate that monoherb therapy with *Withania somnifera* or *Convolvulus pluricaulis* may be effective in reducing symptoms of anxiety neurosis (Malviya 1976; R.H. Singh and Mehta 1977). Open trial data (Boral et al. 1989; Chakraborty 1983; Shah et al. 1990) support the potential anxiolytic and adaptogenic effects of Geriforte, a proprietary polyherb formula whose main ingredient is *chyavanprash,* a traditional rasayana of multiple medhya herbs. In one double-blind, placebo-controlled study of Geriforte (Shah et al. 1993), 40 subjects meeting ICD-10 (World Health Organization 1992) criteria for mixed anxiety-depressive disorder were randomized to receive Geriforte or placebo tablets for 4 weeks; Geriforte was significantly better than placebo in improving anxiety, but not depressive, symptoms. No significant side effects with Ayurvedic herbs were observed in any of these studies.

Cognitive Dysfunction

The results of numerous clinical trials support the traditional use of medhya herbs to improve cognitive function in people with diverse sources of cognitive disability. Individuals with mental retardation, children with attention-deficit/hyperactivity disorder (ADHD) and adults with age-associated memory impairment (AAMI) or age-related cognitive decline are among the most studied populations. Just among these three populations, at least 11 randomized, double-blind, placebo-controlled trials have examined the cognitive effects of Ayurvedic herbs.

Individuals with mental retardation may experience cognitive improvement with *Centella asiatica, Bacopa monnieri,* or Mentat. In a double-blind, placebo-controlled study involving 30 children with mental retardation, subjects receiving *Centella* for 12 weeks showed a significant increase in the Binet-Kamat Scale of Intelligence and outperformed control subjects on measures of cooperation, concentration, attention, and overall adjustment (Appa Rao et al. 1973); furthermore, the positive findings persisted at 6 months (Appa Rao et al. 1977). In a single-blind, placebo-controlled study involving 286 adults with mild, moderate, and severe mental retardation, subjects with mild-to-moderate mental retardation who received *Bacopa* daily for 1 year showed significant improvement in concentration, memory span, and overall cognitive ability (Agrawal et al. 1993); subjects with severe mental retardation showed no improvement with *Bacopa* or placebo. Mentat improved cognitive performance and behavioral abnormalities in children with mild-to-moderate mental retardation, as shown in a 6-month open trial with 30 subjects (Trivedi 1999); a 1-year single-blind, placebo-controlled trial with 60 subjects (Dixit et al. 1992); and a 12-week double-blind, placebo-controlled trial with 20 subjects (Dave et al. 1993).

Children with ADHD may obtain significant cognitive benefits from *Bacopa monnieri* and Mentat. In a randomized, double-blind, placebo-controlled study of 36 school-age children meeting DSM-IV (American Psychiatric Association 1994) criteria for ADHD, subjects receiving *Bacopa monniera* for 12 weeks outperformed controls on 3 of 10 cognitive tests: sentence repetition, logical memory, and paired associate learning (Negi et al. 2000). These results were replicated in a second study of identical design but with a larger subject population of 86 children (Srivastava et al. 2002). The efficacy of Mentat in treating ADHD has been demonstrated in three randomized double-blind, placebo-controlled clinical trials (D'Souza and Chavda 1991; Kalra et al. 2002; R. B. Patel and Pereira 1991). In the study by Kalra et al. (2002), 60 children meeting DSM-IV criteria for ADHD were randomized equally to receive daily Mentat or daily placebo; at the end of 6 months, subjects receiving Mentat showed significant improvement of ADHD symptoms as measured by the Conners Parent and Teacher Rating Scales.

Finally, there is growing evidence that older adults with mild cognitive dysfunction may obtain benefits from *Bacopa monnieri* and Memorin. Using the AAMI criteria promulgated by the National Institutes of Health, a double-blind, placebo-controlled study was conducted (Srivastava et al. 2003) in which 30 subjects with AAMI were randomized to receive *Bacopa* or placebo for 12 weeks; the *Bacopa* group showed significant improvement on four of six cognitive tests from the Weschler Memory Scale: mental control, logical memory, digit span forward, and paired associate learning. A nearly identical pattern of cognitive improvement was obtained in another 12-week randomized, double-blind, placebo-controlled study of *Bacopa* in subjects with AAMI (H. Singh et al. 2004). Memorin may also improve cognitive dysfunction in older adults, as shown in a randomized, double-blind, placebo-controlled trial involving 45 men and women meeting DSM-IV criteria for age-related cognitive decline (Andrade et al. 1998); at the end of 3 months, men and women in the Memorin group significantly outperformed the placebo group on most neuropsychological measures of cognition. However, only men in the Memorin group showed significant improvement over the placebo group on tests specifically assessing memory; the age of the subjects did not account for this sex difference.

Cognitive Enhancement

Medhya herbs have been traditionally used in Ayurveda not only to ameliorate cognitive decline or disability but also to preserve and enhance healthy cognitive function. Results from at least eight randomized, double-blind, placebo-controlled trials lend some support to the traditional use of medhya herbs as cognitive enhancers. There is an important methodological issue to confront when evaluating these positive clinical trials: Are the positive findings "real" or simply attributable to chance? When healthy subjects are used in a clinical trial of a putative cognitive enhancer, outcome measures for detecting cognitive improvement may not be as obvious as with subjects who have a specific disorder (e.g., ADHD). Therefore, researchers may administer a wide array of tests before and after the intervention to capture the impact of the intervention on the maximum number of cognitive parameters. However, they must also make an educated guess before the trial takes place about the cognitive improvements they expect to see. This is important because the more cognitive parameters they test, the more likely it is that chance alone will lead to a positive (but coincidental) association between the intervention and one of the tested parameters. However, if multiple positive findings emerge, it is less likely that the results are due to chance. If only one or two positive findings emerge or if the findings are not what the researchers predicted based on previous data, then the results must be replicated by other studies before they can be considered meaningful.

Among Ayurvedic herbs, *Bacopa monnieri* has been the one most frequently studied as a possible cognitive enhancer in healthy individuals. One of the first scientific studies of *Bacopa monnieri*'s cognitive effects in healthy subjects was a single-blind, placebo-controlled trial with 40 healthy Indian schoolchildren (R. Sharma and Chaturvedi 1987). At the end of 3 months, subjects in the *Bacopa* group significantly outperformed the placebo group on two of four cognitive tasks: visual-motor discriminative learning and immediate verbal memory. In this study, the selective use of only four cognitive measures was a relative strength; however, the major limitation was that raters were not blind to the subjects' group assignment.

The results of three subsequent randomized, double-blind, placebo-controlled trials support the use of *Bacopa* as a cognitive enhancer in healthy individuals. In the first such study, Abhang (1993) randomly assigned 110 healthy schoolchildren to receive *Bacopa* or placebo daily for 9 months. The *Bacopa* group significantly outperformed the placebo group on tests of arithmetic and direct verbal memory based on the results of a wide battery of cognitive measures. Because such a wide array of tests was used, it is unclear how much significance to attach to the positive findings. In the second study (Stough et al. 2001), 46 healthy adults were randomly assigned to receive *Bacopa* or placebo daily for 12 weeks; the *Bacopa* group had significantly reduced anxiety compared with the placebo group and outperformed the placebo group on 4 of 15 cognitive measures: speed of visual information processing, verbal learning rate, retention of verbal information, and overcoming proactive interference with learning. The enhanced processing of visual information among *Bacopa* users in this study seems congruent with the superior visual-motor discriminative learning reported by R. Sharma and Chaturvedi (1987); likewise, the improved retention of verbal information among *Bacopa* users in this study seems to be consistent with the improved verbal memory reported by Abhang (1993). In a third randomized double-blind, placebo-controlled study involving 76 healthy adults (Roodenrys et al. 2002), subjects receiving *Bacopa* for 12 weeks performed significantly better than the placebo group on the retention of new information, perhaps consistent with earlier findings that *Bacopa* improves verbal memory (Abhang 1993) and retention of verbal information (Stough et al. 2001). However, Roodenrys et al. (2002) found no significant differences between the *Bacopa* and placebo groups on any other measures of verbal or visual memory. In summary, there are intriguing positive results from clinical trials investigating the potential nootropic effects of *Bacopa*; however, the interpretation of these results has been limited by the use of large batteries of cognitive tests within a given trial, substantial variation in cognitive tests used among different trials, and inconsistency of findings among trials.

There have also been three randomized double-blind, placebo-controlled trials that examined the cognitive effects of *Bacopa* in healthy individuals and reported only negative findings. In two of these trials (Maher et al. 2002; Nathan et al. 2001), only a one-time dose of *Bacopa* was used in assessing cognitive benefits, and in the third trial (Nathan et al. 2004), *Bacopa* was used for only 2–4 weeks. The negative findings in all three trials were not surprising; in traditional Ayurvedic practice, it is understood that cognitive enhancement occurs only after *Bacopa* has been taken for several weeks or months. Previous trials showing some cognitive benefits of *Bacopa* were conducted for at least 12 weeks. Thus, it is likely that these three negative trials of *Bacopa* were of too short a duration to detect any potential cognitive benefits.

Ayurvedic herbs other than *Bacopa monnieri* have also been studied for their purported nootropic effects. For example, in one randomized, double-blind, placebo-controlled trial with 57 psychiatrically healthy schoolchildren (Kuppurajan et al. 1978), subjects treated with a daily dose of *Centella asiatica* for 1 year showed significant improvement in their IQ compared with control subjects, who received placebo for the same duration. In another randomized, double-blind, placebo-controlled study (Karnick 1991), 30 psychiatrically healthy adults were randomly divided into three groups and assigned to receive *Withania somnifera*, *Panax ginseng*, or placebo for 6 weeks. At the end of the study, the *Withania* and *Panax* groups outperformed the control group in tests of mental arithmetic and psychomotor function; the *Withania* group outperformed the *Panax* group in measures of integrated sensorimotor function and auditory reaction time.

Among Ayurvedic polyherb formulas, several have shown promise in enhancing cognitive function in healthy subjects. In an open trial with 50 adults ages 50–70 years (R.H. Singh and Sinha 1979), Geriforte was shown to decrease anxiety and mental fatigue while increasing immediate memory span. In a 6-week randomized, double-blind, placebo-controlled study with 50 schoolchildren (Kaur et al. 1998), the group taking a daily dose of a six-herb Ayurvedic formula containing *Bacopa* and *Centella* showed significant improvement in attention compared with the placebo group. In another 6-week randomized, double-blind, placebo-controlled study with 48 men (Gelderloos et al. 1990), the group taking Maharishi Amrit Kalash outperformed the placebo group on a visual discrimination task measuring alertness. In a third randomized, double-blind, placebo-controlled study involving 24 schoolchildren (Koti 1991), subjects taking Mentat for 4 months had the highest overall annual exam scores, followed by subjects taking Mentat plus placebo for 2 months; subjects taking placebo for 4 months had the lowest scores among the three groups. In a fourth randomized, double-blind, placebo-controlled study with 50 psychiatrically healthy adults (Agrawal 1991), subjects taking Mentat for 3 months showed a small but significant increase in short-term memory span and a decrease in fluctuation of attention.

Substance Abuse

Alcoholism, or *madatyaya,* is well described in the ancient Ayurvedic texts. Alcoholism is traditionally treated with a multimodal approach that includes panchakarma, herbs, behavioral changes, nutritional therapy, yoga, and psychospiritual interventions. Herbs are used for hepatoprotective effects as well as to ameliorate the psychological and cognitive damage resulting from alcohol abuse. However, there are few scientific data on the use of Ayurvedic herbs in treating alcoholism. In one small open trial (Trivedi 1999), 21 alcoholic subjects received Mentat tablets daily as an adjuvant to outpatient behavioral treatment; after 6 months, subjects reportedly showed improvement in social adaptability and personality. However, because there was no control group, it is unclear how much of the improvement was attributable to Mentat rather than to outpatient behavioral treatment alone.

Insomnia

Two herbs in the *Valerian* family, *Valeriana jatamansi* and *Nardostachys jatamansi,* have been traditionally used as soporific agents in Ayurveda. The use of *Valeriana* species for treating insomnia has been supported by several randomized, placebo-controlled studies (Donath et al. 2000; Leathwood and Chauffard 1985; Leathwood et al. 1982; Trevena 2004; Ziegler et al. 2002). In a small study of subjects with chronic insomnia, an Ayurvedic polyherb formula of *Nardostachys jatamansi, Rauwolfia serpentina,* and *Tinospora cordifolia* produced electrocardiographic improvements in sleep latency, quality, and duration (Rani and Naidu 1998).

Ayurvedic Herbs for General Medical Conditions

Ayurvedic herbs have potential benefit in a wide range of medical disorders (Table 10–2). It is beyond the scope of this chapter to enumerate all the medical disorders in which Ayurvedic herbal remedies have been studied; interested readers are referred to the comprehensive textbook edited by Mishra (2004), which synthesizes and critically reviews the scientific literature on Ayurvedic herbs in medical treatment. In a concise journal article, Khan and Balick (2001) summarized clinical studies on the therapeutic activity of 166 plant species from the Ayurvedic pharmacopoeia. Over the past 50 years, several large compendia of Indian medicinal plants have been published containing detailed research data on phytochemistry, pharmacological activity, and therapeutic indications for more than 5,000 plants (Chatterjee and Pakrashi 1991–1997; Rastogi and Mehrotra 1960–1994; Warrier et al. 1993–1996).

RESEARCH ON YOGA INTERVENTIONS

After herbal medicines, yoga interventions have the largest representation in the Ayurvedic research database. Yoga interventions include *asanas* (bodily postures), *pranayama* (breathing exercises), and *dhyana* (meditation). Both yoga and Ayurveda originate in the ancient Vedic culture of India and share the view that a healthy body and mind are important preparatory steps in the journey toward spiritual enlightenment. Although the early stages of yoga emphasize techniques for optimizing physical and mental health through asanas and pranayama, the later stages of yoga focus on spiritual development through increasingly sophisticated meditative practices. Ayurveda dedicates itself to creating the optimal somatopsychic foundation for advanced yoga practice and other intensive spiritual pursuits. To this end, Ayurveda incorporates therapeutic aspects of asana, pranayama, and dhyana from yoga but greatly expands the conceptual framework and repertoire of therapies for promoting health and healing.

When yoga was introduced to the West, the integral connection between Ayurveda and yoga was virtually lost. Indeed, within many yoga schools, instruction in the more physical practices of asana and pranayama—sometimes called *hatha yoga*—often became disconnected from instruction in dhyana (meditation). Thus, in most clinical trials, the therapeutic aspects of hatha yoga and meditation have been studied separately from one another and from an overall

TABLE 10–2. Clinical use of Ayurvedic herbs for some general medical conditions

Medical condition	Ayurvedic herbs	Supporting evidence	Evidence rating	Comments
Diabetes	*Gymnema sylvestre Coccinia indica Trigonella foenum*	Elder 2004 Hardy et al. 2001 Yeh et al. 2003	2	Most subjects had type 2 diabetes
Hypercholesterolemia	*Commiphora mukul Trigonella foenum*	Thompson and Ernst 2003 Urizar and Moore 2003	2	Several positive Indian trials, one negative U.S. trial
Congestive heart failure and angina	*Terminalia arjuna*	Bharani et al. 2002; A.L. Miller 1998	2	None
Hepatitis	*Phyllanthus* species	Liu et al. 2001; Martin and Ernst 2003; Thyagarajan et al. 2002	2	Negative studies may be underreported
Parkinson's disease	*Mucuna pruriens*	Katzenschlager et al. 2004; Manyam and Sanchez-Ramos 1999	2	None
Osteoarthritis	*Withania somnifera, Curcuma longa, Boswellia serrata*	Chopra 2000; Kulkarni et al. 1991	2	All three herbs given together in polyherb formula
Irritable bowel syndrome	*Bacopa monnieri, Aegle marmaelos*	Yadav et al. 1989	2	Herbs given together in polyherb formula

Ayurvedic approach. Although there are literally hundreds of clinical studies demonstrating the physiological and psychological effects of hatha yoga and meditation, these studies have not attempted to match specific asana, pranayama, or meditative practices to the unique tri-dosha constitutions of the subjects. Therefore, the full therapeutic potential of these interventions within a traditional Ayurvedic framework has not been investigated.

Yoga for Psychiatric Conditions

In Chapter 16 of this volume, Brown and Gerbarg have written an excellent review of many clinical applications of yoga in psychiatry. In other yoga-related literature reviews, transcendental meditation and mindfulness meditation are reported to have benefits in psychiatric conditions. Transcendental meditation has been used to reduce alcohol and substance abuse (Alexander et al. 1994; Gelderloos et al. 1991) as well as treat symptoms of depression, posttraumatic stress disorder, and other anxiety disorders (Brooks and Scarano 1985; Eppley et al. 1989; Glueck and Stroebel 1975). Mindfulness meditation is said to reduce symptoms of anxiety (Kabat-Zinn et al. 1992; J. J. Miller et al. 1995) and help prevent the relapse of depressive symptoms when combined with cognitive-behavioral therapy (Ma and Teasdale 2004; Teasdale et al. 2000).

Yoga for General Medical Conditions

A number of randomized, controlled trials have provided level 2 evidence for the efficacy of meditation in treating general medical conditions. Although promising, these findings must be replicated in larger independent studies before meditation can be considered to be a primary form of medical therapy. Meditation may be effective in treating hypertension (Alexander et al. 1996; Barnes et al. 2004), atherosclerosis (Castillo-Richmond et al. 2000), irritable bowel syndrome (Keefer and Blanchard 2001), epilepsy (Panjwani et al. 1996), premenstrual and menopausal symptoms (Goodale et al. 1990; Irvin et al. 1996), and sleep disturbance in patients with cancer (Cohen et al. 2004; Shapiro et al. 2003).

Randomized controlled trials also support the use of the other yoga practices, such as asanas and pranayama, in the treatment of medical conditions. However, the fact that studies supporting these yoga practices sometimes involve significant co-interventions makes it difficult to gauge the specific contribution of yoga practices to the subjects' overall improvement. With this caveat, it has been shown that asanas and pranayama may be beneficial in treating hypertension (Murugesan et al. 2000; C. Patel et al. 1985), atherosclerosis (Manchanda et al. 2000), and hyperlipidemia (Mahajan et al. 1999). Asanas and pranayama play a clearer role in improving irritable bowel syndrome (Taneja et al. 2004), carpal tunnel syndrome (Garfinkel et al. 1998; O'Connor et al. 2003), and arthritis (Garfinkel et al. 1994; Haslock et al. 1994). After several randomized controlled trials, conflicting results have emerged on the efficacy of yoga interventions for asthma patients (Ernst 2000; Holloway and Ram 2004; Steurer-Stey et al. 2002).

RESEARCH ON PANCHAKARMA

Panchakarma refers to special Ayurvedic cleansing procedures intended to correct toxic effects of dosha imbalance and enhance the efficacy of subsequent Ayurvedic treatments (Gerson 2001). Common panchakarma procedures include whole-body massage with medicinal oils (*abhyanga*), streaming of medicinal oils on the forehead (*shirodara*), herbalized steam treatment (*svedana*), nasal administration of medicinal oils (*nasya*), emesis (*vamana*), purgation (*virechana*), and enemas (*basti*). The specific components and duration of panchakarma therapy vary by individual, medical condition, and the extent of dosha imbalance.

Panchakarma for Psychiatric Conditions

Panchakarma procedures have been traditionally used in the Ayurvedic treatment of many psychiatric conditions. However, scientific study supporting such use is minimal. In one study with psychiatrically healthy individuals (Schneider et al. 1990), 62 consecutive subjects presenting to an Ayurvedic panchakarma facility were tested with the Profile of Mood States before and after several days of panchakarma procedures. As a control condition, 71 subjects participating in didactic classes were also tested with the same instrument before and after several days of classroom lectures. The results showed that the panchakarma group had significant decreases in anxiety, depression, and overall distress compared with the control group. Limitations of the study included the potential rater bias and self-selection bias of the subjects; in addition, it is unclear whether improvements in mood would be seen in a psychiatric population.

Panchakarma for General Medical Conditions

In the *Scientific Basis for Ayurvedic Therapies* (Mishra 2004), the results from several open trials (A. Gupta 1999; A. Sharma 2001; R.H. Singh and Chaturvedi 1967) demonstrating the efficacy of isolated panchakarma modalities in treating medical conditions such as peptic ulcers, rheumatoid arthritis, and bronchial asthma are summarized. A small number of open clinical trials have also shown the benefits of multimodal panchakarma therapies in decreasing risk factors for cardiovascular disease (H.M. Sharma et al. 1993), improving liver function (MacIntosh and Ball 2000), and reducing serum levels of toxic agrochemicals (Herron and Fagan 2002). In one study of people with Parkinson's disease, subjects receiving both panchakarma and an Ayurvedic herbal remedy exhibited much more improvement in neurological symptoms than did a small control group receiving only the herbal remedy (Nagashayana et al. 2000).

OTHER AYURVEDIC TREATMENTS

Ayurvedic therapies beyond herbs, yoga, and panchakarma have received minimal attention from researchers, despite their great importance in traditional Ayurvedic healing. For example, dosha-specific nutritional changes are an essential component of every Ayurvedic treatment plan, given that the tastes and intrinsic qualities of different foods are said to affect Vata, Pitta, and Kapha in specific and profound ways (Zisman et al. 2003). Yet scientific research on Ayurvedic nutritional therapy is virtually nonexistent. In another example, research on the whole system of Ayurvedic care rather than one specific Ayurvedic modality is rare. To date, only two open clinical trials have been undertaken to show that constitution-specific, multimodal Ayurvedic treatment may be of significant benefit to people with chronic medical illness (Janssen 1989; Nader et al. 2000), and only two randomized controlled trials have investigated (and affirmed) traditional claims that Ayurvedic lifestyle changes may prevent medical illness and optimize health (Fields et al. 2002; Pelletier 2000).

Serious study of constitution-specific Ayurvedic remedies is not likely to be undertaken until there is some scientific validation of the tri-dosha theory. A few scattered attempts have been made to correlate dosha predominance with a specific pattern of symptom presentation or clinical outcome in medical illness (Chandola et al. 1994; Kar et al. 1997; Shanbhag 1988). However, observer bias and other methodological limitations have been significant in such studies. The recent development of a validated instrument to quantify Vata, Pitta, and Kapha in study subjects should enhance research efforts to investigate the clinical utility of this core Ayurvedic concept (R.R. Joshi 2004).

SAFETY ISSUES

Ayurvedic Herbal Medicine

Ancient Ayurvedic texts assert that the toxicity or medicinal value of a given substance depends entirely on its correct preparation and application: "A potent poison may be converted into an excellent medicine by the correct method of preparation, while even the best medicine becomes a potent poison if used badly" (Charaka 1949, I 1.126). Toxicology (*Agada Tantra*) and the conversion of poisons into medicinal agents comprise a core branch of traditional Ayurvedic knowledge. The importance of following traditional Ayurvedic detoxification procedures is exemplified by *Aconitum ferox*. The rhizome of this Ayurvedic plant was historically considered to be quite toxic, and modern investigation has confirmed its toxicity by isolating a lethal aconitine alkaloid. Ancient Ayurvedic physicians converted this toxic rhizome into a valuable anti-inflammatory and analgesic agent through an elaborate detoxification process (Gogtay et al. 2002). This process involved first boiling the rhizome in two parts cow urine and then in two parts cow milk, each for 7 hours per day on 2 consecutive days; afterward, the rhizome was thoroughly washed in warm water and then cut, dried, and ground according to special instructions. A modern animal study has demonstrated that when these detoxification steps are followed in their entirety and in the correct sequence, the lethal aconitine alkaloid is converted to a substance with an extremely wide margin of safety (Thorat and Dahanukar 1991). However, when proper detoxification does not occur, the aconitine alkaloid may cause life-threatening cardiac toxicity and fatalities (Chan et al. 1993).

Traditional Ayurvedic medicines called *bhasmas* contain not only herbs but also minerals and gems such as copper, iron, zinc, mercury, arsenic, lead, gold, silver, diamond, and pearl. As with aconitine, these substances must be converted from toxic into therapeutic agents via elaborate Ayurvedic detoxification procedures. For example, in the Ayurvedic detoxification of lead (Thatte et al. 1993), unprocessed lead is first heated until it glows, then dipped thrice in a mixture of sesame oil, buttermilk, cow urine, and three herbs. Next, the lead is heated again and dipped in a powder of tamarind and hot pepper. Finally, the lead is mixed with arsenic sulfide and heated at a fixed temperature in a wrapping of betel leaf. This entire detoxification procedure is repeated 30 times before the lead is rendered safe for use in a bhasma. Ancient Ayurvedic texts describe tests to ensure that various bhasmas have been properly prepared and detoxified; for example, if a bhasma containing copper added to yogurt causes discoloration a few hours later, it is considered to still be impure (D. Joshi 1998).

Traditional Ayurvedic physicians carefully prepared their herbal remedies by hand. Herbs were cultivated in specific soils and harvested at particular times of day and in specific seasons to enhance their purity and efficacy. Elaborate methods for detoxifying certain ingredients were meticulously observed. Ingredients and dosage were adjusted to suit the tri-dosha constitution of the patient. Specific dietary recommendations and panchakarma practices were used to modulate pharmacological effects. This fastidious and individualized approach to the manufacturing and use of Ayurvedic remedies minimized the risk of adverse effects while maximizing their healing powers (Gogtay et al. 2002; Thatte et al. 1993).

As Ayurveda becomes more popular and the global demand for Ayurvedic medicine increases, mass production of over-the-counter Ayurvedic herbal remedies has become common. In this context, the responsibility for ensuring proper preparation and use of Ayurvedic remedies has shifted from individual Ayurvedic physicians to manufacturing companies or regulatory agencies that may be less adherent to correct Ayurvedic practice. For example, generic Ayurvedic remedies may now be sold directly to a patient without regard for the patient's unique tri-dosha constitution and without consultation from an Ayurvedic physician. Plant materials contaminated by pesticides or pollutants may be used in herbal preparations. Herbs may be misidentified and substituted in tra-

TABLE 10–3. Some Ayurvedic herbs and medicinal ingredients with potential adverse interactions with allopathic drugs

Herb or ingredient	Allopathic drug	Adverse interaction	References
Shankhapushpi[a]	Phenytoin	↓ Phenytoin level ↓ Antiepileptic efficacy	Dandekar et al. 1992
Mentat[a]	Phenytoin, carbamazepine	↑ Antiepileptic drug levels	M. Tripathi et al. 2000
Valerian species	Barbiturates	↑ Sedation ↓ Respiratory drive	L.G. Miller 1998
Areca catechu (Betel nut)	Typical antipsychotics	↑ Extrapyramidal symptoms	Deahl 1989
Capsicum species (Chili pepper)	Angiotensin-converting enzyme inhibitors	Recurrent cough	Hakas 1990
Carica papaya (Papaya)	Warfarin	↑ International normalized ratio	Shaw et al. 1997
Madhu (Honey)	Carbamazepine	↓ Bioavailable carbamazepine	Koumaravelou et al. 2002
Glycyrrhiza glabra (Licorice)	Prednisolone Digoxin Thiazide diuretic	↑ Plasma drug level ↑ Digoxin sensitivity Hypokalemia	Chen et al. 1991 A.L. Miller 1998 L.G. Miller 1998

[a]Polyherb formulas, listed by traditional Sanskrit name or by proprietary name, as appropriate.

ditional Ayurvedic formulas. Traditional, time-consuming detoxification procedures may be circumvented. Herbs may be combined into new formulations not described in traditional texts. In addition, patients may combine Ayurvedic remedies with allopathic pharmaceuticals unknown to the ancient practitioners; adverse interactions have been reported between some allopathic drugs and Ayurvedic medicinal ingredients (Table 10–3).

Thus, safeguards inherent in the traditional preparation and prescription of Ayurvedic medicines have been weakened in modern times, leading to the potential for significant toxicities and adverse reactions. There have been several recent reports of heavy metal toxicities related to the use of some Ayurvedic medicines (Centers for Disease Control and Prevention 2004; Ernst 2002; Saper et al. 2004). These toxicities appear to be largely the result of contamination or improper processing and preparation of Ayurvedic medicinal ingredients; in some cases, patients are using the remedies in higher doses or for a longer duration than recommended. As of December 2002, stringent good manufacturing practices (GMPs) for Ayurvedic medicines went into effect in India (Gogtay et al. 2002). Most large-scale Indian manufacturers of Ayurvedic medicines have demonstrated compliance with these GMPs, but small manufacturers may escape regulatory attention and still produce improperly prepared Ayurvedic products for consumption in India and abroad. New GMP requirements for imported and domestic herbal products are awaiting final approval in the United States; once implemented, the new GMPs will protect consumers from exposure to toxic herbal products.

Ayurvedic herbs are currently classified as dietary supplements under the U.S. Dietary Supplement Health and Education Act of 1994 (DSHEA). Some critics argue that this classification endangers public health because the regulation of herbs under DSHEA is not as stringent as it would be under the Federal Drug Act. In response, advocates of the current classification point out that the U.S. food supply is closely regulated under DSHEA; with implementation and enforcement of new DSHEA GMPs for herbal products, Ayurvedic medicines will be as safe for consumption as is the U.S. food supply. In addition, advocates point out that most Ayurvedic herbs have a centuries-old empirical record of safety and efficacy; public access to these valuable herbs may be hindered unduly if the herbs must undergo the same costly testing for safety and efficacy required under the Federal Drug Act as newly synthesized pharmaceutical agents.

Panchakarma

Panchakarma should be initiated only after consultation with an experienced Ayurvedic physician. It is advisable for a person considering panchakarma to also consult an allopathic physician. The components and duration of panchakarma will depend on an individual's unique constitution and the extent of any dosha imbalance or illness. Some panchakarma practices, especially purgation and emesis, are contraindicated for individuals with acute febrile illness, acute gastrointestinal illness, alcohol or drug withdrawal, very low body weight, an eating or metabolic disorder, diabetes, hypertension, hypothyroidism, cancer, an immune deficiency state, alcohol or drug withdrawal, or recent surgery. Panchakarma is also contraindicated in children, elderly adults, and pregnant women.

Yogic Interventions

When yogic interventions are undertaken with supervision from an experienced yoga teacher, the adverse effects are minimal. When performing asanas (bodily poses), individuals are encouraged to master the pose gradually over time to avoid injury. Adjustments to asanas are made for individuals with specific musculoskeletal problems, such as chronic back pain. *Pranayama* (breathing exercises) may be modified or withheld for pregnant women and individuals with seizure disorders, migraines, high blood pressure, cardiovascular disease, or severe pulmonary disease. Meditation may lead to a state of heightened self-awareness that can sometimes be overwhelming for psychologically fragile individuals unaccustomed to paying close attention to internal sensations, perceptions, and images. Thus, meditation must be used cautiously in people who show impaired reality testing, poor ego boundaries, or a rigid, overcontrolling personality style.

GUIDELINES FOR CLINICAL USE OF AYURVEDIC THERAPIES

In the United States, Ayurveda is not currently recognized as an independent health care discipline, and there is no state licensure to regulate its practice. However, in several states (e.g., New York, California), health care providers already licensed to practice medicine, nursing, physical therapy, nutrition, chiropractic, or massage may incorporate Ayurvedic principles into their existing professional activities. Ayurvedic physicians formally trained in India may continue to practice Ayurveda in the United States but under a much narrower scope of activity that cannot be represented to the public as the practice of allopathic medicine; for example, symptoms must not be discussed with patients in terms of allopathic medical diagnoses but instead as dosha imbalances. In several regions of the United States, Ayurvedic organizations have developed curricula for training Ayurvedic practitioners. Dialogue has begun on the task of setting statewide and national standards to demonstrate training and competency in Ayurvedic health care. Ayurvedic organizations also have begun the process of lobbying state legislatures for recognition and licensure of Ayurvedic practice.

When working with patients interested in an Ayurvedic approach to healing, an allopathic physician may consider three broad responses: 1) *confirm* the efficacy of Ayurvedic therapies that have a favorable risk–benefit ratio, as established in scientific studies; 2) *co-follow* (jointly monitor) patients seeing Ayurvedic practitioners for therapies that are scientifically untested but traditionally considered to be useful; and 3) *caution* against Ayurvedic therapies that have an unfavorable risk–benefit ratio, as established in scientific studies (Table 10–4). All three responses involve gaining familiarity with the evidence base on Ayurvedic therapies and assessing the patient's motivations and expectations about pursuing Ayurvedic treatment. Allopathic physicians considering an Ayurvedic approach should consult with a network of colleagues experienced in providing Ayurvedic health care.

TABLE 10–4. Clinical considerations in using Ayurvedic therapies

	Data issues	Patient issues
Confirm	Ayurvedic therapy has scientific evidence demonstrating good efficacy and low risk.	Patient is willing and able to adhere to specific protocols of the Ayurvedic therapy.
Co-Follow	Traditional use indicates that an Ayurvedic therapy may be helpful and safe for your patient, but there is a lack of scientific evidence.	Patient is willing to stay in close contact with you so that you can monitor the course of Ayurvedic treatment together.
Caution	Ayurvedic therapy has known harmful effects, especially in patients similar to yours.	Patient is abandoning effective conventional treatment with low risk of side effects because of misinformation or interpersonal conflict with providers.

The following case example illustrates the importance of the personalized approach intrinsic to proper Ayurvedic health care.

Alice, Bella, and Carrie are three sisters from a very close-knit Midwestern family. After a family gathering one winter night, Carrie drives home on an icy road and dies in a tragic car accident. Alice and Bella are heartbroken. Over the next 6 months, each of the surviving sisters neglects herself and becomes quite debilitated in her own particular way.

Prior to the loss of her sister, Alice was a slender, active woman working in a graphic design firm; she was known for her creativity and quick wit, and she kept a rather erratic eating and sleeping schedule as she raced to make her deadlines. After Carrie's death, Alice lost her appetite entirely; her already slender frame became gaunt and dangerously thin. She slept only 2–3 hours per night, often spending a great deal of time tossing and turning. She felt exhausted during the day and could not keep up with the demands of her job; she eventually chose to take a leave of absence. However, even when given the opportunity to rest, she was unable to do so; she was tense, anxious, and constantly moving. She ruminated on her sister's death and was plagued by a sense of guilt about letting her sister drive alone on the night of the accident. She telephoned family members often in an attempt to seek solace, but could not really focus on their responses.

Bella was another story altogether. She was always the "steady one" in the family, and her ample, solid build and frequent hugs made people feel warm and welcome. She relished her role as a mother and homemaker, taking pride in cooking big, festive meals. After Carrie's death, Bella felt numb and apathetic. She lost interest in caring for her children, withdrawing instead to her bedroom. She slept 10–12 hours each day. She no longer cooked for her family and overate "comfort foods" such as ice cream and chocolate. She rarely spoke, and when she did, her speech was painfully slow and sparse. Her movements appeared leaden. She described herself as being paralyzed by her sister's loss.

In allopathic psychiatry, both Alice and Bella would likely receive the same diagnosis: major depressive disorder. They might be tried on the same antidepressant medications or undergo the same cognitive-behavioral therapy. In an Ayurvedic approach, however, the diagnosis for each woman was quite different: Alice suffered from Vata excess, whereas Bella showed clear signs of Kapha excess. Each woman was prescribed a series of very different Ayurvedic interventions designed to pacify the aggravated dosha.

For Alice, an Ayurvedic physician recommended Vata-lowering panchakarma procedures such as hot steam baths. Her diet was filled with warm, moist, and protein-rich foods. She was encouraged to perform yoga asanas that calm and soothe the nervous system. She underwent massage with Vata-lowering medicinal oils and was given teas with cardamom and other Vata-pacifying herbs. She was cautioned against traveling to Vata-stimulating environments such as windy, mountainous regions and was advised to wear Vata-lowering colors, fragrances, and gems.

For Bella, an Ayurvedic physician recommended Kapha-lowering panchakarma procedures such as therapeutic emesis. Her diet was switched to light, spicy foods with lots of greens and salads. She was encouraged to perform yoga asanas that invigorate the nervous system. She underwent massage with Kapha-lowering medicinal oils and was given teas with ginger and other Kapha-lowering herbs. She was cautioned against traveling to Kapha-stimulating environments such as the foggy, overcast Pacific Northwest and was advised to wear Kapha-lowering colors, fragrances, and gems.

The goal of these Ayurvedic treatments was to create the right context for each woman to regain her own unique doshic equilibrium so her body–mind–spirit could once again effectively metabolize and heal from life stressors and challenges.

REFERENCES

Abhang R: Study to evaluate the effect of a micro (*suksma*) medicine derived from Brahmi on students of average intelligence. Journal of Research in Ayurveda and Siddha 14:10–24, 1993

Agrawal A, Dubey ML, Dubey GP: Effect of Mentat on memory, anxiety scores and neuroticism index in normal subjects in three age groups. Probe 30:257–261, 1991

Agrawal A, Gupta U, Dixit SP, et al: Management of mental deficiency by an indigenous drug Brahmi. Pharmacopsychoecologia 6:1–5, 1993

Alexander C, Robinson P, Rainforth M: Treating and preventing alcohol, nicotine, and drug abuse through transcendental meditation: a review and statistical meta-analysis. Alcohol Treat Q 11:13–87, 1994

Alexander CN, Schneider RH, Staggers F, et al: Trial of stress reduction for hypertension in older African Americans, II: sex and risk subgroup analysis. Hypertension 28:228–237, 1996

American Psychiatric Association: Diagnostic and Statistical Manual of Mental Disorders, 4th Edition. Washington, DC, American Psychiatric Association, 1994

American Psychiatric Association: Diagnostic and Statistical Manual of Mental Disorders, 4th Edition, Text Revision. Washington, DC, American Psychiatric Association, 2000

Andrade C, Gowda S, Chaturvedi SK: Treatment of age-related cognitive decline with an herbal formulation: a double-blind study. Indian J Psychiatry 40:240–246, 1998

Appa Rao MVR, Srinivasan K, Koteswara Rao T: The effect of mandookaparni (*Centella asiatica*) on the general mental ability (medhya) of mentally retarded children. Journal of Research in Indian Medicine 8:9–16, 1973

Appa Rao MVR, Srinivasan K, Koteswara Rao T: Effect of *Centella asiatica* on the general mental ability of mentally retarded children. Indian J Psychiatry 19:54–59, 1977

Bacher NM, Lewis HA: Lithium plus reserpine in refractory manic patients. Am J Psychiatry 136:811–814, 1979

Barnes VA, Treiber FA, Johnson MH: Impact of transcendental meditation on ambulatory blood pressure in African American adolescents. Am J Hypertens 17:366–369, 2004

Berlant JL: Neuroleptics and reserpine in refractory psychoses. J Clin Psychopharmacol 6:180–184, 1986

Bharani A, Ganguli A, Mathur LK, et al: Efficacy of *Terminalia aruna* in chronic stable angina. Indian Heart Journal 54:170–175, 2002

Bodeker G: Evaluating Ayurveda. J Altern Complement Med 7:389–392, 2001

Boral GC, Bandopadyaya G, Boral A, et al: Geriforte in anxiety neurosis. Indian J Psychiatry 31:258–260, 1989

Bradwejn J, Zhou Y, Koszycki D, et al: A double-blind, placebo-controlled study on the effects of Gotu Kola (*Centella asiatica*) on acoustic startle response in healthy subjects. J Clin Psychopharmacol 20:680–684, 2000

Brooks JS, Scarano T: Transcendental meditation in the treatment of the post-Vietnam adjustment. J Couns Dev 64:212–215, 1985

Castillo-Richmond A, Schneider RH, Alexander CN, et al: Effects of stress reduction on carotid atherosclerosis in hypertensive African Americans. Stroke 31:568–573, 2000

Centers for Disease Control and Prevention: Lead poisoning associated with Ayurvedic medications: five states, 2000–2003. MMWR Morb Mortal Wkly Rep 53:582–584, 2004

Chakraborty S: Geriforte in psychosomatic psychological disorders in adults. Probe 23:31–33, 1983

Chan TY, Tomlinson B, Critchley JA: Acontine poisoning following the ingestion of Chinese herbal medicines: a report of eight cases. Aust N Z J Med 23:268–271, 1993

Chandola HM, Tripathi SN, Udupa KN: Variations in the progression of maturity onset diabetes according to body constitution. Ancient Science of Life 13:293–301, 1994

Charaka: Charaka Samhita, Vols I–VI. Translated by Shree Gulab Kunverba Ayurvedic Society. Jamnagar, India, Shree Gulab Kunverba Ayurvedic Society, 1949

Chatterjee A, Pakrashi SC (eds): The Treatise on Indian Medicinal Plants, Vols 1–5. New Delhi, NISCOM, 1991–1997

Chen MF, Shimada F, Kato H, et al: Effect of oral administration of *Glycyrrhizin* on the pharmacokinetics of prednisolone. Endocrinol Jpn 38:167–174, 1991

Chopra A: Ayurvedic medicine and arthritis. Rheum Dis Clin North Am 26:133–144, 2000

Choudhuri O: Development of an Ayurvedic regimen for the management of residual schizophrenia. MD thesis (Kayachikitsa), Banaras Hindu University, Varanasi, India, 2001

Christison GW, Kirch DG, Wyatt RJ: When symptoms persist: choosing among alternative somatic treatments for schizophrenia. Schizophr Bull 17:217–245, 1991

Cohen L, Warneke C, Fouladi RT, et al: Psychological adjustment and sleep quality in a randomized trial of the effects of a Tibetan yoga intervention in patients with lymphoma. Cancer 100:2253–2260, 2004

Colabawalla HM: A preliminary report on the lack of toxicity of a preparation of total Rauwolfia alkaloids. J Neurochem 21:213–215, 1958

Cott J, Misra R: Medicinal plants: a potential source for new psychotherapeutic drugs, in Herbal Medicines for Neuropsychiatric Diseases: Current Developments and Research. Edited by Kanba S, Richelson E. Philadelphia, PA, Brunner/Mazel, 1999, pp 51–70

Damle VB, Gore AG: Treatment of involutional depression in males with Geriforte: an indigenous drug (study of 25 cases). Indian Pract 35:73–76, 1982

Dandekar UP, Chandra RS, Dalvi SS, et al: Analysis of a clinically important interaction between phenytoin and shankapushpi, an Ayurvedic preparation. J Ethnopharmacol 35:285–288, 1992

Danino M, Sujata N: The Invasion That Never Was. Delhi, India, Voice of India, 1996

Das S, De Sousa A: Mentat (BR-16A) in schizophrenia. Journal of Community Psychiatry 12:15–16, 1989

Dash SC, Tripathi SN, Singh RH: Clinical assessment of medhya drugs in the management of psychosis (*unmada*). Ancient Science of Life 3:77–81, 1983

Dave U, Chauhan V, Dalvi J: Evaluation of Mentat in cognitive and behavioural dysfunction of mentally retarded children: a placebo-controlled study. Indian J Pediatr 60:423–428, 1993

De Sousa A, Gangdev P, Manoj Agrawal M, et al: Geriforte in depression (dysthymic disorder). Journal of Community Psychiatry 12:12–13, 1989

Deahl M: Betel nut-induced extrapyramidal syndrome: an unusual drug interaction. Mov Disord 4:330–332, 1989

Dixit SP, Agrawal A, Dubey GP: Effect of Mentat on language and learning disabilities in children with mild mental deficiencies. Indian Pract 45:1067–1070, 1992

Donath F, Quispe S, Diefenbach K, et al: Critical evaluation of the effect of valerian extract on sleep structure and sleep quality. Pharmacopsychiatry 33:47–53, 2000

D'Souza B, Chavda KB: Mentat in hyperactivity and attention deficiency disorders: a double-blind, placebo-controlled study. Probe 30:227–232, 1991

Elder C: Ayurveda for diabetes mellitus: a review of the biomedical literature. Altern Ther Health Med 10:44–50, 2004

Eppley K, Abrams AI, Shear J: The differential effects of relaxation techniques on trait anxiety: a meta-analysis. J Clin Psychol 45:957–974, 1989

Ernst E: Breathing techniques: adjunctive treatment modalities for asthma? a systematic review. Eur Respir J 15:969–972, 2000

Ernst E: Heavy metals in traditional Indian remedies. Eur J Clin Pharmacol 57:891–896, 2002

Feuerstein G, Subhash K, Frawley D: In Search of the Cradle of Civilization. Wheaton, IL, Quest Books, 1995

Fields JZ, Walton KG, Schneider RH, et al: Effect of a multimodality natural medicine program on carotid atherosclerosis in older subjects: a pilot trial of Maharishi Vedic Medicine. Am J Cardiol 89:952–958, 2002

Filliozat J: The expansion of Indian medicine abroad, in India's Contributions to World Thought and Culture. Edited by Chandra L. Madras, India, Vivekananda Memorial Committee, 1970, pp 67–70

Frawley D: Ayurveda and Mind. Twin Lakes, WO, Lotus Press, 1997

Frederiksen PK: Baclofen in the treatment of schizophrenia (letter). Lancet 1(7908):702, 1975

Garfinkel MS, Schumacher HR Jr, Husain A, et al: Evaluation of a yoga-based regimen for treatment of osteoarthritis of the hands. J Rheumatol 21:2341–2343, 1994

Garfinkel MS, Singhal A, Katz WA, et al: Yoga-based intervention for carpal tunnel syndrome: a randomized trial. JAMA 280:1601–1603, 1998

Gelderloos P, Ahlstrom HHB, Orme-Johnson DW, et al: Influence of a Maharishi Ayurvedic herbal preparation on age-related visual discrimination. Int J Psychosom 37:25–29, 1990

Gelderloos P, Walton KG, Orme-Johnson DW, et al: Effectiveness of the transcendental meditation program in preventing and treating substance misuse: a review. Int J Addict 26:293–325, 1991

Gerson S: Ayurvedic medicine: antitoxification versus detoxification. Alternative and Complementary Therapies 7:233–239, 2001

Ghosh S: The History of Education in Ancient India. New Delhi, India, Munshiram Manoharlal, 2001

Glueck BC, Stroebel CF: Biofeedback and meditation in the treatment of psychiatric illnesses. Compr Psychiatry 16:303–321, 1975

Gogtay NJ, Bhatt HA, Dalvi SS, et al: The use and safety of non-allopathic Indian medicines. Drug Saf 25:1005–1019, 2002

Goodale IL, Domar AD, Benson H: Alleviation of premenstrual syndrome symptoms with the relaxation response. Obstet Gynecol 75:649–655, 1990

Gupta A: Study to evaluate the efficacy of Basti therapy in rheumatoid arthritis. MD thesis, National Institute of Ayurveda, Jaipur, India, 1999

Gupta S: The Indus-Saraswati Civilization. Delhi, India, Pratibha Prakashan, 1996

Gupta SK, Singh RH: A clinical study on depressive illness and its Ayurvedic management. Journal of Research in Ayurveda and Siddha 23:82–93, 2002

Gupta SP: Psychopathology in Indian Medicine (Ayurveda), With Special Reference to Its Philosophical Bases. Aligarh, India, Ajaya, 1977

Gupta SPK: Rustom Jal Vakil (1911–1974): father of modern cardiology. Journal of the Indian Academy of Clinical Medicine 3(1):100–104, 2002

Hakas JF: Topical capsaicin induces cough in patient receiving ACE inhibitor. Ann Allergy 65:322–323, 1990

Halbfass W: India and Europe: An Essay in Understanding. Albany, NY, State University of New York Press, 1988

Haldipur CV: Madness in ancient India: concept of insanity in Charaka Samhita. Compr Psychiatry 25:335–344, 1984

Hardy ML, Coulter I, Venuturupalli S, et al: Ayurvedic interventions for diabetes mellitus: a systematic review. Evid Rep Technol Assess (Summ) Jun (41):2p, 2001

Harle JC: The "Indian" terracottas from ancient Memphis, in South Asian Archaeology, 1989, in Papers From the Tenth International Conference of South Asian Archaeologists in Western Europe. Edited by Jarrige C, Gerry JP, Meadow RH. London, Prehistory Press, 1992

Haslock I, Monro RE, Nagarathna R, et al: Measuring the effects of yoga in rheumatoid arthritis. Br J Rheumatol 33:787–788, 1994

Hauben DJ: Sushruta Samhita (Sushruta'a Collection) (800–600 B.C.?): pioneers of plastic surgery. Acta Chir Plast 26:65–68, 1984

Herron RE, Fagan JB: Lipophil-mediated reduction of toxicants in humans: an evaluation of an Ayurvedic detoxification procedure. Altern Ther Health Med 8:40–51, 2002

Holloway E, Ram FS: Breathing exercises for asthma. Cochrane Database Syst Rev (1): CD001277, 2004

Ifrah G: The Universal History of Numbers: From Prehistory to the Invention of the Computer. Translated by Bellos D, Harding EF, Wood S, et al. New York, Wiley, 2000

Irvin JH, Domar AD, Clark C, et al: The effects of relaxation response training on menopausal symptoms. J Psychosom Obstet Gynaecol 17:202–207, 1996

Jaggi OP: Indian System of Medicine. Delhi, India, Atma Ram, 1981

Janssen G: The Maharishi Ayur-Veda treatment of 10 chronic diseases. Nederlands Tijdschrift voor Integrale Geneeskunde 5:56–94, 1989

Jee BS: Aryan Medical Science: A Short History (1895). Delhi, India, Low Price Publications, 1993

Joshi D: Rasamritam, 1st Edition. Varanasi, India, Chaukhambha Sanskrit Bhawan, 1998

Joshi RR: A biostatistical approach to Ayurveda: quantifying the tridosha. J Altern Complement Med 10:879–889, 2004

Kabat-Zinn J, Massion AO, Kristeller J, et al: Effectiveness of a meditation-based stress reduction program in the treatment of anxiety disorders. Am J Psychiatry 149:936–943, 1992

Kak S: Indic ideas in the Graeco-Roman world. Indian Historical Review, 1999. Available at: www.ece.lsu.edu/kak/ihr.pdf

Kak S: Ayurveda, in Gale Encyclopedia on India. Edited by Wolpert S. New York, Macmillan-Scribners-Gale, 2005a

Kak S: Greek and Indian cosmology: review of early history, in History of Science, Philosophy and Culture in Indian Civilization, Vol 1, Part 4: A Golden Chain. Edited by Pande GC. Delhi, India, Centre for Studies in Civilizations, 2005b, pp 871–894

Kalra V, Zamir H, Kulkarni KS: A randomized double-blind, placebo-controlled drug trial with Mentat in children with attention deficit hyperactivity disorder. Neurosciences Today 6:223–227, 2002

Kar CA, Upadhyay BN, Ojha D: Prognosis of prameha on the basis of insulin level. Ancient Science of Life 16:277–283, 1997

Karnick CR: A double-blind, placebo-controlled clinical study on the effects of *Withania somnifera* and *Panax ginseng* extracts on psychomotor performance in healthy Indian volunteers. Indian Medicine (Vijayawada) 3:1–5, 1991

Katzenschlager R, Evans A, Manson A, et al: *Mucuna pruriens* in Parkinson's disease: a double-blind clinical and pharmacological study. J Neurol Neurosurg Psychiatry 75:1672–1677, 2004

Kaur BR, Adhiraj J, Pandit PR, et al: Effect of an Ayurvedic formulation on attention, concentration and memory in normal school-going children. Indian Drugs 35:200–203, 1998

Kaushik A, Singh R: Clinical evaluation of medhya rasayana compound in cases of non-depressive anxiety neurosis. Ancient Science of Life 2:11–16, 1982

Keay J: India: A History. London, HarperCollins, 2000

Keefer L, Blanchard EB: The effects of relaxation response meditation on the symptoms of irritable bowel syndrome: results of a controlled treatment study. Behav Res Ther 39:801–811, 2001

Khan S, Balick MJ: Therapeutic plants of Ayurveda: a review of selected clinical and other studies for 166 species. J Altern Complement Med 7:405–515, 2001

Khor M, Lin LL (eds): Promotion of indigenous systems of medicine in India, in Good Practices and Innovative Experiences in the South, Vol 2. Penang, Malaysia, United Na-tions Development Programme and Third World Network, 2001. Available at: http://tcdc.undp.org/experiences/vol4/Promotion%20of%20indigenous%20systems.pdf. Accessed October 6, 2004.

Kline NS: Use of *Rauwolfia serpentina Benth.* in neuropsychiatric conditions. Ann N Y Acad Sci 59:107–132, 1954

Koirala RR: Clinical and behavioural study of Medhya drugs on brain functions. MD thesis, Banaras Hindu University, Varanasi, India, 1992

Koti ST: Effect of Mentat on school students' performance: a double-blind, placebo-controlled study. Probe 30:250–252, 1991

Koumaravelou K, Adithan C, Shashindran CH, et al: Effect of honey on carbamazepine kinetics in rabbits. Indian J Exp Biol 40:560–563, 2002

Kulkarni RR, Patki PS, Jog VP, et al: Treatment of osteoarthritis with a herbomineral formulation: a double-blind, placebo-controlled, crossover study. J Ethnopharmacol 33:91–95, 1991

Kuppurajan K, Srinivasan K, Janaki K: A double-blind study on the effect of mandooka-parni on the general mental ability of normal children. Journal of Research in Indian Medicine 13:37–41, 1978

Kushwaha HK, Sharma KP: Clinical evaluation of shankhpushpi syrup in the management of depressive illness. Sacitra Ayurveda 45:45–50, 1992

Lad V: The Textbook of Ayurveda. Albuquerque, NM, Ayurvedic Press, 2002

Lal BB: The Earliest Civilization of South Asia: Rise, Maturity and Decline. New Delhi, India, Aryan Books, 1997

Leathwood PD, Chauffard F: Aqueous extract of valerian reduces latency to fall asleep in man. Planta Med 2:144–148, 1985

Leathwood PD, Chauffard F, Heck E, et al: Aqueous extract of valerian root (*Valeriana officinalis L.*) improves sleep quality in man. Pharmacol Biochem Behav 17:65–71, 1982

Lele RD: Ayurveda and Modern Medicine. Bombay, India, Bhartiya Vidya Bhavan, 1986

Litman RE, Hong WW, Weissman EM, et al: Idazoxan, an alpha2 antagonist, augments fluphenazine in schizophrenic patients: a pilot study. J Clin Psychopharmacol 13:264–267, 1993

Liu J, Lin H, McIntosh H: Genus *Phyllanthus* for chronic hepatitis B virus infection: a systematic review. J Viral Hepat 8:358–366, 2001

Lopez-Munoz F, Bhatara V, Alamo C, et al: Historical approach to reserpine discovery and its introduction in psychiatry [in Spanish]. Actas Esp Psiquiatr 32:387–395, 2004

Ma SH, Teasdale JD: Mindfulness-based cognitive therapy for depression: replication and exploration of differential relapse prevention effects. J Consult Clin Psychol 72:31–40, 2004

MacIntosh A, Ball K: The effects of a short program of detoxification in disease-free individuals. Altern Ther Health Med 6:70–76, 2000

Mahajan AS, Reddy KS, Sachdeva U: Lipid profile of coronary risk subjects following yogic lifestyle intervention. Indian Heart J 51:37–40, 1999

Mahal AS, Ramu NG, Chaturvedi DD: Double-blind controlled study of brahmyadiyoga and tagara in the management of various types of *unmada* (schizophrenia). Indian J Psychiatry 18:283–292, 1976

Maher BF, Stough C, Shelmerdine A, et al: The acute effects of combined administration of *Ginkgo biloba* and *Bacopa monniera* on cognitive function in humans. Hum Psychopharmacol 17:163–164, 2002

Malhotra SK: A study of the efficacy of Geriforte in depressive disorders. The Medicine and Surgery 6:21, 1986. Available at: http://himalayahealthcare.com/pdf_files/geriforte098.pdf

Malviya PC: Studies on Cittodvega vis-à-vis anxiety neurosis and its treatment with the Rasayana drug Asvagandha (*Withania somnifera dunal*). Thesis, Banaras Hindu University, Varanasi, India, 1976

Manchanda SC, Narang R, Reddy KS, et al: Retardation of coronary atherosclerosis with yoga lifestyle intervention. J Assoc Physicians India 48:687–694, 2000

Manyam BV, Sanchez-Ramos JR: Traditional and complementary therapies in Parkinson's disease. Adv Neurol 80:565–574, 1999

Martin KW, Ernst E: Antiviral agents from plants and herbs: a systematic review. Antivir Ther 8:77–90, 2003

McDowell F: The Source Book of Plastic Surgery. Baltimore, MD, Williams & Wilkins, 1977, pp 65–85

Miller AL: Botanical influences on cardiovascular disease. Altern Med Rev 3:422–431, 1998

Miller JJ, Fletcher K, Kabat-Zinn J: Three-year follow-up and clinical implications of a mindfulness meditation–based stress reduction intervention in the treatment of anxiety disorders. Gen Hosp Psychiatry 17:192–200, 1995

Miller LG: Herbal medicinals: selected clinical considerations focusing on known or potential drug-herb interactions. Arch Intern Med 158:2200–2211, 1998

Mishra LC (ed): Scientific Basis for Ayurvedic Therapies. Boca Raton, FL, CRC Press, 2004

Mookerji R: Ancient Indian Education: Brahmanical and Buddhist. London, Motilol Banarsidass, 1947

Murugesan R, Govindarajulu N, Bera TK: Effect of selected yogic practices on the management of hypertension. Indian J Physiol Pharmacol 44:207–210, 2000

Nader T, Rothenberg S, Averbach R, et al: Improvements in chronic diseases with a comprehensive natural medicine approach: a review and case series. Behav Med 26:34–46, 2000

Nagashayana N, Sankarankutty P, Nampoothiri MR, et al: Association of L-dopa with recovery following Ayurveda medication in Parkinson's disease. J Neurol Sci 176:124–127, 2000

Nathan PJ, Clarke J, Lloyd J, et al: The acute effects of an extract of *Bacopa monniera* (Brahmi) on cognitive function in healthy normal subjects. Hum Psychopharmacol 16:345–351, 2001

Nathan PJ, Tanner S, Lloyd J, et al: Effects of a combined extract of *Ginkgo biloba* and *Bacopa monniera* on cognitive function in healthy humans. Hum Psychopharmacol 19:91–96, 2004

Negi KS, Singh YD, Kushwaha KP, et al: Clinical evaluation of memory-enhancing properties of Memory Plus in children with attention deficit hyperactivity disorder. Indian J Psychiatry 42 (suppl), 2000

O'Connor D, Marshall S, Massy-Westropp N: Nonsurgical treatment (other than steroid injection) for carpal tunnel syndrome. Cochrane Database Syst Rev (1): CD003219, 2003

Panjwani U, Selvamurthy W, Singh SH, et al: Effect of Sahaja yoga practice on seizure control and EEG changes in patients of epilepsy. Indian J Med Res 103:165–172, 1996

Patel C, Marmot MG, Terry DJ, et al: Trial of relaxation in reducing coronary risk: 4-year follow-up. Br Med J (Clin Res Ed) 290:1103–1106, 1985

Patel RB, Pereira L: Experience with Mentat in hyperkinetic children. Probe 30:271–274, 1991

Pelletier K: Ayurvedic medicine and yoga, in The Best Alternative Medicine: What Works? What Does Not? New York, Simon & Schuster, 2000, pp 240–243

Possehl G (ed): Harrapan Civilization. New Delhi, Oxford, and IBH Publishing, 1982

Rajaram N, Frawley D: Vedic Aryans and the Origins of Civilization. St Hyacinthe, Canada, World Heritage Press, 1995

Ramu MG, Senapati HM, Jankiramaiah N, et al: A pilot study on role of brahmyadiyoga on chronic *unmada* (schizophrenia) patients. Ancient Science of Life 2:205–207, 1983

Ramu MG, Chaturvedi DD, Venkataram BS, et al: A double-blind controlled study of the role of brahmyadiyoga and tagara in chronic schizophrenia, in Ayurvedic Management of Unmada. New Delhi, India, Central Council for Research in Ayurveda and Siddha, 1999, pp 77–88

Rana RE, Arora BS: History of plastic surgery in India. J Postgrad Med 48:76–78, 2002

Rani PU, Naidu MUR: Subjective and polysomnographic evaluation of a herbal preparation in insomnia. Phytomedicine 5:253–257, 1998

Rao SR: Dawn and Devolution of the Indus Civilization. Delhi, India, Aditya Prakashan Press, 1991

Rastogi RP, Mehrotra BN (eds): Compendium of Indian Medicinal Plants, Vols 1–5. New Delhi, India, PID Press; Lucknow, India, CDRI Press, 1960–1994

Rawlinson HG: Early contacts between India and Europe, in A Cultural History of India. Edited by Basham AL. New Delhi, India, Oxford University Press, 1975, pp 425–441

Roodenrys S, Booth D, Bulzomi S, et al: Chronic effects of Brahmi (*Bacopa monnieri*) on human memory. Neuropsychopharmacology 27:279–281, 2002

Saper RB, Kales SN, Paquin J, et al: Heavy metal content of Ayurvedic herbal medicine products. JAMA 292:2868–2873, 2004

Schneider RH, Cavanaugh KL, Kasture HS, et al: Health promotion with a traditional system of natural health care: Maharishi Ayurveda. J Soc Behav Pers 5:1–27, 1990

Sen G, Bose KC: *Rauwolfia serpentina*. Indian Medical World 2:194–201, 1931

Shah LP, Mazumdar K, Nayak PR, et al: Clinical evaluation of Geriforte in patients with generalised anxiety disorders. Bombay Hospital Journal 32:29–31, 1990

Shah LP, Nayak PR, Sethi A: A comparative study of Geriforte in anxiety neurosis and mixed anxiety-depressive disorders. Probe 32:195–201, 1993

Shanbhag V: The role of Sankha-Bhasma (an Ayurvedic medicine) in the treatment of acne vulgaris. MD thesis, University of Poona, Pune, India, 1988

Shapiro SL, Bootzin RR, Figueredo AJ, et al: The efficacy of mindfulness-based stress reduction in the treatment of sleep disturbance in women with breast cancer: an exploratory study. J Psychosom Res 54:85–91, 2003

Sharma A: Clinical evaluation of the role of Samsodhana and Bhargee Sarkara in the management of bronchial asthma. PhD thesis, National Institute of Ayurveda, Jaipur, India, 2001

Sharma HM, Nidich SI, Sands D, et al: Improvement in cardiovascular risk factors through Panchakarma purification procedures. Journal of Research and Education in Indian Medicine 12:2–13, 1993

Sharma KP, Kushwaha HK, Sharma SS: A placebo-controlled trial on the efficacy of Mentat in managing depressive disorders. Probe 33:26–31, 1993

Sharma R, Chaturvedi C, Tewari PV: Efficacy of *Bacopa monnieri* in revitalising intellectual functions in children. Journal of Research and Education in Indian Medicine 6:1–10, 1987

Shaw D, Leon C, Kolev S, et al: Traditional remedies and food supplements: a 5-year toxicological study (1991–1995). Drug Saf 17:342–356, 1997

Singh B: The Vedic Harappans. Delhi, India, Aditya Prakashan Press, 1995

Singh H, Singh S, Dalal PK, et al: Bacopa monniera extract in elderly subjects with age-associated memory impairment. Indian J Psychiatry 46:66, 2004

Singh RH, Chaturvedi GN: Therapeutic value of Snehapana in the management of peptic ulcer syndrome. Nagurjuna 11:572–578, 1967

Singh RH, Mehta AK: Studies on psychotropic effect of the medhya rasayana drug, shankapushpi (*Convolvulus pluricaulis*), I: clinical studies. Journal of Research in Indian Medicine 12:18–25, 1977

Singh RH, Singh L: Studies on the anti-anxiety effect of the Medhya Rasayana drug Brahmi (*Bacopa monniera Wet.*), part 1. Journal of Research on Ayurveda and Siddha 1:133–148, 1980

Singh RH, Sinha BN: Further studies on the effect of an indigenous compound Rasayana drug on physical and mental disability in aged persons. Journal of Research in Indian Medicine, Yoga and Homeopathy 14:45–50, 1979

Singh RH, Shukla SP, Mishra BK: The psychotropic effect of medhya rasayana drug mandukaparni (*Hydrocotyle asiatica*): an experimental study, part II. Journal of Research in Ayurveda and Siddha 2:1–10, 1981

Singhal DP: India and World Civilization. Ann Arbor, MI, Michigan University Press, 1969

Srivastava JS, Asthana OP, Gupta RC, et al: Double blind placebo controlled randomised study of standardized *Bacopa monniera* extract in children with attention deficit hyperactivity disorder. Indian J Psychiatry 44:28, 2002

Srivastava JS, Asthana OP, Gupta RC, et al: Randomised controlled trial of standardised *Bacopa monniera* extract in subjects with age-associated memory impairment. Indian J Psychiatry 45:49, 2003

Steurer-Stey C, Russi EW, Steurer J: Complementary and alternative medicine in asthma: do they work? Swiss Med Wkly 132:338–344, 2002

Stough C, Lloyd J, Clarke J, et al: The chronic effects of an extract of *Bacopa monniera* (Brahmi) on cognitive function in healthy human subjects. Psychopharmacology (Berl) 156:481–484, 2001

Subbarayappa BV: India's contributions to the history of science, in India's Contribution to World Thought and Culture. Edited by Chandra L. Madras, India, Vivekananda Memorial Committee, 1970, pp 47–66

Svoboda RE: Ayurveda: Life, Health and Longevity. New York, Arkana/Penguin Books, 1992

Svoboda R, Lade A: Tao and Dharma: Chinese Medicine and Ayurveda. Twin Lakes, WI, Lotus Press, 1995

Talageri S: The Rigveda: A Historical Analysis. Delhi, India, Aditya Prakashan Press, 2000

Taneja I, Deepak KK, Poojary G, et al: Yogic versus conventional treatment in diarrhea-predominant irritable bowel syndrome: a randomized control study. Appl Psychophysiol Biofeedback 29:19–33, 2004

Teasdale JD, Segal ZV, Williams JM, et al: Prevention of relapse/recurrence in major depression by mindfulness-based cognitive therapy. J Consult Clin Psychol 68:615–623, 2000

Telner JI, Lapierre YD, Horn E, et al: Rapid reduction of mania by means of reserpine therapy (letter). Am J Psychiatry 143:1058, 1986

Thatte UM, Rege NN, Phatak SD, et al: The flip side of Ayurveda. J Postgrad Med 39:179–182, 1993

Thompson Coon JS, Ernst E: Herbs for serum cholesterol reduction: a systematic review. J Fam Pract 52:468–478, 2003

Thorat S, Dahanukar S: Can we dispense with Ayurvedic samskaras? J Postgrad Med 37:157–159, 1991

Thyagarajan S, Jayaram S, Gopalakrishnan V, et al: Herbal medicines for liver diseases in India. J Gastroenterol Hepatol 17 (suppl 3):S370–S376, 2002

Torsegno M, Zucchi M: Treatment of mental patients with a preparation of the total alkaloids of *Rauwolfia serpentina benth*. Minerva Med 46:604–607, 1955

Trevena L: Sleepless in Sydney: is valerian an effective alternative to benzodiazepines in the treatment of insomnia? ACP J Club A14–A16, 2004

Tripathi JS, Singh RH: Clinical evaluation of smriti sagar rasa in cases of residual schizophrenia. Journal of Research in Ayurveda and Siddha 15:8–16, 1994

Tripathi M, Sundaram R, Rafiq M, et al: Pharmacokinetic interactions of Mentat with carbamazepine and phenytoin. Eur J Drug Metab Pharmacokinet 25:223–226, 2000

Tripathi RK, Singh RH: A clinical study on the management of depressive neurosis with rasayana-vajikarna drugs. Ancient Science of Life 2:220–226, 1983

Trivedi BT: A clinical trial on Mentat. Probe 38:226–228, 1999

Upadhyay SK, Saha A, Bhatia BD, et al: Evaluation of the efficacy of Mentat in children with learning disability: a placebo-controlled double-blind clinical trial. Neurosciences Today 6:184–188, 2002

Urizar NL, Moore DD: GUGULIPID: a natural cholesterol-lowering agent. Annu Rev Nutr 23:303–313, 2003

Vaidya AB, Vaidya RA, Nagaral SI: Ayurveda and a different kind of evidence: from Lord Macaulay to Lord Walton (1835 to 2001 AD). J Assoc Physicians India 49:534–537, 2002

Warrier PK, Nambiar VPK, Ramankutty C (eds): Indian Medicinal Plants: A Compendium of 500 Species, Vols 1–5. Hyderabad, India, Orient Longman, 1993–1996

World Health Organization: International Classification of Diseases, 9th Edition. Geneva, World Health Organization, 1975

World Health Organization: International Classification of Diseases, 10th Edition. Geneva, World Health Organization, 1992

World Health Organization: Traditional Medicine Strategy 2002–2005 (Publ No WHO/ EDM/TRM/2002.1). Geneva, Switzerland, World Health Organization, 2002. Available at: http://hinfo198.tempdomainname.com/medicinedocs/library.fcgi?e=d-0edmweb--00-1-0--010---4----0--0-10l--1en-5000---50-about-0---01131-0011q%28XUy4Jk46bbed8a0000000043ff2b9f-0utfZz-8-0-0&a=d&c=edm-web&cl=CL1.1.11.2&d=Js2297e. Accessed October 6, 2004.

Yadav SK, Jain AK, Tripathi SN, et al: Irritable bowel syndrome: therapeutic evaluation of indigenous drugs. Indian J Med Res 90:496–503, 1989

Yeh GY, Eisenberg DM, Kaptchuk TJ, et al: Systematic review of herbs and dietary supplements for glycemic control in diabetes. Diabetes Care 26:1277–1294, 2003

Ziegler G, Ploch M, Miettinen-Baumann A, et al: Efficacy and tolerability of valerian extract LI 156 compared with oxazepam in the treatment of nonorganic insomnia: a randomized, double-blind, comparative clinical study. Eur J Med Res 7:480–486, 2002

Zisman S, Goldberg D, Veniegas M: Nutritional theory of Ayurveda. Alternative and Complementary Therapies 9:191–197, 2003

Lifestyle and Women's Issues

11

Nutrition

Melanie Hingle, M.P.H., R.D.

A wise healer once said, "Let food be thy medicine and medicine be thy food." This "food as medicine" philosophy of Hippocrates has largely been neglected in modern Western medicine, where a physician's tools are often limited to expertise in advanced surgical techniques and a prescription pad. Although many doctors agree that food choices play an important role in the prevention and treatment of disease, nutrition as a healing modality remains largely overlooked by the conventional medical practitioner.

However, this situation may be about to change. The obesity epidemic and its associated health risks are leading to a revived interest in the role of nutrition in health and well-being. In addition, there is a growing demand for practitioners who are able to offer sound, practical advice to their patients regarding optimal dietary choices in addressing their medical or psychiatric problems. An extensive body evidence supports the role of nutrition in the prevention and treatment of many diseases that are leading causes of morbidity and mortality in industrialized countries, including cardiovascular disease, stroke, diabetes, and cancer. A growing body of scientific evidence also recognizes the use of nutrition therapy in the prevention and management of mental illness.

DIETARY TRENDS AND DISEASE

Most readers will be familiar with the maxim "You are what you eat." This most basic argument for healthy eating rings especially true in today's world of expanding food choices and diminishing food quality. The past century has seen major changes in the way food is produced, processed, and distributed, all of which influence food quality, food choices, and our health. During the twentieth century, a significant increase in the lifetime risk of major psychiatric disorders was observed, a trend that cannot be completely explained by new diagnostic criteria, changes in attitude toward mental illness, reporting bias, or another artifact (Logan 2003; Rogers 2001; Silvers and Scott 2000). However, this increased risk may correlate with a population-wide shift to a more processed and refined diet, suggesting that changes in dietary habits may be causally related to the increased prevalence of many psychiatric disorders. If this hypothesis is borne out, identifying influential dietary factors is an important step in reducing the risk of developing many psychiatric disorders.

THE CONNECTION BETWEEN PHYSICAL AND MENTAL HEALTH

For most medical illnesses, research findings suggest that good nutrition is an effective means of reducing symptoms or slowing disease progression. Despite these findings, the role of diet in the treatment of mental illness remains poorly defined. Researchers have noted that psychiatric illness is often accompanied by physical illness. For example, obesity is common in mentally ill populations. As a result, when treating mentally ill patients, clinicians must consider the health of the patients' body in addition to that of their mind (Rogers 2001). Although mental health problems are clearly related to medical illness and both have known dietary risk factors, the nature of this relation is less clear (i.e., Does poor diet contribute to physical decline, leading to mental illness, or vice versa?). Because physical comorbidities may precede mental illness or occur as direct or indirect results of mental illness, a reasonable approach is to treat physical and psychiatric symptoms concurrently (Rogers 2001).

IDENTIFYING DIETARY RISK FACTORS

The most compelling evidence to date supporting the role of specific nutrients in maintaining mental health is derived from epidemiological and correlational studies, the results of which suggest that certain dietary factors play a key role in mental health, including essential fatty acids (EFAs), carbohydrates, proteins, alcohol, B vitamins, and caffeine. Research findings also point to a strong correlation between obesity and mental health problems. The following sections review these findings and provide guidelines for the application of nutritional counseling in the clinical setting.

Fats and Oils

Adequate intake of fat is essential for survival. Fat has many crucial functions in the body, including facilitation of fat-soluble vitamin absorption, regulation of cholesterol metabolism, maintenance of cell membrane structure, and regulation of the immune response. These last two functions are believed to be the mechanisms by which fats exert their influence on mental health. The main compo-

TABLE 11–1. Dietary sources of essential fatty acids

	α-Linolenic acid (omega-3 family): choose more often	Linoleic acid (omega-6 family): choose less often
Fats and oils	Canola oil, soybean oil, walnuts, flaxseeds, omega-3–enriched margarine	Corn oil, soybean oil, cottonseed oil, sunflower oil, safflower oil, margarine
Proteins	Fish, animals fed omega-3–enriched grains, eggs, grains	Meat, eggs
Carbohydrates	Leafy greens, soybeans and soybean products, fortified cereals	Foods processed with omega-6–rich fats and oils (e.g., chips, cookies, crackers, pastries)

Source. Logan AC: "Neurobehavioral Aspects of Omega-3 Fatty Acids: Possible Mechanisms and Therapeutic Value in Major Depression." *Alternative Medicine Review* 8:410–425, 2003.

nents of all fats are *fatty acids,* which may be saturated, monounsaturated, or polyunsaturated, depending on the presence of carbon-to-carbon double bonds. The body is able to manufacture most of the fats it requires, making it unnecessary for humans to obtain them from their diet. However, two polyunsaturated fatty acids (PUFAs), linoleic acid (LA) and α-linolenic acid (ALA), are termed "essential" because they cannot be manufactured de novo and must therefore be obtained from the diet to prevent deficiency states (Emsley et al. 2003; see also Table 11–1). LA and ALA are the parent molecules of the omega-6 and omega-3 fatty acids, respectively. Both are further metabolized within the body by desaturase enzymes to yield their functional derivatives: ALA is elongated to form eicosapentaenoic acid (EPA) and docosahexanoic acid (DHA), and LA is converted to arachidonic acid (AA) (Silvers and Scott 2002). (See Chapter 7, "Omega-3 Essential Fatty Acids," for a more in-depth discussion of the putative role of EFAs in the prevention and treatment of psychiatric disorders.)

Dietary Trends

The typical North American diet is low in all omega-3 fatty acids, including those derived from fish, leafy green vegetables, soy products, and nuts and seeds, and is high in processed foods, meats, and dairy (Logan 2003). Over the past few decades, this dietary pattern, coupled with a "fat is harmful" mind-set, has led to a population-wide substitution of fat with carbohydrates, resulting in an unfavorable shift in the omega-6–to–omega-3 ratio (Logan 2003; Yehuda 2003) to a current ratio in Western countries of approximately 20:1. This is far from the recommended ratio of 4:1 (or even 1:1) suggested by most researchers and nutritionists and may contribute to the increased incidence of cardiovascular disease, inflammatory disorders, and possibly also certain psychiatric disorders seen in recent decades (Rogers 2001; Simopoulos 2002; Yehuda 2003).

Role in Membrane Structure and Function and Effects on Cognitive Function

Dietary PUFAs—specifically, the EFAs ALA, LA, EPA, and DHA—are the primary determinants of neuronal membrane structure and function. Changes in fatty acid intake, either through an imbalance in the ratio of omega-6 to omega-3 fatty acids consumed or inadequate intake of fats that are metabolized to these fatty acids, have the potential to significantly alter membrane lipid fluidity and thus neuronal function (Logan 2003). Omega-3 and omega-6 EFAs are metabolically distinct in their actions and have opposing physiological effects (Simopoulos 2002). Omega-3 EFAs displace cholesterol from cell membranes, resulting in increased membrane fluidity, whereas omega-6 EFAs redistribute cholesterol, resulting in decreased fluidity (Logan 2003; Yehuda 2003). The relative degree of neuronal membrane fluidity is believed to affect functioning at the level of neurotransmitter receptors. Thus a higher ratio of omega-6 to omega-3 fatty acids is associated with less fluid neuronal membranes and may interfere with normal functioning of neurotransmitter receptors, adversely affecting cognitive functioning and general psychological health (Rogers 2001; Simopoulos 2002). Omega-6 and omega-3 fatty acids are metabolized by the same enzymes; thus the balance of end products, including prostaglandins and their precursors EPA, DHA, and AA, depends on the type and ratio of fats consumed (Silvers and Scott 2002; Simopoulos 2002). In general, a high dietary omega-6–to–omega-3 ratio will result in significant depletion of longer chain omega-3 PUFAs (including EPA and DHA), whereas increased intake of omega-3 relative to omega-6 fatty acids will favor their production (Silvers and Scott 2002).

Carbohydrates and Protein

Research findings and anecdotal reports confirm that individuals with a range of mental health problems typically alter their dietary intake toward increased consumption of carbohydrates (Christensen 1997).

Self-Medication Theory

Several theories have been advanced in efforts to explain the effects of increased carbohydrate consumption on mood; however, few studies support these models. The earliest and most often widely accepted model is the "self-medication" hypothesis (Wurtman and Wurtman 1989). Many researchers have reported an association between the intake of carbohydrate-rich meals or snacks and acute relief of depressed mood (Christensen 1997; Rogers 2001; Wurtman and Wurtman 1989). On the basis of these findings, investigators have theorized that increased carbohydrate intake might represent an individual's attempts to self-medicate in an effort to relieve depressive symptoms (Rogers 2001). The putative mechanism for this effect hinges on evidence suggesting that increased carbohydrate intake increases the synthesis and release of serotonin, which plays a primary regulatory role in mood and behavior (Christensen 1997). Wurtman and Wurtman (1989) proposed that the consumption of proteins and carbohydrates at specific ratios influences brain serotonin levels by altering the availability of tryptophan (the amino acid precursor of serotonin) for uptake into the brain (Rogers 2001). This hypothesis was based on research in tryptophan supplementation and depletion studies in rats and the observation that diet-induced alterations of the ratio of plasma tryptophan to long-chain neutral amino acids led to behavioral changes. High carbohydrate intake was observed to increase this ratio, thus increasing the synthesis of serotonin (Christensen 1997).

The results of human studies on mood-altering effects of tryptophan supplementation or depletion in healthy individuals have been mixed, with most studies not demonstrating any antidepressant effects (Christensen 1997). Conversely, the findings of many studies do not support the self-medication hypothesis, which maintains that variations in protein and carbohydrate intake achieved by eating "real" foods do not affect brain serotonin levels. Even very large differences in carbohydrate and protein intake have failed to produce consistent effects on mood or behavior (Christensen 1997; Rogers 2001).

Others have suggested that if carbohydrate craving is due to decreased brain serotonin, then drugs that increase serotonergic activity should diminish cravings. This hypothesis was tested in trials of fenfluramine, a drug that increases brain serotonin activity (Freedman et al. 2001). Fenfluramine was found to be efficacious in decreasing carbohydrate intake, but its effect was not specific for carbohydrate craving as protein intake was also decreased (Freedman et al. 2001).

Sugar Cravings

Another commonly reported finding in patients who report mental health problems is sugar craving. Many psychiatric patients are overweight or obese because of excessive consumption of refined sugar. These individuals describe frequent, powerful cravings for foods rich in simple carbohydrates, especially refined sugar. This observation has led to speculation about "addictive" carbohydrates and the suggestion that excessive insulin production in some overweight or obese individuals prevents a rise in brain serotonin with carbohydrate intake, thus preventing normal feelings of satiation and resulting in excessive carbohydrate consumption (Freedman et al. 2001). The resulting cycle of craving, consumption, and hyperinsulinemia may be the underlying cause of obesity in psychiatric populations. Although this is a plausible explanation, there are probably many mechanisms by which carbohydrate consumption affects mood. Despite limited data supporting this hypothesis, many individuals describe themselves as "carbohydrate cravers," with some even stating that they have a "natural, overwhelming desire for carbohydrate that doesn't correlate with hunger—a genetic predisposition to carbohydrate craving, which can be reduced by a low-carb diet" (Freedman et al. 2001, p. 16S). Although there is no doubt that the ingestion of carbohydrates diminishes mood symptoms, there is no evidence to support the hypothesis of a genetic predisposition to carbohydrate "craving." Therefore, using this approach to categorize individuals in this manner is unsubstantiated.

A countertheory by Benton and Donohoe (1999) suggests that increased carbohydrate consumption is reinforced by endorphin release after carbohydrate intake, and perhaps even more so after chocolate intake. This hypothesis has been supported by results from animal and human studies, in which the intake of sweets has been shown to be increased by opiate agonists and decreased by antagonists (Benton and Donohoe 1999). Endogenous opiates seem to regulate food intake by modulating the intensity of pleasure associated with good-tasting foods. This mechanism may play a role in eating behavior during periods of stress (Benton and Donohoe 1999). In an interesting finding, regulatory effects of carbohydrate intake on mood have been reported in depressed patients and emotionally stressed individuals (Benton and Donohoe 1999; Christensen 1997).

In summary, many studies have shown that increased carbohydrate intake is associated with improved mood. An alternative theory is that depressed mood stimulates increased consumption of nutrient dense "comfort foods" that are often high in refined sugar and fat (Benton and Donohoe 1999). Although some individuals may be predisposed to craving certain foods, the mechanism by which increased carbohydrate consumption may improve depressed mood remains unclear, and widely discussed models are not supported by convincing empirical findings (Christensen 1997).

Alcohol

Alcohol is a macronutrient, similar to fat, protein, and carbohydrates. Providing 7 cal/g, its energy value is greater than that of carbohydrate and protein (4 cal/g) and less than that of fat (9 cal/g) (Mahan and Escott-Stump 2000). Research findings suggest that alcohol is associated with both negative and positive effects on mental health, depending on the amount of alcohol consumed. Moderate alcohol consumption is associated with decreased risk for cardiovascular disease, and moderate drinkers appear to be at decreased risk for developing dementia later in life (Letenneur et al. 2004). Complete abstinence is associated with slightly increased risk of cardiovascular disease, whereas heavy alcohol use greatly increases risk of developing this type of disease (Letenneur et al. 2004). The definition of "moderate" consumption differs slightly with each study but usually means no more than one drink per day in women and no more than two drinks per day in men.

Mechanism(s) of Action Related to Cognitive Function and Mental Health

It has been suggested that alcohol decreases the risk of developing dementia through its actions on the cardiovascular system, including inhibition of platelet aggregation and beneficial changes in serum lipid profiles (Letenneur et al. 2004). A more direct effect on brain functioning has also been suggested, through the release of acetylcholine in the hippocampus, that facilitates learning and memory (Letenneur et al. 2004).

Alcohol as an Obesity-Inducing Macronutrient

Because of its high energy density and minimal effect on satiety, alcohol consumption may contribute greatly to total caloric intake and is considered by some to be the macronutrient most directly associated with obesity (Saris and Tarnopolsky 2003). Little research evidence supports the view that reducing food intake can compensate for the high levels of calories ingested with alcohol. Alcohol suppresses fatty acid oxidation, increases short-term thermogenesis, and stimulates several neurotransmitters and metabolic pathways implicated in appetite control, perhaps contributing further to overconsumption (Saris and Tarnopolsky 2003). Because of the potential for addiction, individuals who do not consume alcohol should not be encouraged to drink moderately just to obtain its health benefits, and those who drink moderately should not be discouraged from doing so. Moderate drinking has not been shown to be beneficial for mental health problems (Letenneur et al. 2004).

B Vitamins

The hypothesis that a vitamin B deficiency might increase the risk of developing neuropsychiatric problems dates back to the 1950s, when Osmond and Smythies theorized that abnormal methylation reactions taking place in the nervous system were the cause of schizophrenia (Morris 2002). Despite these early observations, prior to the 1980s, few reports appeared in the scientific literature pertaining to a possible relation between vitamin B deficiency and changes in mental status (Morris 2002). More recently, suboptimal intake of B vitamins has been linked to psychiatric syndromes, including minor or severe depressive episodes (Benton and Donohoe 1999). If this relation proves to be valid, current micronutrient recommendations may not adequately prevent poor mental health outcomes.

Recommended Levels of Intake

Dietary reference intakes (DRIs) are recommended levels of intake for essential nutrients. These reference values are an umbrella term that includes recommended dietary allowances, adequate intake, and tolerable upper limit. DRIs are specific to age, stage of life, and sex. These reference values are based on extensive research over many years, the goal of which was to provide the lowest continuing level of intake needed to maintain adequate human nutrition (Food and Nutrition Information Center 2004). It is important to note that these reference values are set to prevent deficiency states in healthy populations and not intended to prevent or treat disease. Therefore, in patients with diagnosed psychiatric disorders, the DRIs should be used as minimum starting points for any diet therapy (Table 11–2). Ensuring adequate intake of essential nutrients by encouraging consumption of foods rich in the specific nutrients is the best place to begin while considering a dietary supplement for the purposes of reaching therapeutic levels on a case-by-case basis. (See Chapter 6, "Nutritional Supplements," for recommendations on nutritional supplementation.)

Mechanism(s) of Action Related to Cognitive Function and Mental Health

The B vitamins (specifically, folate, B_{12}, and B_6) are essential for proper brain function, as they are necessary for one-carbon metabolism reactions in the synthesis of thymidylate and purines (used for nucleic acid synthesis) and methionine (used for protein synthesis and biological methylations) that are crucial biosynthetic pathways for the production of essential neurotransmitters (Selhub et al. 2000). Two separate lines of research regarding B vitamins and affective and cognitive functioning have developed within the last decade: one focusing on the consequences of low folate status and the other on the effects of high blood levels of homocysteine, an endogenously produced, sulfur-containing amino acid (Morris 2002).

There is an association between folate and homocysteine: folate (specifically, N-methyltetrahydrofolate) disposes of homocysteine via remethylation to methionine, a reaction catalyzed by vitamin B_{12} (Morris 2002). The reaction of methionine and adenosinetriphosphatase, catalyzed by the enzyme S-adenosylmethionine synthase, results in the formation of S-adenosyl-L-methionine (SAMe), a universal methyl donor in many biosynthetic reactions essential to normal brain function, including reactions that yield the neurotransmitters norepinephrine, serotonin, and dopamine as well as phospholipids and myelin

(Morris 2002). Therefore, chronic low folate levels can result in a buildup of homocysteine in the blood and neurological and psychological dysfunction due to impaired methylation, leading to decreased production of SAMe (Selhub et al. 2000). Elevated homocysteine levels are also an independent risk factor for atherosclerosis in coronary, cerebral, and peripheral arteries (Rogers 2001). In addition, hyperhomocystinemia has been linked with increased systemic inflammation, an established risk factor in depression and Alzheimer's disease. Because homocysteine is a precursor of the excitotoxic amino acids cysteine and homocysteic acid, it may directly affect neurons, thereby accelerating degeneration (Rogers 2001). To date, results from studies of the possible associations among folate, homocysteine, and psychiatric conditions have served mainly to emphasize the complexity of these relationships and generate hypotheses about mechanisms of action. Limited clinical trial data demonstrate causal relations between folate deficiency and disease states. However, many positive research findings point to the potential mental health benefits of folate (and other B vitamin) supplementation beyond doses traditionally indicated for the prevention of deficiency (Alpert et al. 2000; Morris 2002).

Caffeine

Dietary Sources of Caffeine

Caffeine is often unintentionally omitted from a patient's dietary list unless he or she is specifically asked about caffeine intake. Caffeine is found primarily in beverages, and liquids are generally not considered to be in the same category as solid foods (although they may contain a significant number of calories). It is estimated that over 80% of adults in North America consume caffeine regularly, with an average intake of 200–250 mg/day (the equivalent of a strong 8-oz cup of coffee) (Carrillo and Benitez 2000). The major dietary sources of caffeine are coffee, tea, and colas, although the level of caffeine in these beverages differs depending on the particular bean or leaf used and the method of preparation (Table 11–3).

Mechanism(s) of Action Related to Cognitive Function and Mental Health

Caffeine's significance with regard to mental health problems stems from its generalized excitatory effect on the central nervous system (CNS) and its potential to interact with selected pharmaceuticals. (Although caffeine affects several organ systems, including the cardiovascular, renal, and gastrointestinal systems, the following review focuses only on caffeine's effects on the CNS.) A pharmacological dose of caffeine is considered to be greater than or equal to 200 mg (Carrillo and Benitez 2000). Common side effects at this dose include increased agitation, anxiety, headache, insomnia, irritability, tremor, restlessness, and sensory

TABLE 11–2. Dietary reference intakes and food sources of selected micronutrients

Micronutrient	Dietary reference intake	Upper limit	Food sources
Folate	Men, age 18+ years: 400 µg/day Women, age 18+ years: 400 µg/day Pregnant women: 600 µg/day Lactating women: 500 µg/day	1,000 µg/day	Dark, leafy green vegetables (e.g., spinach, kale, mustard greens, arugula), oranges, lentils, pinto beans, garbanzo beans, asparagus, broccoli, cauliflower, liver, brewer's yeast
Vitamin B$_{12}$	Men, age 18+ years: 2.4 µg/day Women, age 18+ years: 2.4 µg/day Pregnant women: 2.6 µg/day Lactating women: 2.8 µg/day	Not established	Fortified cereal grains and soy products, meat, fish, and poultry
Vitamin B$_6$	Men, age 18+ years: 1.3 mg/day Men, age 50+ years: 1.7 mg/day Women, age 18+ years: 1.3 mg/day Pregnant women: 1.9 mg/day Lactating women: 2.0 mg/day	100 mg/day	Widely distributed; greatest concentrations in meat, especially organ meats, whole grain products or fortified grains, vegetables (potatoes, avocado, brussels sprouts, cauliflower, tomatoes), selected fruits (bananas, prunes, orange juice, apples, dried apricots), selected nuts and seeds (peanuts and peanut butter, sunflower seeds), and fortified soy products
Thiamine	Men, age 18+ years: 1.2 mg/day Women, age 18+ years: 1.1 mg/day Pregnant women: 1.4 mg/day Lactating women: 1.4 mg/day	Not established	Enriched, fortified, or whole grain products; bread and bread products; mixed foods whose main ingredient is grain; ready-to-eat cereals

TABLE 11–2. Dietary reference intakes and food sources of selected micronutrients *(continued)*

Micronutrient	Dietary reference intake	Upper limit	Food sources
Riboflavin	Men age 18+ years: 1.3 mg/day Women age 18+ years: 1.1 mg/day Pregnant women: 1.4 mg/day Lactating women: 1.6 mg/day	Not established	Organ meats, milk, bread, and fortified cereals

Source. Food and Nutrition Information Center 2004; Hendler and Rorvik 2001; Mahan and Escott-Stump 2000.

TABLE 11–3.   Caffeine content of selected foods and beverages

	Caffeine content	Beverage quantity
Coffee		
Decaffeinated	<8 mg	8 oz (liquid)
Ground (brewed)	112–208 mg	
Instant	80–112 mg	
Tea		
Iced	43–50 mg	8 oz (liquid)
Instant	40–56 mg	
Leaf or bag	48–80 mg	
Chocolate		
Chocolate milk	5 mg	1 oz (weight)
Cocoa/hot chocolate	6 mg	
Milk chocolate	6 mg	
Soft drinks		
Coca Cola/Diet Coke	45 mg	12 oz (can)
Dr. Pepper	40 mg	
Diet Rite	36 mg	
Mountain Dew	54 mg	
Pepsi Cola/Diet Pepsi	38 mg	
Royal Crown Cola	36 mg	
Tab	45 mg	
Shasta Cola	44 mg	

Source.   Adapted from Carrillo JA, Benitez J: "Clinically Significant Pharmacokinetic Interactions Between Dietary Caffeine and Medications." *Clinical Pharmacokinetics* 39:127–153, 2000.

disturbances (Carrillo and Benitez 2000). Individuals respond differently to caffeine: some exceed the dose without experiencing adverse effects (thus exhibiting a naturally high tolerance) whereas others report adverse effects at much lower doses. These different response patterns relate to individual levels of the cytochrome enzyme P450 (CYP) 1A2, which metabolizes caffeine and other clinically important drugs, including certain selective serotonin reuptake inhibitors and antipsychotics. Drugs that are metabolized by or bind to the same CYP enzyme have a higher potential for pharmacokinetic interactions due to the inhibition of drug metabolism. Therefore, interactions at the CYP 1A2 enzyme level may cause toxic effects when caffeine is consumed with certain drugs. Because excessive caffeine intake has been observed in psychiatric patients in general, it is important to consider dietary caffeine intake when planning or assessing a patient's response to conventional drug therapy (Carrillo and Benitez 2000). Although caffeine toxicity is rare, it does occur. Signs of toxicity are simply an extension of its pharmacological effects, with the most serious CNS effects including moderately increased heart rate, severe cardiac arrhythmia, and, rarely, delirium and seizures (Carrillo and Benitez 2000).

OBESITY

Relation of Obesity to Cognitive Function and Mental Health

Obesity is common among patients diagnosed with a psychiatric disorder. Potential complications of obesity, including type 2 diabetes, insulin resistance, hyperinsulinemia, dyslipidemia, atherosclerosis, hypertension, and stroke, are among the leading causes of morbidity and mortality in industrialized nations (Rogers 2001). In addition to the adverse effects of obesity on physical health, complications of obesity also include impaired cognitive functioning and diminished psychological well-being. Many studies have established an association between physical health and mental function: Atherosclerosis has been associated with increased risk of cerebral ischemia and stroke, hypo- and hyperglycemic episodes occurring in type 2 diabetes adversely impact acetylcholine neurotransmitter function, hypertension in mid-life is linked with an increased risk of dementia 15–20 years later, and depression is both the strongest predictor of coronary heart disease and a common psychological consequence of obesity (Rogers 2001; Silvers and Scott 2002). Taken together, these data indicate the importance of weight management as a major preventive strategy against cognitive and psychological decline.

Weight Gain With Psychotropic Medications

Most contemporary psychiatric medications cause weight gain, and ultimately obesity, in susceptible individuals (Keck and McElroy 2003; Schwartz et al. 2004) (Table 11–4). On average, psychotropics lead to an average weight gain of 2–17 kg over the course of clinical treatment; however, most of that weight gain is preventable with lifestyle (nutrition and physical activity) modifications (Schwartz et al. 2004). Many studies have shown that the weight gain associated with mood stabilizers, antipsychotics, and antidepressants contributes to medication noncompliance and increased incidence of potentially serious comorbid medical problems, including hypertension, type 2 diabetes, osteoarthritis, stroke, dyslipidemia, atherosclerosis, and sleep apnea (Keck and McElroy 2003; Schwartz et al. 2004). Although antipsychotics and mood stabilizers are associated with the greatest weight gain, antidepressants cause most weight-related

TABLE 11–4.   Average weight gain from psychotropic medications

Medication type	Patients who gain weight (%)	Average weight gain (kg)
Antipsychotics	0–70	0–31
Antidepressants	10–40	5–10
Mood stabilizers	8–71	1–15

Source.   Adapted from Schwartz TL, Nihalani N, Jindal S, et al.: "Psychiatric Medication-Induced Obesity: A Review." *Obesity Review* 5:115–121, 2004.

medical problems in the general population because anxiety and depression are much more common than schizophrenia or bipolar illness. Of the antidepressants, tricyclic antidepressants and monoamine oxidase inhibitors are more likely to cause weight gain than selective serotonin reuptake inhibitors or other newer antidepressants (Schwartz et al. 2004).

Several different mechanisms are thought to contribute to the weight gain associated with psychiatric medications, including direct stimulation of the appetite center of the hypothalamus, indirect insulin-like effects on carbohydrate metabolism, increased thirst (which may be quenched by high-calorie beverages), increased fluid retention and/or edema, and impaired fatty acid metabolism (Keck and McElroy 2003). In summary, clinicians should expect patients to gain weight when they are taking most conventional psychotropic medications, and they should inform their patients of the potential medical risks of increased weight and provide them with basic recommendations about improved nutrition and physical activity.

EVIDENCE SUPPORTING THE USE OF NUTRITION IN PSYCHIATRIC TREATMENT

Major Depressive Disorder

Most data on dietary factors that are related to major depression are obtained from epidemiological studies. Cumulative results suggest that several key nutrients (EFAs, carbohydrates, and folate) may have protective effects.

Omega-3 Essential Fatty Acids

Essential fatty acids play a central role in physical and mental health. This section is a brief summary of current research evidence for the importance of dietary omega-3 EFAs in mental health. (A more thorough review of this subject is provided in Chapter 7, "Omega-3 Essential Fatty Acids.")

Population studies indicate significant differences in the prevalence of major depression across countries that also reflect cross-national trends in mortality from cardiovascular causes. This finding suggests that common dietary risk factors may play a role in both diseases (Hibbeln 1998; Noaghiul and Hibbeln 2003). An analysis of national dietary patterns in relation to international variations in prevalence suggests that an important common dietary risk factor is the intake of fish and other foods rich in omega-3 fatty acids (Peet 2004). Epidemiological studies suggest that fish consumption worldwide is inversely correlated with the prevalence of depression (Silvers and Scott 2002); however, the data are inconsistent (Hakkarainen et al. 2004). Fish consumption is also negatively correlated with the risk of seasonal affective disorder and postpartum depression and predicts improved mental health status in general (Hibbeln 1998; Logan 2003). Although these findings do not prove causation, the hypothesis that fish intake plays a role in reducing the risk of depression is supported by results of clinical studies showing that higher levels of DHA in red-blood cell membranes and higher serum EPA-to-AA ratios are inversely correlated with severity of depressive symptoms (Hibbeln 1998; Noaghiul and Hibbeln 2003). Causal links between certain EFAs and depression are poorly defined, and it is unclear whether changes in lipids are etiologically related to depression or are a result of the neurobiological changes that take place during depression (Bruinsma and Taren 2000). In summary, research findings suggest that regular consumption of omega-3 EFAs (found in fish, soy, leafy greens, and nuts and seeds) should be encouraged in depressed patients (see Table 11–5 for recommendations on fish intake).

Carbohydrates and Proteins

Carbohydrate intake is associated with improved mood in all individuals, and depressed mood often stimulates the consumption of "comfort foods," which are usually rich in carbohydrates and fat (Benton and Donohoe 1999; Christensen 1997). Many theories have been advanced in an effort to explain the possible physiological mechanisms of behavioral effects associated with carbohydrate consumption in humans, but to date there have been no definitive findings (Christensen 1997). If increased carbohydrate intake is beneficial for mood in general, recommendations for carbohydrate consumption probably apply to the public at large (see Table 11–6 for recommendations).

Folate

Epidemiological studies have confirmed earlier observations that folate plays a significant role in mood regulation. A meta-analysis of population studies showed that low folate status is common among depressed patients and that serum folate levels in these patients are significantly lower than those in patients with other psychiatric disorders or in healthy individuals (Morris 2002; Rogers

TABLE 11–5.   Recommended intake of fish based on mercury levels

Fish to avoid	Fish to limit to 1 meal (6–8 oz) per month	Fish to limit to 1 meal (6–8 oz) per week	Fish to limit to 2 meals (6–8 oz) per week
King mackerel, shark, swordfish, tilefish, fish caught in local lakes (unless local advisories have released safety information)	Halibut, marlin, northern lobster, orange roughy, pollock, red snapper, saltwater bass, tuna steaks, wild trout	Cod, crab, haddock, herring, mahi mahi, tuna (canned, white or albacore), whitefish	Clams, crawfish, flounder, oysters, perch, salmon, sardines, scallops, shrimp, sole, tilapia, tuna (canned, "light" and yellowfin)

Note.   Although fish are an important part of a healthy diet and the regular consumption of fish may help to decrease the incidence and severity of mental illness, nearly all fish and shellfish contain traces of mercury. Some fish contain higher amounts of mercury and may be harmful if consumed in excess.
Source.   Santerre 2004; U.S. Environmental Protection Agency 2004.

2001). Elderly and substance-abusing populations are at greatest risk for folate (and other B vitamin) deficiency because of age-related gastric atrophy and inadequate intake, respectively (Selhub et al. 2000). Although it is unclear whether low folate status actually causes depression, antidepressant trials have demonstrated that increasing serum folate levels in depressed patients improves the efficacy of antidepressants and increases response in previously refractory patients (Alpert 2000; Morris 2002). These findings support the view that low folate status is widespread in depressed individuals and that changes in psychological functioning (including changes in mood) are an important indicator of low folate (Benton and Donohoe 1999).

Bipolar Disorder

As with major depressive disorder, there is a robust correlation between increased seafood consumption and reduced prevalence rates of bipolar disorder, thus reinforcing the link between mental health and omega-3 fatty acids (Allison and Weber 2003). Epidemiological studies examining lifetime prevalence rates of bipolar I and bipolar II disorder in several countries have found an association between greater seafood consumption and lower lifetime prevalence rates of all types of bipolar disorder (Noaghiul and Hibbeln 2003). Consistent with these findings, investigators have found lower plasma concentrations of EPA and DHA

TABLE 11–6.   Key dietary recommendations for optimizing mental health

	Recommended quantity	Common food sources	Increase or maintain	Decrease or eliminate
Fats	<30% of total daily calories	Plant and fish oils, animal fats, nuts and seeds, avocados	All sources of omega-3 fats, omega-9 fats (olives, olive oil, avocados), and select omega-6 fats (nuts and seeds, soybean oil)	Refined oils (including corn, sunflower, safflower, and cottonseed oils and margarine) and foods processed with these oils; partially hydrogenated oils; saturated fats from animal foods and palm kernel oil; fried foods
Carbohydrates	45%–65% of total daily calories	Vegetables, fruits, milk, yogurt, legumes, sugar, and sweetened beverages	Whole, minimally processed vegetables, fruits, grains (e.g., high-fiber bread, oats, brown and wild rice, pasta al dente); low-fat, low-sugar dairy and dairy alternatives	Refined carbohydrates, including sugar and processed carbohydrates (pretzels, cookies, chips, crackers, processed baked goods, sweetened cereals and yogurts, sweetened beverages, including most juices and flavored milks)
Protein	10%–30% of total daily calories	Meat, poultry, fish, cheese, eggs, nuts and seeds, legumes	Lean protein (skinless poultry, lean cuts of meat), fish (two times/week), egg whites, low-fat cheese, plant proteins (soy; legumes)	Processed and cured meats (e.g., hot dogs, bologna, salami, pastrami), high-fat cuts of meat, poultry with skin, full-fat dairy, >4 egg yolks/ week

TABLE 11–6. Key dietary recommendations for optimizing mental health *(continued)*

	Recommended quantity	Common food sources	Increase or maintain	Decrease or eliminate
B vitamins	Eat a variety of foods each day to meet or exceed recommended levels of intake for essential nutrients	Various foods and supplements	See Table 11–2 for foods high in B vitamins	None
Antioxidants	Varies	Brightly colored vegetables and fruit, tea, cocoa, olive oil	Brightly colored vegetables and fruit, tea, cocoa, olive oil	None
Alcohol	None to moderate intake (<1 drink/day for women, <2 drinks/day for men[a])	Beer, wine, distilled spirits	No recommendation	Not recommended for those who do not already drink or who have a history of substance abuse
Caffeine	None to moderate intake (<200 mg/day)	Coffee, tea, selected soft drinks, and chocolate	No recommendation	Not recommended for those with sensitivity to caffeine or anxiety disorders

TABLE 11–6. Key dietary recommendations for optimizing mental health *(continued)*

	Recommended quantity	Common food sources	Increase or maintain	Decrease or eliminate
Meal patterns	3–4 meals/snacks per day	Varies	Regular and adequate meals, with emphasis on portion control and macronutrient balance; plan ahead	Skipping meals or inadequate intake; number of meals away from home

aEqual to 12 oz of beer, 5 oz of wine, or 1½ oz distilled spirits.

in patients diagnosed with bipolar disorder compared with in healthy adults. There is limited clinical trial evidence suggesting that the frequency of severe affective episodes is reduced when serum ratios of dietary fatty acids are balanced in favor of omega-3 fatty acids (Noaghiul and Hibbeln 2003; Simopoulos 2002).

Schizophrenia and Other Psychotic Disorders

Few studies have been conducted on dietary factors related to schizophrenia. One ecological analysis of the relation of national dietary patterns and variations in prevalence rates of schizophrenia revealed better long-term outcomes in countries where the average diet is rich in PUFAs (specifically, those from marine and plant sources) compared with countries where saturated fatty acids (from red meat and poultry) are the major sources of fat (Emsley et al. 2003). Other epidemiological data show that higher national dietary intake of refined sugar and dairy products, which are also high in saturated fatty acids, correlated with poor 2-year outcomes in schizophrenic patients (Peet 2004). Case reports and several open-label clinical trials have provided limited support for the putative benefits of omega-3 fatty acids from marine sources (Emsley et al. 2003). To date, much of the research on fatty acids and schizophrenia has been hampered by methodological problems.

Alzheimer's Disease and Other Dementias

Nutrition may play a protective role in Alzheimer's type and other dementias. The associations among dietary factors, vascular health, and dementia are well documented, suggesting that maintaining good physical health throughout life is protective (Selhub et al. 2000). In addition, several specific risk factors are preventable to a certain degree through dietary modifications.

B Vitamin Status

Epidemiological investigations of dietary factors related to dementia show positive correlations between serum levels of certain B vitamins and improved cognitive function (Morris 2002). Population studies have demonstrated correlations between cognitive skills and B vitamin concentration in the serum, leading to the hypothesis that poor B vitamin status may be partially responsible for the cognitive decline frequently seen in elderly individuals (Selhub et al. 2000). However, the role of suboptimal vitamin status in elderly patients in impaired cognitive functioning is unclear (Selhub et al. 2000). Serum homocysteine levels may also be a useful functional indicator of B vitamin status. Abnormally high homocysteine levels correlate with low B_{12} levels and are associated with increased risk of vascular disease, stroke, and thrombosis (Selhub et al. 2000). More recent studies on homocysteine and vascular disease suggest that in addition to increasing risk for vascular disease, homocysteine exerts an independent toxic effect on neurons (Selhub et al. 2000). Taken together, these findings suggest that B vitamin status plays a central role in normal cognitive function. A specific concern among elderly individuals is the high prevalence (20%–50%) of atrophic gastritis with hypochlorhydria, which impairs release of B_{12} from food and interferes with its absorption, resulting in increased homocysteine levels (Selhub et al. 2000). Low levels of several B vitamins (especially B_{12}) result in reduced synthesis of methionine and SAMe, which indirectly interferes with the biosynthesis of myelin, several neurotransmitters (including dopamine, norepinephrine, and serotonin), and membrane phospholipids (Nourhashemi et al. 2000).

Oxidative Stress

Some research findings suggest that oxidative stress and free radicals play a significant role in the pathophysiology of dementia by increasing lipid peroxidation and accelerating neuronal degeneration (Nourhashemi et al. 2000). Population studies have demonstrated correlations between preserved cognitive functioning in elderly subjects and intake of antioxidants—specifically, vitamin C, vitamin E, folate, beta-carotene, and various flavonoids. These antioxidants are found in abundance in colorful vegetables, fruits, nuts, seeds, and tea (Rogers 2001). Clinical trials on the protective effects of antioxidants have been inconclusive, and potentially therapeutic doses are not clearly defined.

Inflammation

Autopsy studies suggest that inflammation is an important factor contributing to neuronal loss. Many population studies suggest that regular use of anti-inflammatory drugs reduces the risk for Alzheimer's disease. Further, increased omega-3 fatty acid intake is associated with reduced cardiovascular disease risk (including reduced risk of thrombosis, reduced inflammatory responses, reduced blood pressure, and improved insulin sensitivity) and general beneficial effects on cognitive functioning (Nourhashemi et al. 2000; Rogers 2001).

Alcohol

Moderate alcohol consumption (especially red wine) is probably protective against both Alzheimer's type and other dementias, although more studies are needed to confirm the strength of this association (Letenneur et al. 2004; Nourhashemi et al. 2000). The J-shaped curve representing alcohol consumption and dementia incidence looks similar to that depicting the relationship between alcohol consumption and cardiovascular risk. Cohort studies examining alcohol and dementia risk in elderly individuals suggest that the most significant risk reduction takes place in light-to-moderate drinkers (1–3 drinks per day) compared with those who do not drink (Letenneur et al. 2004).

Treatment of Obesity and Overweight Patients

Most Americans are trying to lose or maintain weight (Freedman et al. 2001). Despite this fact, the percentage of obese Americans continues to increase at an alarming pace. Reasons for the obesity epidemic are believed to be primarily environmental: increased availability of high-energy foods combined with decreased physical activity. Restaurant portions have also grown noticeably larger within the past decade, and more of today's income is spent on eating food away from home (Peters et al. 2002). Relatively ineffective biological mechanisms have evolved in humans to protect them against overeating. Therefore, maintaining optimal body weight often requires deliberate planning and motivation. Many who do not invest considerable time and energy experience gradual weight gain (Peters et al. 2002).

Research findings suggest that several simple approaches may help reverse the trend in obesity. Palatability and energy density are the major determinants of energy intake in animals and humans (McCrory et al. 2000; Saris and Tarnopolsky 2003). Energy density is based largely on energy content per gram of ingredients and water content of the food product; thus low-energy, high-water foods (e.g., vegetables, fruits, whole grains) typically have the desired effects on satiety without the extra calories. Dietary variety also is a predictor of relative body fat, but the strength of the association depends on which food groups are consumed for variety (e.g., fruits and vegetables are associated with decreased body fat, whereas sweets, snacks, condiments, entrees, and refined carbohydrates are associated with increased body fat) (McCrory et al. 2000). These findings suggest that diets that are abundant in vegetables and fruit but include few other foods may reduce total energy intake and ultimately prevent obesity or reduce weight in obese people. How often meals are consumed outside of the home is correlated with relative body fat independently of educational level, smoking status, alcohol intake, and physical activity (McCrory et al. 2000).

Research findings indicate that factors such as appearance and physical comfort play a central role in determining personal weight goals; this is significant because most clinicians emphasize desired changes in a medical condition or weight as the main motivator over these personal factors (Freedman et al. 2001). It is essential to choose a treatment approach that is in line with the patient's expectations. Data documenting successful long-term and clinically meaningful weight loss are available, most notably from the Diabetes Prevention Program and the National Weight Control Registry. The Diabetes Prevention Program has provided compelling evidence for the health benefits of "small" weight losses (5%–10% of total body weight), previously dismissed as trivial by many health practitioners. Subjects who lost less than 8 kg of body weight (and on average maintained less than 4 kg of body weight loss) experienced a 58% reduction in the incidence of new-onset diabetes (Allison and Weber 2003). The National

Weight Control Registry is a good example of a cohort that is at risk for weight gain while maintaining healthy weight. The registry tracks individuals who have succeeded in maintaining at least a 13.6-kg weight loss for at least 1 year and is an excellent observational data set pertaining to individuals who maintain weight loss. Although there are many approaches to weight loss, most programs share several common features, including training directed at deliberately restricting food intake, adopting a low-fat diet, and engaging in moderate to high levels of physical activity on a regular basis (Peters et al. 2002).

CONCLUSION: WRITING A DIETARY PRESCRIPTION

Optimal nutritional status can be thought of as a balance between nutrient requirements and nutrient intake. Each person has unique nutrient requirements, and there is no "one-size-fits-all" approach when advising patients about appropriate changes in nutrition. Nutritional requirements are influenced by many factors, including physiological stressors (e.g., infection, disease, fever, trauma), psychological stressors, stage of life (e.g., pregnancy, growth), genetics, physical activity, and body composition (Mahan and Escott-Stump 2000). Individual choices in nutrient intake are also influenced by socioeconomic status, learned eating behaviors, emotional state, cultural influences, and overall health status (Mahan and Escott-Stump 2000). In view of these issues, when recommending specific dietary changes, it is important to consider the patient's nutrient requirements and preferred intake patterns.

Generally speaking, there is no single best "diet" for optimal health; instead, a reasonable pattern of eating that includes an abundance of fresh vegetables and whole grains, low-to-moderate amounts of unrefined fats and oils, and lean protein choices should be encouraged. The Mediterranean pattern of eating meals rich in vegetables, fruit, legumes, whole grains, lean meats, and fish and using heart-healthy fats and oils, with only a moderate consumption of animal fats and sweets, has been widely embraced as the gold standard. Dietary advice should emphasize the importance of obtaining adequate amounts of omega-3 fatty acids from oily fish, flaxseed oil, and other plant sources while decreasing the relative intake of omega-6 fatty acids, saturated fats, and trans fatty acids (found mostly in animal foods, processed foods, and refined oils). Weight management recommendations should ideally focus on realistic dietary goals that are acceptable to the patient and, whenever possible, include increased physical activity (see Chapter 12, "Physical Activity, Exercise, and Mental Health," for recommendations).

The findings reviewed in this chapter suggest that several important dietary factors significantly impact mental health and that dietary changes probably improve outcomes in many cases. All long-term dietary recommendations must be acceptable to the patient and should be tailored to the patient's unique lifestyle and personal preferences. When advising patients about dietary changes in the context of addressing a mental health problem, it is reasonable to begin with a few basic dietary recommendations (see Table 11–6). When there is not enough time to thoroughly evaluate a patient's nutritional status and discuss with the patient implications of poor nutrition on mental health, a referral to a registered dietitian or other health professional trained in the clinical management of nutrition will ensure that the patient will be informed about important nutritional factors affecting his or her mental health and will be provided with a realistic dietary plan.

REFERENCES

Allison DB, Weber MT: Treatment and prevention of obesity: what works, what doesn't work, and what might work. Lipids 38:147–155, 2003

Alpert JE, Mischoulon D, Nierenberg AA, et al: Nutrition and depression: focus on folate. Nutrition 16:544–581, 2000

Benton D, Donohoe RT: The effects of nutrients on mood. Public Health Nutr 2:403–409, 1999

Bruinsma KA, Taren DL: Dieting, essential fatty acid intake, and depression. Nutr Rev 58:98–108, 2000

Carrillo JA, Benitez J: Clinically significant pharmacokinetic interactions between dietary caffeine and medications. Clin Pharmacokinet 39:127–153, 2000

Christensen L: The effect of carbohydrates on affect. Nutrition 13:503–514, 1997

Emsley R, Oosthuizen P, van Rensburg SJ: Clinical potential of omega-3 fatty acids in the treatment of schizophrenia. CNS Drugs 17:1081–1091, 2003

Food and Nutrition Information Center: Dietary Reference Intakes (DRI) and Recommended Dietary Allowances (RDA). Available at: www.nal.usda.gov/fnic/etext/000105.html. Accessed August 11, 2004.

Freedman MR, King J, Kennedy E: Popular diets: a scientific review. Obes Res 9 (suppl 1): 1S–40S, 2001

Hakkarainen R, Partonen T, Haukka J, et al: Is low dietary intake of omega-3 fatty acids associated with depression? Am J Psychiatry 161:567–569, 2004

Hendler SS, Rorvik D (ed): PDR for Nutritional Supplements, 1st Edition. Montvale, NJ, Thomson PDR, 2001

Hibbeln JR: Fish consumption and major depression. Lancet 351:1213, 1998

Keck PE, McElroy SL: Bipolar disorder, obesity, and pharmacotherapy-associated weight gain. J Clin Psychiatry 64:1426–1435, 2003

Letenneur L, Larrieu S, Barberger-Gateau P: Alcohol and tobacco consumption as risk factors of dementia: a review of epidemiological studies. Biomed Pharmacother 58:95–99, 2004

Logan AC: Neurobehavioral aspects of omega-3 fatty acids: possible mechanisms and therapeutic value in major depression. Altern Med Rev 8:410–425, 2003

Mahan LK, Escott-Stump S (eds): Krause's Food Nutrition and Diet Therapy, 10th Edition. Pennsylvania, PA, WB Saunders, 2000

McCrory MA, Fuss PJ, Saltzman E, et al: Dietary determinants of energy intake and weight regulation in healthy adults. J Nutr 130:276S–279S, 2000

Morris MS: Folate, homocysteine, and neurological function. Nutr Clin Care 5:124–132, 2002

Noaghiul S, Hibbeln JR: Cross-national comparisons of seafood consumption and rates of bipolar disorders. Am J Psychiatry 160:2222–2227, 2003

Nourhashemi F, Gillette-Buyonnet S, Andrieu S, et al: Alzheimer disease: protective factors. Am J Clin Nutr 71 (suppl):643S–649S, 2000

Peet M: International variations in the outcome of schizophrenia and the prevalence of depression in relation to national dietary practices: an ecological analysis. Br J Psychiatry 184:404–408, 2004

Peters JC, Wyatt HR, Donahoo WT, et al: From instinct to intellect: the challenge of maintaining healthy weight in the modern world. Obes Rev 3:69–74, 2002

Rogers PJ: A healthy body, a healthy mind: long-term impact of diet on mood and cognitive function. Proc Nutr Soc 60:135–143, 2001

Santerre CR: Fish for your health. Family Nutrition Program, Purdue University, Indiana Fishing Advisory. Available at: http://fn.cfs.purdue.edu/anglingindiana. Accessed August 19, 2004.

Saris WHM, Tarnopolosky MA: Controlling food intake and energy balance: which macronutrient should we select? Curr Opin Clin Nutr Metab Care 6:609–613, 2003

Schwartz TL, Nihalani N, Jindal S, et al: Psychiatric medication-induced obesity: a review. Obes Rev 5:115–121, 2004

Selhub J, Bagley LC, Miller J, et al: B vitamins, homocysteine, and neurocognitive function in the elderly. Am J Clin Nutr 71 (suppl):514S–520S, 2000

Silvers KM, Scott KM: Fish consumption and self-reported physical and mental health status. Public Health Nutr 5:427–431, 2002

Simopoulos AP: Omega-3 fatty acids in inflammation and autoimmune diseases. J Am Coll Nutr 21:495–505, 2002

U.S. Environmental Protection Agency: What You Need to Know About Mercury in Fish and Shellfish. Available at: www.epa.gov/waterscience/fishadvice/advice.html. Accessed August 11, 2004.

Wurtman RJ, Wurtman JJ: Carbohydrates and depression. Scientific American 260:50–57, 1989

Yehuda S: Omega-6/omega-3 ratio and brain-related functions, in Omega-6/Omega-3 Essential Fatty Acid Ratio: The Scientific Evidence. Edited by Simopoulos AP, Cleland LG. World Review of Nutrition and Dietetics, Vol 92. Basel, Switzerland, Karger, 2003, pp 37–56

12

Physical Activity, Exercise, and Mental Health

Robert B. Lutz, M.D., M.P.H.

The interdependent roles of the mind and the body in health and illness have been recognized for thousands of years. Although Renaissance philosophy postulated an artificial separation between mind and body that influenced medical thought and practice into modern times, in more recent times there has been renewed appreciation of their interconnectivity. In 1947, the World Health Organization (WHO) proposed a working definition of health as "a state of complete physical, social and mental well-being, and not merely the absence of disease or infirmity" (World Health Organization 1947). The WHO Ottawa Charter on Health Promotion modified this definition to a more functional working one: "Health is a resource for everyday life, not the object of living. It is a positive concept emphasizing social and personal resources as well as physical capabilities" (World Health Organization 1986, p. 1). Further parsing of this concept has seen the term *wellness* come into common use. Wellness has been defined as a "multidimensional state of being describing the existence of positive health in an individual as exemplified by quality of life and a sense of well-being" (Corbin and Pangrazi 2001). Experts agree that both physical and mental health are fundamental to achieving this state.

Research on the health-related benefits of physical activity and exercise has historically focused primarily on the physiological benefits of exercise. It is widely acknowledged that exercise lowers risk for cardiovascular disease, ischemic stroke, type 2 diabetes, some cancers (e.g., colon cancer, breast cancer), osteoporosis, depression and anxiety, and fall-related injuries. Additional benefits include improved muscular strength, flexibility, and agility; increased bone density; improved lipid profiles; enhanced immune function; and improved insulin

301

levels (U.S. Department of Health and Human Services 1996). The multidimensional nature of health, however, requires a broader interpretation of the potential benefits of physical activity and exercise. Attending to emotional, mental, and spiritual health is just as important as—and, for some, more important than—addressing physical health. This interpretation of health provides a conceptual foundation for evaluating the role of physical activity and exercise in mental health and is consistent with the guiding philosophy of integrative medicine that "engages the mind, spirit, and community as well as the body...to stimulate the body's innate healing" (Gaudet 1998, p. 67).

Nonetheless, it is important to acknowledge that current models of the relation between exercise and mental health are limited. Research conducted over the past two decades has addressed this issue in mostly broad terms (Fox 1999); research that examines a specific kind of physical activity will probably not provide an adequate understanding of an individual's health and well-being. Healthy and unhealthy behaviors are linked in every person to affect overall physical and mental health. *Healthy lifestyles,* currently defined as including physical activity, good diet, no smoking, moderation of alcohol use, and safe sexual practices, could also include stress management, spiritual practices, and social connection, to name a few. To date, minimal research has looked at complex healthy and unhealthy behaviors and their combined influence on health. The acknowledged importance of physical activity and exercise for general good health and well-being makes this an important area of continuing research, with the goal of improving the quality of life of all individuals affected by mental illness.

PHYSICAL ACTIVITY AND MENTAL HEALTH DISORDERS

Research into the relation of physical activity and exercise to mental health has explored a number of possible biological mechanisms; it is likely that any association is multifactorial. In integrative medicine, which follows a whole-person approach to health care, physical activity and exercise recommendations are often important components of interventions aimed at improving the health and well-being of individuals who have a mental illness.

The health benefits of physical activity and exercise have historically been researched from a physiological and/or a medical viewpoint, with recommendations being presented as health and fitness guidelines. Although these recommendations may lead to physical benefit for those who follow them, they may not adequately address the whole person or may fail to take into account the context or "behavior setting" in which a patient is being encouraged to undertake a new health-promoting behavior. As such, most health and fitness guidelines are inherently limited in their beneficial effect and often fall short of providing the necessary stimulus for behavior change.

A challenge confronting exercise researchers is identifying the specific aspects of physical activity that provide the recognized benefits. Questions such as the optimal type of activity (aerobic versus resistance), quantity or dose (frequency, intensity, duration), quality of exercise, and appropriate stage of an individual's life to perform certain types of physical activities (life stage versus lifelong) continue to be the focus of research. It is therefore not surprising that research defining the relation between exercise and mental health continues to evolve as new information comes to light.

To date, the mental health benefits of exercise have been identified with regard to aerobic activities as well as resistance and flexibility training forms of activity (Dunn et al. 2001). These effects appear to be independent of the fitness level achieved (Craft and Landers 1998). Research suggests that continuous activity of moderate intensity (e.g., 30 minutes/day) may be more beneficial for mental health than intermittent bouts of physical activity (e.g., three periods of 10 minutes/day) (Osei-Tutu and Campagna 1998). However, it is important to keep in mind that the general health-related benefits of exercise can be achieved through the current public health guidelines (a cumulative total of 30 minutes or more of moderate-intensity physical activity on most, and preferably all, days of the week) (U.S. Department of Health and Human Services 1996). Estimates of health-related quality of life, as indicated by the number of days in the past month during which mental and physical health were not good, roughly correspond to these general recommendations. Individuals who have achieved these goals have reported fewer "unhealthy" days compared with inactive or insufficiently active people. However, daily exercising and participation in short bouts (less than or equal to 20 minutes/day) or extended bouts of exercise (more than or equal to 90 minutes/day) have been associated with poorer quality of life (Brown et al. 2004). These data speak of the methodological problems inherent in efforts to determine a dosage-response relation between physical activity and depression (i.e., Is there a relation between lower levels of depression and higher levels of physical activity?) (Dunn et al. 2001; Farmer et al. 1988; Paffenbarger et al. 1994).

Epidemiological research generally supports an association of physical activity and exercise with mental health (Paluska and Schwenk 2000). This link has been most clearly identified in mood disorders (i.e., mild-to-moderate depression and anxiety). However, there is currently little available research that has looked at the effect of exercise, whether for preventive or therapeutic purposes, in other types of mental illness. In a single intervention study, patients with schizophrenia, bipolar disorder, or major depression were compared with waiting list control subjects and light exercisers; those individuals who ran three times per week demonstrated decreased depression and improved fitness. However, the researchers did not analyze the results by subgroup to differentiate response (Hannaford and Harrell 1988). In theory, most patients would benefit from being physically active, as low fitness levels are commonly found in individuals with mental illness (Paluska and Schwenk 2000). In addition, if the proposed neurobiochemical mechanisms are the primary mediators for the mood-enhancing effects of exercise, then physical activity would be beneficial in patients with many mental illnesses, as they often demonstrate dysregulation of these neurotransmitters (Meyer and Broocks 2000).

Physical Activity and Mood Disorders

In research on exercise and depression, intervention studies have used various study designs for both intervention and measurement of the effect of exercise on depression levels. Although such studies often yield evidence of the positive effect of exercise, they have been plagued by methodological weaknesses that challenge their interpretation (Craft and Landers 1998; Lawlor and Hopker 2001). Different groups of researchers have studied clinically depressed and nonclinically depressed individuals and have likewise looked at different exercise modalities (i.e., aerobic versus resistance), leading to a wide array of findings. The limitations of these studies must be recognized when reviewing the available literature.

Depressed individuals are commonly less active and have poorer fitness levels than nondepressed individuals. Therefore, it is not surprising that cross-sectional studies looking at physically inactive or sedentary individuals have often demonstrated an inverse relation with incidence rates of depression (Farmer et al. 1988). Depression may serve as an explanation for physical inactivity in some individuals. Conversely, individuals who become inactive may demonstrate a greater likelihood of experiencing depression (Camacho et al. 1991).

For individuals with a mood disorder, most of the research has focused on mild-to-moderate depression. Some research has suggested that the benefits of exercise may be equally or more effective than those of pharmaceuticals as well as more rapid in the onset of effects (Babyak et al. 2000; Blumenthal et al. 1999). Likewise, a classic study by Greist et al. (1978) suggested that exercise was equally as effective as psychotherapy for treating depression. In the few studies looking at major depression, rating scales (e.g., Hamilton Rating Scale for Depression [Ham-D)], Beck Depression Inventory) rather than clinical measures have been used to define outcomes (Babyak et al. 2000). A meta-analysis looking at individuals of varying ages and both sexes found significantly decreased depressive symptoms reported after short and prolonged exercise (Craft and Landers 1998). These results were most significant in patients with the most severe depression and/or those receiving psychological therapy.

Recently published findings by Dunn et al. (2005) demonstrated that regular aerobic exercise performed at levels consistent with public health recommendations significantly improved mood in mild and moderate depression. In this 12-week intervention study, men and women ages 20–45 years were randomized to one of four exercise protocols that varied in total energy expenditure and frequency. All participants had been diagnosed with major depressive disorder and met criteria for mild or moderate depressed mood based on the 17-item Ham-D. At the end of the intervention, 46% of the individuals who achieved public health guideline levels of exercise (exercising 3 or 5 days per week, with total energy expenditure equivalent to 17.5 kcal [chempoint] kg^{-1} [chempoint] $week^{-1}$) demonstrated a greater than 50% reduction in their Ham-D scores and 42% achieved complete remission of their depressive symptoms. The finding that both 3 and 5 days of activity produced similar results suggests that total energy expenditure during aerobic activity is the most important factor in symptom reduction and remission.

Physical activity and exercise may benefit diverse populations of depressed individuals (Shepard 1995). Adolescents have been found to demonstrate positive affective responses to exercise (Calfas and Taylor 1994; Steptoe and Butler 1996). Likewise, research has demonstrated that older adults who are active may experience less depression (King et al. 1993). Cross-sectional data from a 5-year ancillary study of older individuals who participated in the Alameda County Study, a longitudinal study of health and mortality that followed a cohort of more than 6,000 individuals from 1965, demonstrated a protective effect of physical activity on depression. This association was identified even in subjects who had physical disabilities, as do many elderly individuals. No differences in the association between physical activity and depression were identified by age or ethnicity (Strawbridge et al. 2002). Three community-based longitudinal studies, however, found no preventive benefits from physical activity related to risk for depression (Cooper-Patrick et al. 1997; Lennox et al. 1990; Weyerer 1992); two of these studies (Cooper-Patrick et al. 1997; Lennox et al. 1990) reported results in only men. In addition, in one study (Weyerer 1992), exercise was defined as "sports," which would underreport the amount of activity by failing to capture participation in physical activities such as walking and gardening that are commonly found to be performed by large numbers of senior citizens.

Bhui and Fletcher (2000) suggested that physical activity has different effects on mood based on a person's sex. In that study, the researchers found that although the unadjusted analysis identified a strong inverse association between physical activity for both men and women, adjustment for demographic confounders (age, disability, medication, smoking status, income, and employment status) found statistically significant results for only men. Specifically, men who were regularly active in low-level exercise for periods in excess of an average of 92 minutes per day demonstrated lower odds of self-reported depression than women who were similarly active. The authors, in recognizing the limitations of their cross-sectional study, found their female cohort to be less physically active overall and to participate in lower-intensity activities, consistent with what has been previously reported in the literature. A randomized, controlled study of sedentary premenopausal women enrolled in a 15-week moderate aerobic exercise program reported improvements in global well-being but no improvement in mood as measured by the Profile of Mood States (Cramer et al. 1991).

Physical Activity and Anxiety Disorders

Both acute and chronic exercise have been evaluated for their effects on acute (state) and chronic (trait) anxiety, with most researchers focusing on aerobic activity. As noted with research in major depression, outcome measures have often been reported using rating scales (Profile of Mood States, Spielberger State-Trait Anxiety Inventory) rather than clinical measures. Study results have indicated that acute bouts of activity are associated with moderate benefits for state anxiety symptoms (Paluska and Schwenk 2000). Causality has not been determined, however (Petruzzello et al. 1991). Aerobic activity has demonstrated a larger effect than resistance or flexibility training programs (Paluska and Schwenk 2000). Exercise programs of varying durations have been shown to have a moderate effect on acute and chronic forms of anxiety (Osei-Tutu and Compagna 1998). Exercise interventions lasting for more than 20 minutes per session for a minimum of 10 weeks affected trait anxiety, with a maximum benefit being seen after 40-minute sessions (Osei-Tutu and Compagna 1998; Petruzzello 1991).

Individuals with panic disorder have historically been discouraged from participating in exercise programs due to the belief that aerobic activity could trigger panic attacks. Exercise avoidance has been an important component of panic disorder treatment; interviews with panic disorder patients have indicated that these patients are concerned that exercise could precipitate a heart attack or other serious cardiac problems (Zimetbaum and Josephson 1998). However, controlled exercise programs have been found to be equally efficacious to medication therapy in this population (Brooks et al. 1998). Although there has been minimal research in this area, the available evidence suggests that exercise and physical activity improve the symptoms of panic disorder without necessarily triggering attacks.

Physical Activity and Cognitive Impairment

The aging of the American population has led to increased rates of cognitive impairment on a continuum from mild senescent forgetfulness to Alzheimer's disease. This demographic trend renders efforts to prevent cognitive impairment of great importance. The role of physical activity and exercise in the prevention of cognitive decline is an area of considerable research interest. Hippocampal degeneration is associated with cognitive decline and especially memory loss (MacQueen et al. 2003); it may also be associated with mood disorders, including major depressive disorder, a common finding in cognitively impaired individuals (Sheline et al. 2003). Animal models have demonstrated many benefits of exercise on brain function (Gomez-Pinilla et al. 1998), including stimulation of neural growth factors in the hippocampus (Gomez-Pinilla 1997). Increased cerebral blood flow has also been postulated as the physiological basis for the potential benefits of exercise on cognitive functioning (Singh 2004). Cardiovascular and peripheral vascular disease decrease cerebral blood flow and cerebral oxygenation and thus increase the risk of ischemic cerebrovascular accidents (stroke).

To date, the research evidence for a relation between physical activity and improved cognitive functioning is mixed (Larson and Wang 2004). However, recent findings are encouraging. Data from the Canadian Study of Health and Aging, a large prospective, longitudinal study, showed that physical activity is correlated with lower rates of cognitive impairment with no dementia, Alzheimer's disease, and dementia of any type. After adjustment for age, sex, and education, a trend was noted between higher levels of physical activity and the absence of cognitive impairment with no dementia (odds ratio [OR] = 0.58, 95% confidence interval [CI] = 0.41–0.83), Alzheimer's disease (OR = 0.50, 95% CI = 0.28–0.90), and dementia of any type (OR = 0.63, 95% CI = 0.40–0.98). This finding was most robust for women; the same trend was also observed in men, but did not reach statistical significance (Laurin et al. 2001). The Monongahela Valley Independent Elders Survey evaluated the association between physical activity and cognitive decline by examining the relation of self-reported exercise levels and results from the Mini-Mental State Examination. Volunteers were followed longitudinally, with data being collected at 2-year intervals. Using a multiple regression model (adjusted for age, sex, education, previous level of cognitive function, and self-rated health), the researchers found an inverse relation between physical activity and cognitive decline. Compared with no exercise, there was an inverse relation between exercise frequency and cognitive decline in individuals who engaged in physical activity at least 5 days/week (as suggested by the U.S. Surgeon General's guidelines) (Lytle et al. 2004).

Exercise training also benefits depressed elderly individuals without dementia (Blumenthal et al. 1999; Mather et al. 2002). Because of the high comorbidity of depression with dementia, the added benefits of increased physical activity for these individuals are very significant. Teri et al. (2003) demonstrated that a program combining exercise training with caregiver behavioral management techniques effectively improved physical health measures and depressive symptoms in individuals with Alzheimer's disease.

The benefits of physical activity and exercise on health and well-being are widely acknowledged. In view of the above research findings on the benefits of increased activity in cognitively impaired individuals, it is reasonable to conclude that regular physical activity has many health-related benefits. The knowledge that simple activities (e.g., walking) may lessen cognitive impairment (Teri et al. 2003) should encourage health care providers to routinely recommend increased physical activity to their patients.

POSSIBLE MECHANISMS FOR BENEFICIAL EFFECTS OF PHYSICAL ACTIVITY

Different psychological and physiological mechanisms have been suggested to explain the indirect and direct benefits of physical activity on mental health and general well-being. However, to date, research has not satisfactorily determined the exact nature of this relation. It is likely that multiple etiologies interact synergistically and have varying influences on mental health on a case-by-case basis. Likewise, the intensity and duration of activity as well as environmental factors probably play important roles.

The well-recognized benefits of exercise on physical health, such as lowering the risk of developing cardiovascular disease and type 2 diabetes, probably result in an improved sense of health that positively affects overall quality of life and an individual's subjective sense of well-being. However, improved fitness that is achieved through exercise has not been demonstrated to have a strong relation to changes in mood (Craft and Landers 1998). A perceived sense of physical improvement that is experienced as an individual's body appearance changes (e.g., weight loss, increased muscle tone) has been shown to affect self-esteem and self-perception, which in turn has positive influences on mental health (Fox 1997). Reviews suggest an inconsistent relation between physical activity and global self-esteem and underscore the notion that self-esteem is affected by multiple factors (Spence and Poon 1997).

The "distraction hypothesis" suggests that an individual who is distracted from unpleasant situations through exercise may experience enhanced mood. Although this hypothesis has been challenged (Yeung 1996), it may account for some of the psychological short-term benefits achieved with exercise.

Bandura's self-efficacy theory has also been suggested as contributing to the relation of physical activity and an improved sense of well-being (Marcus et al. 1992). Self-efficacy for being active may enhance an individual's mood by giving individuals the sense that they can successfully handle the physical challenges that confront them. Although self-efficacy is behavior specific, it has been suggested that achieving improved self-perception may enhance well-being (Petruzzello et al. 1991).

Social support and interaction may positively affect an individual's mood. Although studies have not consistently found that social interaction is a significant contributor to the relation between activity and mental health (Glenister 1996), it probably plays a role. For example, for a person who is just beginning to exercise but lacks self-motivation, encouragement from others may be very helpful.

An important indirect benefit of physical activity is improved sleep. Poor sleep quality significantly impacts mental health and is strongly associated with poor work performance and diminished psychological resiliency (National

Commission on Sleep Disorders Research 1993). Epidemiological data have suggested that daylight exercise is the behavior most closely associated with improved sleep quality (Youngstedt et al. 1997). Although it is a common perception that vigorous physical activity close to bedtime adversely affects sleep, this has not been borne out by surveys and observational reports (Urponen et al. 1988; Youngstedt et al. 1999).

Much has been written about the endorphin hypothesis and its role in exercise (Thoren et al. 1990). Although many athletes search for the "runner's high," this experience is rarely felt by most people who exercise (Dishman 1997). Prolonged exercise may enhance the release of endorphins (Dishman 1997), but how endorphins affect mood states has not yet been clearly defined. Challenging this putative mechanism is the finding that endorphin antagonists (e.g., naloxone) do not alter exercise-induced improvements in mood (Yeung 1996). It is possible that methodological issues, different criteria used to define the "runner's high," and the measurement of peripheral rather than central endorphin levels have confounded research findings in this area.

Another group of neurotransmitters that has been studied in relation to exercise is the monoamines: norepinephrine, dopamine, and serotonin. All three neurotransmitters play an important role in mood regulation. The "monoamine hypothesis" proposes that exercise enhances the release of monoamines, thus increasing arousal and attentiveness (Chaouloff 1997; Dishman 1997). This hypothesis is supported by studies demonstrating that urinary excretion of amines is increased after exercise (Dunn and Dishman 1991). Although this hypothesis is plausible, it requires further research including direct measurement of brain monoamines.

INTEGRATIVE RECOMMENDATIONS

At present, there is limited evidence to suggest that counseling by health care providers has beneficial effects on physical activity performance (U.S. Preventive Services Task Force 2004). However, there is considerable evidence supporting the statement that physical activity and exercise positively affect morbidity and mortality associated with chronic disease and may serve as a first-line therapy and protection against many chronic health conditions (Chakravarthy et al. 2002; U.S. Department of Health and Human Services 1996). Physical activity and exercise recommendations should always be tailored to individual health status and personal lifestyle choices (U.S. Preventive Services Task Force 1996).

The belief that physical activity and exercise positively affect health at multiple levels is consistent with a basic tenet of integrative medicine that this approach "engages the mind, spirit, and community as well as the body...to stimulate the body's innate healing" (Gaudet 1998, p. 67). Physical activity is a key component of any recommendation aimed at promoting good health; developing healthy lifestyles, which are also fundamental to integrative medicine, is integral to achieving good health. Lifestyle recommendations encourage individuals to take an active role in their health by eating nutritiously, identifying coping strategies for addressing stressors, appreciating the role that spirituality or religion plays in their lives, and recognizing that social connection is an important element of well-being.

In this regard, it is important for psychiatrists and other mental health professionals to create opportunities for patients to be "naturally active" in contrast to relying on the formula-based exercise prescription that has historically been used (see Appendix 12-A). This is not to say that the traditional exercise prescription does not have a role, but rather that it should not be used as the only basis for recommending physical activity. For example, Meyer and Broocks (2000) based their exercise prescription recommendations for individuals with psychiatric disorders on their clinical experience. They recommended that clinicians first determine a patient's baseline fitness level and then have the patient 1) engage in moderate-intensity aerobic activity for 30 minutes or longer two to four times per week, 2) engage in regularly scheduled training breaks of easy activities between sessions, 3) participate in supplemental resistance training to improve muscle strength and endurance, and 4) maintain an exercise journal. Research supports this shift in emphasis, as lifestyle-focused physical activity has been demonstrated to provide health benefits comparable with some traditional exercise recommendations and increases the likelihood of sustained changes in behavior (Dunn et al. 1999).

As some would suggest, physical activity—like many other health-promoting behaviors—is not as simple as "Just Do It," but rather is a complex, often demanding behavior that is regarded by modern society as unnecessary for survival and also generally unnecessary for livelihood. Exercise is often looked at as an added element in everyday life; it must be experienced as worthwhile before it is practiced on a regular basis. Individuals who begin a program of activity or exercise may sometimes experience discomfort, which can be a strong negative reinforcer for their persisting in the activity. Environmental barriers can often be challenging to overcome. When physical activity is seen as part of the "to-do" list rather than a function of daily living, there is a strong likelihood that other priorities will win out.

Questions that need to be considered when encouraging people to make physical activity a way of life include the following:

- What is the individual's past experience with exercise?
- What are the environmental barriers and supports for engaging in this behavior?
- What medical conditions is the patient currently experiencing or at risk of developing?

- What does the patient hope to accomplish by becoming more active?
- What are his or her expectations?

WHO defined a multidimensional view of health (World Health Organization 1947) that encompasses personal, sociocultural, biological, spiritual, and psychological components, and is a resource for everyday life rather than a goal to be achieved. This framework allows patients to consider health as a means to achieve their aspirations and reach their potential. This concept also shifts the frame of reference for providing and receiving physical activity recommendations. Health now becomes a vital element for achieving *wellness,* a multidimensional state of being that describes the existence of positive health in an individual as exemplified by quality of life and a sense of overall well-being. The focus of this shift is on potential. Proactive individuals engage in practices that support this objective, resulting in a sense of achievement as health and well-being improve. An awareness that being active may enhance an individual's state of well-being and quality of life, even when they are experiencing disease, provides opportunities where previously few may have existed. This approach provides a framework for integrating physical activity and exercise recommendations into the patient's desired lifestyle.

It should also be recognized that health is dynamic—it changes throughout an individual's life, based on his or her particular situation in the context of changes in his or her body and the environment. Therefore, any discussion about physically active lifestyles must consider varying approaches based on an individual's life stage (i.e., childhood, adulthood, senior years) and their environmental (social, cultural, physical, and politicoeconomic) context.

Finally, integrative medicine asks health care providers to examine and explore their own lives, because speaking from experience greatly influences how a physician's messages are received. Incorporating role modeling to demonstrate the personal value of physical activity increases patient willingness to follow through with recommendations (Harsha et al. 1996).

A theoretical framework that provides a contextual approach to behavior change recommendations has been proposed by Laitakari and Asikainen (1998). The following elements are important considerations in assessing an individual's readiness to become active:

1. *Quality of life concerns, goals, and expectations:* This is potentially the most important consideration as it defines the purpose for behavior change. It is necessary to identify and/or assist the individual in identifying his or her reasons for becoming (more) physically active (e.g., relaxation, vitality, health-related benefits such as decreased disease risk, weight loss, feeling well, preparation for an event).
2. *Health status and fitness status:* An individual's current health and fitness status will affect recommendations and provide opportunities to determine how their fitness levels can benefit from increased activity.

3. *Health practices and attitudes:* What is the individual's current level of physical activity? What does he or she regularly do, and why? What new activities may be of interest? What are the skills and what is needed to go forward and/or try something new? How do concurrent behaviors, such as tobacco usage and dietary patterns, affect the patient's current health status or efforts to begin new behaviors?

4. *Life situation and environment:* What is the individual's current employment status and life situation (e.g., married versus single)? What kind of work does he or she perform (e.g., what is the amount of work-related physical activity)? Is the individual's current occupation primarily sedentary and, if so, are there opportunities for adding activity to the work day? Do his or her hobbies involve physical activity? Do significant time constraints need to be addressed and, if so, can potential solutions be identified? What does the individual's physical environment look like (e.g., urban versus suburban versus rural; access to trails, parks, and green spaces; proximity and access to recreation facilities; weather considerations)?

Approaching an individual from this inquiry-based framework allows the practitioner to recommend physical activity and exercise from a fitness-based framework as well as a lifestyle standpoint that addresses the multiple domains of health.

CONCLUSION

The health-related benefits of physical activity and exercise are both direct and indirect. Research has consistently demonstrated that cardiovascular fitness and many chronic conditions benefit from regular physical activity and exercise (U.S. Department of Health and Human Services 1996). In keeping with these findings, public health guidelines have acknowledged that general health benefits may be experienced from moderate activity averaging 30 minutes/day (Pate et al. 1995). Furthermore, subjective feelings of well-being and overall quality of life are enhanced through the awareness that health benefits are derived from physical activity (see Table 12–1).

Integrative medicine emphasizes the primacy of the patient–health care provider relationship and attends to the multidimensional nature of health. Physical activity and exercise are elements of a healthy lifestyle and are a fundamental component of any health promotion recommendation for patients who wish to enhance their health and well-being. When properly recommended, physical activity may benefit everyone, regardless of their health or disease status. This knowledge provides psychiatrists and other mental health professionals with a powerful medicine that can assist patients on their path to achieving important personal goals.

TABLE 12–1. Examples of types of exercise and intensity

Activity	Light (<3 METs or <4 kcal/min)	Moderate (3–6 METs or 4–7 kcal/min)	Vigorous (>6 METs or >7 kcal/min)
Walking	Slow walking (1–2 mph)	Brisk walking (2–4 mph)	Brisk walking uphill or with a load
Cycling	Stationary cycling (<50 Watts)	Cycling (<10 mph)	Cycling (10 mph)
Swimming	Swimming, slow treading	Swimming, moderate effort	Swimming, paced effort
Lawn mowing	Mowing lawn (riding)	Mowing lawn (power)	Mowing lawn (hand–push)
Household chores	Home care, carpet cleaning	Home care, general cleaning	Moving furniture

Note. MET = metabolic equivalent.

REFERENCES

Babyak MA, Blumenthal JA, Herman S, et al: Exercise treatment for major depression: maintenance of therapeutic benefit at 10 months. Psychosom Med 62:633–638, 2000

Bhui K, Fletcher A: Common mood and anxiety states: gender difference in the protective effect of physical activity. Soc Psychiatry Psychiatr Epidemiol 35:28–35, 2000

Blumenthal JA, Babyak MA, Moore KA, et al: Effects of exercise training on older patients with major depression. Arch Intern Med 159:2349–2356, 1999

Brooks A, Bandelow B, Pekrun G, et al: Comparison of aerobic exercise, clomipramine, and placebo in the treatment of panic disorder. Am J Psychiatry 155:603–609, 1998

Brown DW, Brown DR, Heath GW, et al: Associations between physical activity dose and health-related quality of life. Med Sci Sports Exerc 36:890–896, 2004

Calfas KJ, Taylor WC: Effects of physical activity on psychological variables in adolescents. Pediatric Exercise Science 6:406–423, 1994

Camacho TC, Roberts RE, Lazarus NB, et al: Physical activity and depression: evidence from the Alameda County Study. Am J Epidemiol 134:220–231, 1991

Chakravarthy MV, Joyner MJ, Booth FW: An obligation for primary care physicians to prescribe physical activity to sedentary patients to reduce the risk of chronic health conditions. Mayo Clin Proc 77:165–173, 2002

Chaouloff F: The serotonin hypothesis, in Physical Activity and Mental Health. Edited by Morgan WP. Washington, DC, Taylor & Francis, 1997, pp 179–198

Cooper-Patrick L, Ford DE, Mead LA, et al: Exercise and depression in midlife: a prospective study. Am J Public Health 87:670–673, 1997

Corbin CB, Pangrazi RP: Toward a uniform definition of wellness: a commentary. President's Council on Fitness and Sport Research Digest, Series 3, No 15, 2001. Available at: www.fitness.gov/pcpfsdigest1201.pdf

Craft LL, Landers DM: The effect of exercise on clinical depression and depression resulting from mental illness: a meta-analysis. Journal of Sport and Exercise Psychology 20:339–357, 1998

Cramer SR, Neiman DC, Lee JW: The effects of moderate exercise training on psychological well-being and mood state in women. J Psychosom Res 35:437–449, 1991

Dishman RK: The endorphin hypothesis, in Physical Activity and Mental Health. Edited by Morgan WP. Washington, DC, Taylor & Francis, 1997, pp 99–212

Dunn AL, Dishman RK: Exercise and the neurobiology of depression. Exerc Sport Sci Rev 19:41–98, 1991

Dunn AL, Marcus BH, Kampert JB, et al: Comparison of lifestyle and structured interventions to increase physical activity and cardiorespiratory fitness: a randomized trial. JAMA 281:327–334, 1999

Dunn AL, Trivedi MH, O'Neal HA: Physical activity dose-response effects on outcomes of depression and anxiety. Med Sci Sports Exerc 33 (suppl):S587–S597, 2001

Dunn AL, Trivedi MH, Kampert JB, et al: Exercise treatment for depression efficacy and dose response. Am J Prev Med 28:1–8, 2005

Farmer ME, Locke BZ, Moscicki EK, et al: Physical activity and depressive symptoms: the NHANES I epidemiological follow-up study. Am J Epidemiol 128:1340–1351, 1988

Fox KR: The physical self and processes in self-esteem development, in The Physical Self: From Motivation to Well-Being. Edited by Fox KR. Champaign, IL, Human Kinetics, 1997, pp 111–140

Fox KR: The influence of physical activity on mental well-being. Public Health Nutr 2:411–418, 1999

Gaudet TW: Integrative medicine. Integrative Medicine 1:67–73, 1998

Glenister D: Exercise and mental health: a review. J R Soc Health 2:7–13, 1996

Gomez-Pinilla F: Physical exercise induces FGF-2 and its mRNA in the hippocampus. Brain Res 764:1–8, 1997

Gomez-Pinilla F, So V, Kessiak JP: Spatial learning and physical activity contribute to the induction of fibroblast growth factor: neural substrates for increased cognition associated with exercise. Neuroscience 85:53–61, 1998

Greist JH, Klein MH, Eischens RR, et al: Running through your mind. J Psychosom Res 22:259–294, 1978

Hannaford CP, Harrell EH: Psychophysiological effects of a running program on depression and anxiety in a psychiatric population. Psychol Rec 38:37–48, 1988

Harsha DM, Saywell RM, Thygerson S, et al: Physician factors affecting patient willingness to comply with exercise recommendations. Clin J Sport Med 6:112–118, 1996

King AC, Taylor CB, Haskell WL: Effects of differing intensities and formats of 12 months of exercise training on psychological outcomes in older adults. Health Psychol 12:292–300, 1993

Laitakari J, Asikainen TM: How to promote physical activity through individual counseling: a proposal for a practical model of counseling on health-related physical activity. Patient Educ Couns 33:S13–S24, 1998

Larson EB, Wang L: Exercise, aging, and Alzheimer disease. Alzheimer Dis Assoc Disord 18:54–56, 2004

Laurin D, Verreault R, Lindsay J, et al: Physical activity and risk of cognitive impairment and dementia in elderly persons. Arch Neurol 58:498–504, 2001

Lawlor DA, Hopker SW: The effectiveness of exercise as an intervention in the management of depression: systematic review and meta-regression analysis of randomized controlled trials. BMJ 322:1–8, 2001

Lennox SS, Bedell JR, Stone AA: The effect of exercise on normal mood. J Psychosom Res 34:629–634, 1990

Lytle ME, Bilt JV, Pandav RS, et al: Exercise level and cognitive decline: the MoVIES Project. Alzheimer Dis Assoc Disord 18:57–64, 2004

MacQueen GM, Campbell S, McEwen BS, et al: Course of illness, hippocampal function, and hippocampal volume in major depression. Proc Natl Acad Sci U S A 100:1387–1392, 2003

Marcus BH, Selby VC, Niaua RS, et al: Self-efficacy and the stages of exercise behavior change. Res Q 63:60–66, 1992

Mather AS, Rodriguez C, Guthrie MF, et al: Effects of exercise on depressive symptoms in older adults with poorly responsive depressive disorder: randomized controlled trial. Br J Psychiatry 180:411–415, 2002

Meyer T, Broocks A: Therapeutic impact of exercise on psychiatric diseases: guidelines for exercise testing and prescription. Sports Med 30:269–279, 2000

National Commission on Sleep Disorders Research: Wake up America: A National Sleep Alert. Executive Summary and Executive Report. Bethesda, MD, National Heart, Lung, and Blood Institute, 1993, pp 1–76

Osei-Tutu KEK, Campagna PD: Psychological benefits of continuous vs. intermittent moderate intensity exercise (abstract). Med Sci Sports Exerc 30 (suppl 5):S117, 1998

Paffenbarger RS, Lee I-M, Leung R: Physical activity and personal characteristics associated with depression and suicide in American college men. Acta Psychiatr Scand 89(S377):16–22, 1994

Paluska SA, Schwenk TL: Physical activity and mental health. Sports Med 29:167–180, 2000

Pate RR, Pratt M, Blair SN, et al: Physical activity and public health. JAMA 273:402–407, 1995

Petruzzello SJ, Landers DM, Hatfield BD, et al: A meta-analysis of the anxiety-reducing effects of acute and chronic exercise. Sports Med 11:143–182, 1991

Sheline YI, Gado MH, Kraemer HC: Untreated depression and hippocampal volume loss. Am J Psychiatry 160:1516–1518, 2003

Shepard RJ: Physical activity, health and well-being at different life stages. Res Q 66:298–302, 1995

Singh MA: Exercise and aging. Clin Geriatr Med 20:201–221, 2004

Spence JC, Poon P: The effect of physical activity on self-concept: a meta-analysis. Alberta Center for Well-Being: Research Update, Vol 4, No 4, June 1997. Available at: www.centre4activeliving.ca/publications/research_update/1997/JunPg1.pdf

Steptoe A, Butler N: Sports participation and emotional well-being in adolescents. Lancet 347:1789–1792, 1996

Strawbridge WJ, Deleger S, Roberts RE, et al: Physical activity reduces the risk of subsequent depression for older adults. Am J Epidemiol 156:328–334, 2002

Teri L, Gibbons LE, McCurry SM, et al: Exercise plus behavioral management in patients with Alzheimer's disease. JAMA 290:2015–2022, 2003

Thoren P, Floras JS, Hoffman P, et al: Endorphins and exercise: physiological mechanisms and clinical implications. Med Sci Sports Exerc 22:417–428, 1990

Urponen H, Vuiri I, Hasan J, et al: Self-evaluation of factors promoting and disturbing sleep: an epidemiological survey in Finland. Soc Sci Med 26:443–450, 1988

U.S. Department of Health and Human Services: Physical Activity and Health: A Report of the Surgeon General. Atlanta, GA, Centers for Disease Control and Prevention, 1996

U.S. Preventive Services Task Force: Guide to Clinical Preventive Services, 2nd Edition. Baltimore, MD, Williams & Wilkins, 1996. Available at: http://odphp.osophs.dhhs.gov/pubs/guidecps/PDF/Frontmtr.PDF

U.S. Preventive Services Task Force: Physical Activity Counseling. Available at: www.ahrq.gov/clinic/uspstf/uspsphys.htm. Accessed August 1, 2004

Weyerer S: Physical activity and depression in the community: evidence from the upper Bavarian field study. Int J Sports Med 13:492–496, 1992

World Health Organization: Preamble to the Constitution of the World Health Organization as adopted by the International Health Conference, New York, 19 June – 22 July 1946; signed on 22 July 1946 by the representatives of 61 States (Official Records of the World Health Organization, no. 2, p. 100) and entered into force on 7 April 1948

World Health Organization: Ottawa Charter for Health Promotion. Copenhagen, Denmark, World Health Organization, 1986

Yeung RR: The acute effects of exercise on mood state. J Psychosom Res 2:123–141, 1996

Youngstedt SD, O'Connor PJ, Dishman RK: The effects of acute exercise on sleep: a quantitative synthesis. Sleep 20:203–214, 1997

Youngstedt SD, Kripke DF, Elliott JA: Is sleep disturbed by vigorous late-night exercise? Med Sci Sports Exerc 31:864–869, 1999

Zimetbaum P, Josephson ME: Evaluation of patients with palpitations. N Engl J Med 338:1369–1373, 1998

APPENDIX 12-A

Health and Fitness Guidelines and Recommendations

Current Public Health Guidelines Regarding Exercise

Every American should accumulate 30 minutes or more of moderate-intensity physical activity on most, and preferably all, days of the week. Adults who engage in moderate-intensity physical activity (i.e., enough to expend 200 calories/day) can expect many of the health benefits described herein. One way to meet this standard is to briskly walk 2 miles/day. Most adults do not currently meet the standard described (Pate et al. 1995).

Recommendations for Cardiorespiratory Fitness and Body Composition: the FITT Prescription for Exercise

F Frequency of training: 3–5 days/week

I Intensity of exercise: from 55%–65% to 90% of maximum heart rate (HR_{max}; calculated as $208 - 0.7 \times age$) based on aerobic capacity goals and fitness level; lower-intensity values are most applicable for less-fit individuals:
- Light exercise: less than 60% of predicted HR_{max}
- Moderate exercise: 60%–85% of predicted HR_{max}
- Vigorous exercise: greater than 85% of predicted HR_{max}

T Time: 20–60 minutes of continuous or intermittent (minimum of 10-minute bouts accumulated throughout the day) aerobic activity. The duration of exercise is dependent on the intensity: lower-intensity activities should be performed for longer periods of time (30 minutes or more); conversely, higher intensity training may be performed for 20 minutes or more. Because total fitness is enhanced by training periods of longer duration and the risk of injury is increased with more intense training, moderate-intensity activities are recommended for most adults.

T Type: Any activity that uses large muscle groups that can be maintained continuously and is rhythmic in nature (Pollock et al. 1998).

Recommendations for Muscular Strength, Endurance, and Flexibility

- *Strength training*—Resistance training should be progressive, individualized, and work all major muscle groups. One set of 8–10 exercises, consisting of 8–12 repetitions that involve the major muscle groups, performed through the full range of motion, should be performed two to three times per week. Multiple-set regimens may provide greater improvements.
- *Flexibility training*—Flexibility exercises should be incorporated into the overall fitness program sufficient to develop and maintain range of motion. These exercises should stretch the major muscle groups and be performed a minimum of 2–3 days per week. Stretching should include appropriate static and/or dynamic techniques (Pollock et al. 1998).

Recommendations for Prevention of Weight Gain and Health Maintenance

All adults and youths should participate in at least 60–90 minutes of daily moderate-intensity physical activity at the same time as not exceeding caloric requirements (Institute of Medicine 2002).

References

Institute of Medicine: Dietary Reference Intakes for Energy, Carbohydrate, Fiber, Fat, Fatty Acids, Cholesterol, Protein, and Amino Acids (Macronutrients). Washington, DC, National Academies Press, 2002

Pate RR, Pratt M, Blair SN, et al: Physical activity and public health. JAMA 273:402–407, 1995

Pollock ML, Gaesser GA, Butcher JD, et al: The recommended quantity and quality of exercise for developing and maintaining cardiorespiratory and muscular fitness, and flexibility in healthy adults. American College of Sports Medicine Position Stand. Med Sci Sports Exerc 30:975–991, 1998

13

Integrative Medicine Treatments for Depression in Women

Priti Sinha, M.D.
Marlene P. Freeman, M.D.
Rebecca A. Hill, M.B.B.S.(Hon.)

In this chapter, we provide an overview of depression in women across the reproductive life span and discuss selected complementary and alternative medicine (CAM) treatment modalities to treat depression. A concise summary of conventional treatment options is provided in the text and the accompanying table to help clinicians and patients make informed decisions. Two caveats should be noted at the outset of this chapter: before a CAM or conventional treatment is begun, the risks and benefits must be weighed in the context of a woman's unique circumstances; second, each of these modalities deserves further research, especially for purposes of establishing their safety and efficacy in the management of mood disorders in women at different stages of their reproductive lives.

Integrative approaches combining alternative and conventional treatments are becoming increasingly common (Eisenberg et al. 1998). However, physicians often fail to ask patients about their use of alternative therapies, and patients may not be forthcoming about such use. Most physicians lack adequate training in alternative or integrative medical approaches (Corbin Winslow and Shapiro 2002); this is especially problematic for women because women experience depression more often than men (Weissman et al. 1984) and more frequently seek nonconventional treatments (Mackenzie et al. 2003).

To emphasize treatments that are especially relevant to women and highlight treatments for which there is substantial evidence, we have chosen to discuss in detail selected CAM modalities rather than provide an exhaustive review of all nonconventional treatments of depression. We review the evidence for the following nonconventional treatments of mood disorders in women: omega-3 essential fatty acids, St. John's wort (*Hypericum perforatum*), S-adenosylmethionine (SAMe), folate, exercise, acupuncture, and bright light exposure therapy. Many of these treatment modalities are reviewed in detail elsewhere in the book, and this general material is not repeated here. For a comprehensive overview of a particular CAM treatment, the reader is referred to the chapter on that modality.

WOMEN AND DEPRESSION: AN OVERVIEW

Depression During Pregnancy

Mood disorders are more common among women than men in general, and approximately 10% of women report experiencing depressed mood during pregnancy (Nonacs and Cohen 2002). Men more often complete suicide whereas women more often attempt suicide.

Approximately one-third of depressed women experience their first episode of major depression during pregnancy (O'Hara 1994). The occurrence of depression during pregnancy raises several important questions for women as for their clinicians. Should a woman of childbearing age with major depression discontinue conventional or nonconventional treatments before conception or after she discovers she is pregnant? What is the risk of recurrent depression during pregnancy or after childbirth? What are the risks to the fetus and pregnant woman if the woman chooses to discontinue or continue treatment? What risks exist for a baby if the mother is depressed during pregnancy? Clinicians are often challenged to provide adequate care for a pregnant woman who is depressed while minimizing the risks to the woman and fetus.

Untreated depression is common in pregnancy and negatively affects pregnancy outcomes. Pregnancy does not protect against depression, as was demonstrated by a prospective study that found a 13.5% incidence of depression at 32 weeks' gestation (Evans et al. 2001). Diagnosing major depressive disorder during pregnancy is complicated by the fact that decreased energy, insomnia, appetite disturbances, and diminished libido are frequently reported by nondepressed pregnant women. Thyroid abnormalities, anemia, and diabetes associated with pregnancy may also confound efforts to diagnose a psychiatric illness (Klein and Essex 1995). It is always prudent to ask a pregnant woman about thoughts of suicidality, hopelessness, guilt, and anhedonia, symptoms that are more specific indicators of major depression.

Psychiatric illness during pregnancy or the postpartum period carries significant risks for women and their children. Depression during pregnancy increases the risk of poor self-care, poor compliance with prenatal care, decreased appetite, and lower weight gain and is associated with negative pregnancy outcomes

(Zuckerman et al. 1989). Antenatal depression is associated with lower birth weight, preterm birth, abnormal small head circumference, and low Apgar scores (Dayan et al. 2002). Animal studies have demonstrated an association of maternal stress with fetal hypoxia, low birth weight, and miscarriage (Wadhwa et al. 1993). Antenatal depression increases the risk of postpartum depression and may interfere with mother–infant bonding. Infants of depressed mothers are more likely to exhibit behavioral, attachment, and cognitive problems (Weinberg and Tronick 1998).

Clinicians and patients should ideally discuss the risks and benefits of conventional and nonconventional treatment options (including psychotherapy) before conception. The clinician should inform the woman about the risk of teratogenesis, toxicity, or withdrawal symptoms in the neonate and possible neurobehavioral problems if the infant is exposed to a proposed intervention (Wisner et al. 2000). To date, few studies have examined the efficacy of antidepressant medication during pregnancy. The clinician should also discuss nonpharmacological treatment options for women who report depressed mood in the weeks before expected childbirth. A list of the issues to be discussed when considering conventional treatment options in pregnant women is provided in Table 13–1.

Selective serotonin reuptake inhibitors (SSRIs) are frequently used to treat major depression during pregnancy. Neither SSRIs nor tricyclic antidepressants (TCAs) increase the risk of major birth defects or intrauterine death (Wisner et al. 2000). SSRI withdrawal or toxicity syndromes have been reported in neonates exposed to antidepressants in late pregnancy. The U.S. Food and Drug Administration recently added warnings to SSRI and venlafaxine labels about signs of toxicity or withdrawal in newborns. Prospective studies and case reports suggest the possible occurrence of respiratory distress, jitteriness, hypoglycemia, and hypotonia (Costei et al. 2002; Laine et al. 2003; Nordeng et al. 2001; Zeskind and Stephens 2004). The findings suggest that SSRI withdrawal or toxicity syndromes are transient; however, further studies are needed to assess longer-term risks to infants. Perinatal syndromes in infants exposed to TCAs in utero include transient symptoms such as jitteriness, irritability, urinary retention, and functional bowel obstruction. Neonatal withdrawal symptoms from TCAs are transient. Seizures have been reported with the use of clomipramine during pregnancy (Cowe et al. 1982).

Little is known regarding the long-term effects of in utero exposure to antidepressants. In one study of children ages 15–17 months, there were no reports of significant adverse effects on the children's IQs, behavior, language, or temperament after exposure to TCAs or fluoxetine during pregnancy (Nulman et al. 2002). However, in utero exposure to fluoxetine may increase the risk of low birth weight (Chambers et al. 1996; Hendrick et al. 2003). One study on SSRI use in pregnant women suggested an association of the drug with premature birth (Simon et al. 2002); however, the results of larger studies did not support

TABLE 13–1.   Issues requiring discussion when considering conventional treatment options for women with depression

Diagnosis	Conventional treatment options	Issues to discuss with patient
Antenatal depression	SSRIs TCAs Interpersonal therapy	Teratogenesis; toxicity/withdrawal in neonate; possible neurobehavioral problems with infant; birth and pregnancy complications if untreated depression
Postpartum depression (PPD)	SSRIs Cognitive-behavioral therapy Interpersonal therapy	Breast-feeding and medications; mother/infant bond development; infant cognition and behavioral problems if untreated PPD
Premenstrual mood disorder	SSRIs (continuous or luteal phase)	Dysfunction at work, school, home without treatment; medication use during possible future pregnancy/breast-feeding
Perimenopause and menopausal depression	SSRIs TCAs HRT	Controversy regarding HRT and medical conditions (heart disease, stroke, pulmonary emboli, breast cancer)

Note.   HRT = hormone replacement therapy; SSRIs = selective serotonin reuptake inhibitors; TCAs = tricyclic antidepressants.

this finding (Ericson et al. 1999; Kulin et al. 1998). Zeskind and Stephens (2004) found that babies exposed to SSRIs in utero were born 1 week earlier on average compared with control subjects. It is important for clinicians to inform their patients that the long-term effects of conventional antidepressants and nonconventional treatments on an unborn child are unknown. Furthermore, patients should be informed of the risk of untreated maternal depression having negative effects on the course of the pregnancy and child development.

Postpartum Depression

According to DSM-IV (American Psychiatric Association 1994), *postpartum depression* (PPD) is defined as the onset of major depression within 4 weeks of delivery. Risk factors for PPD include a history of depression, previous PPD, a family history of PPD, and depression during pregnancy. The Edinburgh Postnatal Depression Scale is a screening tool that has been used to increase the rate at which PPD is detected in clinical settings (Cox et al. 1987).

PPD not only negatively impacts women but also affects the safety and development of their infants. Depressed women may neglect their own basic needs, and those with PPD are less in tune with the needs of their newborns. Infants of mothers with untreated depression are more likely to develop attachment disorders, have poorer cognitive function, and exhibit more behavioral problems compared with infants of mothers whose depression was treated (Cicchetti et al. 1998). In addition, women with PPD may fail to take measures to provide a safe environment for their babies, such as complying with car seat use and "baby proofing" their homes (McLennan and Kotelchuck 2000).

All clinicians should discuss the risks and benefits of antidepressant treatment and breast-feeding for both the mother and her baby with their patients. Breast-feeding is associated with multiple health benefits for the infant (Rodriguez-Palermo et al. 1999). For mothers, breast-feeding is associated with reduced postpartum blood loss and decreased risk of ovarian and premenopausal breast cancers and may enhance emotional attachment between the mother and her infant (Labbok 1999).

Few placebo-controlled studies have been conducted on conventional antidepressant treatments of PPD. One double-blind trial using fluoxetine (Prozac; Appleby et al. 1997) and another double-blind study using estrogen (Gregoire et al. 1996) suggested these treatments may be effective for PPD. Although high levels of fluoxetine (Prozac) have been detected in the blood of breast-fed infants whose mothers were treated with the drug, most findings have suggested that infants who are breast-fed have low blood levels of TCAs and SSRIs (Llewellyn and Stowe 1998; Weissman et al. 2004; Wisner et al. 1996). In one study, the growth curve of breast-fed infants of mothers treated with fluoxetine during and after pregnancy was significantly lower compared with that of infants of nursing mothers who discontinued fluoxetine after childbirth (Chambers et al. 1999). A few case reports have suggested possible adverse events in infants who are breast-fed by mothers treated with antidepressants, including doxepin (Frey et al. 1999), citalopram (K. Schmidt et al. 2000), estrogen (Ball and Morrison 1999), and bupropion (Wellbutrin; Chaudron and Schoenecker 2004).

The findings of most studies indicate that infant exposure to maternal antidepressants via breast milk is low (Burt et al. 2001); however, many women decline treatment with antidepressants if they are breast-feeding because long-term effects on the infant have not been determined. Psychotherapy is often a first-line treatment option for women with PPD, as it avoids these concerns about risks to the breast-feeding infant. Cognitive-behavioral therapy (CBT) and interpersonal psychotherapy (IPT) have also been reported to be beneficial in PDD. In a randomized controlled trial, the recovery rate of women with PDD was higher in those treated with 5–8 weeks of CBT than in the control group (Chabrol et al. 2002). In a small follow-up study, IPT was efficacious in the treatment of women with antepartum and postpartum depression (Klier et al. 2001). In another randomized controlled trial, women assigned to 12 weeks of IPT showed significantly greater improvement than those assigned to a waiting-list control group (O'Hara et al. 2000). Although more research is needed, the results of currently available studies indicate that CBT and IPT are effective treatments for PPD.

Premenstrual Mood Disorders

Premenstrual syndrome is characterized by behavioral, physical, and minor mood symptoms that remit after menses (E. W. Freeman 2003). Premenstrual mood problems typically start when a woman is in her late 20s or early 30s (E. W. Freeman et al. 1995). Risk factors include a history of major depression, postpartum depression, or bipolar affective disorder; a family history positive for premenstrual problems; and psychosocial stressors (Steiner et al. 2003). Approximately 8% of women experience premenstrual syndrome, and its risk is greater in African American and younger women as well as those who report alcohol consumption, longer menses, and high levels of perceived stress (Deuster et al. 1999).

Unlike premenstrual syndrome, the diagnosis of *premenstrual dysphoric disorder* (PMDD) indicates significant psychiatric morbidity and impairment in work, school, or other activities. According to DSM-IV-TR (American Psychiatric Association 2000), a diagnosis of PMDD is merited when women experience five or more of the following marked symptoms: depression, anxiety, affective lability, irritability, poor concentration, diminished motivation, changes in appetite and sleep, feelings of being overwhelmed, and physical complaints. These symptoms must take place on a regular basis for at least 1 year during the last week of the luteal phase. The most frequently occurring symptoms of PMDD include anxiety, irritability, and mood lability (Bloch et al. 1997). These symptoms generally remit within a few days of onset of the follicular phase or menses and are absent for 1 week after the end of menses.

Women with PMDD have higher rates of mood and anxiety disorders, previously diagnosed PPD (if they have children), and more obsessional personality traits in comparison with women who do not experience PMDD (Critchlow et al. 2001). A thorough psychiatric history is necessary to clearly differentiate PMDD from other mood or anxiety disorders. Documenting daily mood ratings and menses for at least 2 months is a practical way to confirm the diagnosis.

The first-line conventional treatment of PMDD is SSRIs. At the time of this writing, the U.S. Food and Drug Administration has approved sertraline (Zoloft), fluoxetine (Prozac), and paroxetine (Paxil) for the treatment of PMDD for continuous use or administration during the luteal phase only (last 2 weeks of menses). In clinical trials of SSRIs for PMDD, symptoms have been reduced with continuous or luteal phase administration (E. W. Freeman 2004). Estrogen probably ameliorates premenstrual symptoms (Smith et al. 1995); however, progesterone is ineffective and may worsen symptoms (Tiemstra and Patel 1998). The evidence for beneficial effects of oral contraceptives on premenstrual mood symptoms is inconclusive (Andersch and Hahn 1982; Joffe et al. 2003).

Perimenopause and Menopause

Researchers have proposed the *estrogen withdrawal theory,* which postulates that the decrease in estrogen during the menstrual cycle, in the immediate postpartum period, and in perimenopause is correlated with depressive mood symptoms (P. J. Schmidt and Rubinow 1991). Perimenopause is associated with changes in the menstrual pattern that typically occur in women ages 40–55 years (Soares and Cohen 2001). Women in perimenopause may be especially vulnerable to depressive symptoms due to their declining estrogen levels.

Estrogen has been demonstrated to have antidepressant effects (Gregoire et al. 1996; Klaiber et al. 1979). However, the risk–benefit analysis for hormone replacement therapy (HRT), in which women are given estrogen and progestin or just estrogen, has recently become more complicated. In the Women's Health Initiative Study, coronary artery disease, stroke, pulmonary emboli, and invasive breast cancer were reported more frequently in women who received both estrogen and progestin than in women who received placebo (Rossouw et al. 2002). The use of HRT remains controversial, and it is unclear whether this approach is a viable treatment option for perimenopausal depression. The findings of double-blind studies show that SSRIs reduce the severity of vasomotor symptoms in perimenopause. Fluoxetine, paroxetine, and venlafaxine (Effexor) are more effective for the management of hot flashes than placebo (Loprinzi et al. 2000, 2002; Stearns et al. 2003). The findings of one open-label study suggested that citalopram (Celexa) improves depressed mood and vasomotor symptoms in perimenopause (Soares et al. 2003). Additional research on conventional treatments for perimenopausal and menopausal depression and vasomotor symptoms is needed.

COMPLEMENTARY AND ALTERNATIVE TREATMENTS FOR WOMEN WITH DEPRESSION

Omega-3 Fatty Acids

The consumption of foods rich in omega-3 fatty acids has general health benefits (see Chapter 7 for a comprehensive review of the basic research, epidemiological findings, and outcome studies pertaining to omega-3 essential fatty acids in mental health care). Intake of omega-3 fatty acids is especially important during pregnancy and in the postpartum period when certain fatty acids are preferentially transferred to the fetus, resulting in decreased availability to the mother (Min et al. 2000). Omega-3 fatty acids, especially docosahexaenoic acid (DHA), are essential for the development of the central nervous system (Holman et al. 1991). Infants depend on maternal breast milk for fatty acids, including the omega-3s. Infant formulas are now available in the United States with added fatty acids, including DHA. In a double-blind, controlled trial, omega-3 supplementation was associated with lower rates of preterm delivery, with no reports of adverse effects on fetal growth or complications during labor (Olsen et al. 1992). Despite the importance of omega-3 fatty acids in pregnancy and breast-feeding, in the United States the intake of foods and supplements containing omega-3 fatty acids by pregnant and nursing women is inadequate (Benisek et al. 2000). In cross-national studies, there is a decrease in the prevalence of major depression, postpartum depression, and depressive symptoms as the per capita consumption of fish, a source of omega-3 fatty acids, increases (Hibbeln 2002).

One small open-label trial evaluated omega-3 fatty acids as a treatment for depression during pregnancy in 15 women with a history of major depressive episodes. The subjects received an average dose of 1.9 g/day consisting of eicosapentaenoic acid and DHA. The women remained in the trial for an average of 8.3 ± 7.1 weeks (SD). The mean reduction in scores on the Edinburgh Postnatal Depression Scale, a screening tool for detecting depression during pregnancy or postpartum, was 40.9%, and the treatment was well tolerated (M.P. Freeman et al. 2006).

Hypericum Perforatum (St. John's Wort)

The evidence for the efficacy of St. John's wort in treating depressed mood is discussed in detail in Chapter 5, "Western Herbal Medicines." This section briefly reviews important research findings pertaining to St. John's wort and depression while emphasizing mood disorders in women.

St. John's wort interferes with hepatic enzymes (the cytochrome P450 system) that metabolize many drugs (Jorm et al. 2002; Stahl 2000, pp. 442–443), thereby affecting serum levels of SSRIs, immunosuppressant agents, and oral contraceptives (Roby et al. 2000). The consequences of these effects include reduced effectiveness of HRT and increased risk of unplanned pregnancy (Jorm et al. 2002). There has been one case report of lower concentrations of a constituent of St. John's wort in breast milk than in maternal plasma. The same constituent was undetectable in the infant, and no adverse effects were observed (Klier et al. 2002). However, a small prospective study of women taking St. John's wort while breast-feeding concluded that newborns experienced symptoms of colic, drowsiness, and lethargy more often compared with depressed and nondepressed nursing mothers who did not take St. John's wort (Lee et al. 2003). The same study found no differences in milk production, adverse maternal events, or infant weight among groups.

S-Adenosylmethionine

SAMe is a methyl donor that has demonstrated antidepressant benefits. Chapter 6, "Nutritional Supplements," provides a detailed review of research findings on SAMe in the management of depression.

Few studies have been done on SAMe in women with postpartum or postmenopausal depression. In a double-blind, placebo-controlled study of SAMe in women with PPD (Cerutti et al. 1993), depressive scores dropped significantly after 1 month of treatment with SAMe 1,600 mg/day. There was a significant difference between the treatment and placebo groups at 10 days. There is also some evidence of beneficial effects of SAMe on depressed postmenopausal women. The findings of a double-blind, placebo-controlled trial in women 6 months to 3 years after natural or surgical menopause showed significant improvement over placebo in the SAMe-treated women (Salmaggi et al. 1993). The difference in response between the SAMe and placebo groups became significant at 10 days of treatment. A physician considering recommending SAMe to a depressed woman should note that there are no data supporting its use during pregnancy or breast-feeding. Furthermore, one study found that subjects treated with SAMe had significant reductions in serum prolactin levels (Thomas et al. 1987). On the positive side, SAMe apparently prevents adverse changes in serum lipid profiles associated with oral contraceptive use (Di Padova et al. 1984).

Folate

Women may experience a differentially greater benefit from folate compared with men. (See Chapter 6, "Nutritional Supplements," for a general review of folate in mental health care.) One study (Coppen and Bailey 2000) found that female patients treated with fluoxetine 20 mg/day who also received folate 500 mg/day experienced a significantly greater improvement in mood symptoms compared with those who received fluoxetine plus placebo. This difference was not observed in men. Furthermore, there were fewer fluoxetine-related adverse effects in patients receiving folic acid. No adverse effects have been associated with folate. Women who are pregnant or may conceive are advised to take 0.4–1.0 mg of folic acid daily to minimize the risk of serious fetal neural tube defects (McDonald et al. 2003). These facts, combined with the evidence supporting augmentation of conventional antidepressants with folate make folate a supplement that may be broadly recommended in depressed women.

Exercise

The evidence for beneficial effects of exercise on mental health is reviewed in Chapter 12, "Physical Activity, Exercise, and Mental Health." In one study, women with depression were randomized to an aerobic exercise group, relaxation, or no treatment for 10 weeks. Compared with the other two groups, the exercise group showed a greater reduction in depression scores at 10 weeks (McCann and Holmes 1984). Pregnant depressed women may benefit from regular exercise. In a prospective study of pregnant women comparing mood, anxiety and stress levels, and physical activity, those who exercised reported significantly improved mood compared with those who did not exercise in the first and second trimesters but not during the third trimester (Da Cost et al. 2003). The American College of Obstetricians and Gynecologists recommends 30 minutes of moderate exercise daily for women during pregnancy and the postpartum period (Artal and O'Toole 2003), although all pregnant women should consult their physicians before starting an exercise regimen. Another study found significant decreases in anxiety and depression in postpartum women who participated in aerobic exercise or quiet rest (Koltyn and Schultes 1997). Exercise also reduces emotional distress and depressed mood when these symptoms occur premenstrually (Aganoff and Boyle 1994). Exercise has been shown to reduce vasomotor symptoms and to improve mood in perimenopausal women (Slaven and Lee 1997).

Acupuncture

Research findings on acupuncture in mental health care are reviewed in Chapter 8, "Chinese Medical Treatments." In a randomized, double-blind, placebo-controlled study, depressed women were randomized to acupuncture, "sham" acupuncture, or a wait-list condition (Allen et al. 1998). The acupuncture group had a higher remission rate compared with the other groups. In an open study on the effects of acupuncture on stress that enrolled mainly women (16 of 17), depressed mood decreased by 44% using a standardized symptom rating scale after four sessions of acupuncture (Chan et al. 2002).

During pregnancy, women need to take special precautions to avoid uterine stimulation when undergoing acupuncture treatment (Motl 2002). The stimulation of certain acupuncture points has been reported to accelerate cervical dilation, resulting in preterm delivery (Rabl et al. 2001). In addition, there are case reports of uterine contractions induced by stimulation of certain acupoints (Dunn et al. 1989). Thus, it is crucial that practitioners who treat pregnant women be aware of the acupoints that can precipitate uterine contractions and avoid those acupoints. In an open study of menopausal women taking tamoxifen, acupuncture had significant beneficial effects on mood and anxiety symptoms, with no adverse effects being reported (Porzio et al. 2002). Based on research findings to date, certain acupuncture protocols probably have a beneficial effect on anxiety and depressive symptoms in women; however, additional controlled studies are indicated to confirm their benefit.

Light Therapy

In placebo-controlled trials, bright light therapy reduces symptoms of seasonal and nonseasonal depression (Eastman et al. 1998; Kripke et al. 1992; Sumaya et al. 2001; Terman et al. 1989; Yamada et al. 1995). Greater intensity of phototherapy is associated with better efficacy in unipolar and bipolar depression (Beauchemin and Hays 1997). Bright light therapy may hasten the response to antidepressant medication (Benedetti et al. 2003) and augments the antidepressant effects of partial sleep deprivation (Colombo et al. 2000; Neumeister et al. 1996). Light therapy's mechanism of action may involve the serotonergic neurotransmitter system (Avissar et al. 1999; Benedetti et al. 2003). Although bright light therapy is generally well tolerated, there have been rare reports of hypomania in bipolar patients after therapy (Kripke et al. 1992).

Bright light exposure is an attractive alternative therapy to conventional medications for depressed pregnant women. In a small open study, depression rating scores improved by 49% at 3 weeks and 59% at 5 weeks in pregnant women receiving 60 minutes/day of bright light therapy (Oren et al. 2002). Most women in the study reported worsening mood after light therapy was discontinued. In a small double-blind study of 10 depressed pregnant women randomized to bright light therapy versus dim light placebo, one case of hypomania was reported in the bright light exposure group, whereas all other women experienced significant improvements in mood at 10 weeks. After only 5 weeks, though, there were no significant differences in depressive symptoms between the bright light and dim light groups (Epperson et al. 2004).

Bright light exposure may be beneficial in women who experience premenstrual symptoms. In a randomized, double-blind, crossover study, women treated with regular bright light exposure experienced significantly greater mood improvements compared with women exposed to dim red morning light. Bright light therapy has not been studied in postpartum depression, and future studies are needed, especially in women with PPD who want to breast-feed (Lam et al. 1999).

CONCLUSION

Women with mood disorders are increasingly using a range of integrative and alternative treatments. Clinicians should ask their female patients with depression or other mood disorder about their use of nonconventional treatments and become familiar with data on their safety and efficacy and potential interactions with drugs. The effectiveness and safety of most nonconventional treatment modalities in pregnancy are not well understood, and their use is based on limited research findings. Omega-3 fatty acids, folate, and exercise are three treatments shown to be beneficial in treating depressed mood during pregnancy.

These interventions are appropriate when weighing the risks and benefits of nonconventional versus conventional treatment options in depressed women.

A thorough psychiatric and reproductive history is an essential first step when recommending treatment to any woman who reports depressive symptoms. It is important to ask women of child-bearing age if they plan to have a family, and the clinician should always discuss family planning and the risks and benefits of conventional and nonconventional treatments across the reproductive life span with female patients. A clinician should take into account the fact that many pregnancies are unplanned and that a woman's plans for having children may change over the course of treatment. For these reasons, the risks and benefits of conventional medications versus nonconventional treatments in pregnancy must be considered for all women of reproductive age.

This chapter focused primarily on unipolar depression and premenstrual and perimenopausal mood disorders in women; however, many women who present with depressive episodes may have a bipolar disorder. To date, few studies have been done on nonconventional treatments of bipolar disorder, and specific recommendations for the use of nonconventional treatments in women with a bipolar disorder cannot be made.

REFERENCES

Aganoff JA, Boyle GJ: Aerobic exercise, mood states and menstrual cycle symptoms. J Psychosom Res 38:183–192, 1994

Allen JB, Schnyer RN, Hitt SK: The efficacy of acupuncture in the treatment of major depressive disorder in women. Psychol Sci 9:397–401, 1998

American Psychiatric Association: Diagnostic and Statistical Manual of Mental Disorders, 4th Edition. Washington, DC, American Psychiatric Association, 1994

American Psychiatric Association: Diagnostic and Statistical Manual of Mental Disorders, 4th Edition, Text Revision. Washington, DC, American Psychiatric Association, 2000

Andersch B, Hahn L: Premenstrual complaints: influence of oral contraceptives (author's translation). Contracept Fertil Sex (Paris) 10:659–664, 1982

Appleby L, Warner R, Whitton A, et al: A controlled study of fluoxetine and cognitive-behavioral counseling in the treatment of postnatal depression. BMJ 314:932–939, 1997

Artal R, O'Toole M: Guidelines on the American College of Obstetricians and Gynecologists for exercise during pregnancy and the postpartum period. Br J Sports Med 37:6–12, 2003

Avissar S, Schreiber G, Nechamkin Y, et al: The effects of seasons and light therapy on G protein levels in mononuclear leukocytes of patients with season affective disorder. Arch Gen Psychiatry 56:178–183, 1999

Ball DE, Morrison P: Oestrogen transdermal patches for postpartum depression in lactating mothers: a case report. Cent Afr J Med 45:68–70, 1999

Beauchemin KM, Hays P: Phototherapy is a useful adjunct in the treatment of depressed in-patients. Acta Psychiatr Scand 95:424–427, 1997

Benedetti F, Colombo C, Serretti A, et al: Antidepressant effects of light therapy combined with sleep deprivation are influenced by a functional polymorphism within the promoter of the serotonin transporter gene. Biol Psychiatry 54:687–692, 2003

Benisek D, Shabert J, Skornik R: Dietary intake of polyunsaturated fatty acids by pregnant or lactating women in the United States. Obstet Gynecol 95:77–78, 2000

Bloch M, Schmidt PJ, Rubinow DR: Premenstrual syndrome: evidence for symptom stability across cycles. Am J Psychiatry 154:1741–1746, 1997

Burt VK, Suri R, Altshuler L, et al: The use of psychotropic medications during breast-feeding. Am J Psychiatry 158:1001–1009, 2001

Cerutti R, Sichel MP, Perin M, et al: Psychological distress during the puerperium: a novel therapeutic approach using S-adenosylmethionine. Current Therapeutic Research 53:707–716, 1993

Chabrol H, Teissedre F, Saint-Jean M, et al: Prevention and treatment of postpartum depression: a controlled randomized study on women at risk. Psychol Med 32:1039–1047, 2002

Chambers CD, Anderson PO, Thomas RB, et al: Weight gain in infants breastfed by mothers who take fluoxetine. Pediatrics 104:e61, 1999

Chambers CD, Johnson KA, Kick LN, et al: Birth outcomes in pregnant women taking fluoxetine. N Engl J Med 335:1010–1015, 1996

Chan J, Briscomb D, Waterhouse E, et al: An uncontrolled pilot study of HT7 for "stress." Acupunct Med 20:74–77, 2002

Chaudron LH, Schoenecker CJ: Bupropion and breastfeeding: a case of a possible infant seizure. J Clin Psychiatry 65:881–882, 2004

Cicchetti D, Rogosch FA, Toth SL: Maternal depressive disorder and contextual risk: contributions to the development of attachment insecurity and behavioral problems in toddlerhood. Dev Psychopathol 10:283–300, 1998

Colombo C, Lucca A, Benedetti F, et al: Total sleep deprivation combined with lithium and light therapy in the treatment of bipolar depression: replication of main effects and interaction. Psychiatry Res 95:43–53, 2000

Coppen A, Bailey J: Enhancement of the antidepressant action of fluoxetine by folic acid: a randomized, placebo-controlled trial. J Affect Disord 60:121–130, 2000

Corbin Winslow L, Shapiro H: Physicians want education about complementary and alternative medicine to enhance communication with their patients. Arch Intern Med 162:1176–1181, 2002

Costei AM, Kozer E, Ho T, et al: Perinatal outcome following third trimester exposure to paroxetine. Arch Pediatr Adolesc Med 156:1129–1132, 2002

Cowe L, Lloyd DJ, Dawling S: Neonatal convulsions caused by withdrawal from maternal clomipramine. Br Med J (Clin Res Ed) 284:1837–1838, 1982

Cox JL, Holden JM, Sagovsky R: Detection of postnatal depression: development of the 10-item Edinburgh Postnatal Depression Scale. Br J Psychiatry 150:782–786, 1987

Critchlow DG, Bond AJ, Wingrove J: Mood disorder history and personality assessment in premenstrual dysphoric disorder. J Clin Psychiatry 62:688–693, 2001

Da Cost D, Rippen N, Dritsa M, et al: Self-reported leisure-time physical activity during pregnancy and relationship to well-being. J Psychosom Obstet Gynaecol 24:111–119, 2003

Dayan J, Creveuil C, Herlicoviez M, et al: Role of anxiety and depression in the onset of spontaneous preterm labor. Am J Epidemiol 155:293–301, 2002

Deuster PA, Adera T, South-Paul J: Biological, social, and behavioral factors associated with premenstrual syndrome. Arch Fam Med 8:122–128, 1999

Di Padova C, Tritapepe R, Di Padova F, et al: S-adenosyl-L-methionine antagonizes oral contraceptive-induced bile cholesterol supersaturation in healthy women: preliminary report of a controlled randomized trial. Am J Gastroenterol 79:941–944, 1984

Dunn PA, Rogers D, Halford K: Transcutaneous electrical nerve stimulation at acupuncture points in the induction of uterine contractions. Obstet Gynecol 73:286–290, 1989

Eastman CI, Yound MA, Fogg FL, et al: Bright light treatment of winter depression: a placebo-controlled trial. Arch Gen Psychiatry 55:883–889, 1998

Eisenberg DM, Davis RB, Ettner SL, et al: Trends in alternative medicine use in the United States, 1990–1997: results of a follow-up national survey. JAMA 280:1569–1575, 1998

Ericson A, Kallen B, Wiholm B: Delivery outcome after the use of antidepressants in early pregnancy. Eur J Clin Pharmacol 55:503–508, 1999

Evans J, Heron J, Francomb H, et al: Cohort study of depressed mood during pregnancy and after childbirth. BMJ 323:257–260, 2001

Epperson CN, Terman M, Terman JS, et al: Randomized clinical trial of bright light therapy for antepartum depression: preliminary findings. J Clin Psychiatry 65:421–425, 2004

Freeman EW: Premenstrual syndrome and premenstrual dysphoric disorder: definitions and diagnosis. Psychoneuroendocrinology 28 (suppl 3):25–37, 2003

Freeman EW: Luteal phase administration of agents for the treatment of premenstrual dysphoric disorder. CNS Drugs 18:453–468, 2004

Freeman EW, Rickels K, Schweizer E, et al: Relationships between age and symptom severity among women seeking medical treatment for premenstrual symptoms. Psychol Med 25:309–315, 1995

Freeman MP, Helgason C, Hill RA: Selected integrative medicine treatments for depression: considerations for women. J Am Med Womens Assoc 59:216–224, 2004

Freeman MP, Hibbeln JR, Wisner KL, et al: An open trial of omega-3 fatty acids for depression in pregnancy. Acta Neuropsychiatrica 18:21–24, 2006

Frey OR, Scheidt P, von Brenndroff AI: Adverse effects in a newborn infant breast-fed by a mother treated with doxepin. Ann Pharmacother 33:690–693, 1999

Gregoire AJP, Kumar R, Everitt B, et al: Transdermal oestrogen for treatment of severe postnatal depression. Lancet 347:930–933, 1996

Hendrick V, Smith LM, Suri R, et al: Birth outcomes after prenatal exposure to antidepressant medication. Am J Obstet Gynecol 188:812–815, 2003

Hibbeln JR: Seafood consumption, the DHA content of mothers' milk and prevalence rates of postpartum depression: a cross-national, ecological analysis. J Affect Disord 69:15–29, 2002

Holman RT, Johnson SB, Ogburn PL: Deficiency of essential fatty acids and membrane fluidity during pregnancy and lactation. Proc Natl Acad Sci U S A 88:4835–4839, 1991

Joffe H, Cohen LS, Harlow BL: Impact of oral contraceptive pill use on premenstrual mood: predictors of improvement and deterioration. Am J Obstet Gynecol 89:1523–1530, 2003

Jorm AF, Christensen H, Griffiths KM, et al: Effectiveness of complementary and self-help treatment for depression. Med J Aust 176:S84–S96, 2002

Klaiber EL, Broverman DM, Vogel W, et al: Estrogen therapy for severe persistent depressions in women. Arch Gen Psychiatry 36:550–554, 1979

Klein MH, Essex MJ: Pregnant or depressed? the effects of overlap between symptoms of depression and somatic complaints of pregnancy on rates of major depression in the second trimester. Depression 2:308–314, 1995

Klier CM, Muzik M, Rosenblum KL, et al: Interpersonal psychotherapy adapted for the group setting in the treatment of postpartum depression. J Psychother Pract Res 10:124–131, 2001

Klier CM, Schaffer MR, Schmid-Siegel B, et al: St. John's wort (Hypericum perforatum): is it safe during breastfeeding? Pharmacopsychiatry 35:29–30, 2002

Koltyn KF, Schultes SS: Psychological effects of an aerobic exercise session and a rest session following pregnancy. J Sports Med Phys Fitness 37:287–291, 1997

Kripke DF, Mullaney DJ, Klauber MR, et al: Controlled trial of bright light for nonseasonal major depressive disorders. Biol Psychiatry 31:119–134, 1992

Kulin NA, Pastuszak A, Sage SR, et al: Pregnancy outcome following maternal use of the new selective serotonin reuptake inhibitors: a prospective controlled multicenter study. JAMA 279:609–610, 1998

Labbok MH: Health sequelae of breastfeeding for the mother. Clin Perinatol 26:491–503, 1999

Laine K, Heikkinen T, Ekblad U, et al: Effects of exposure to selective serotonin reuptake inhibitors during pregnancy on serotonergic symptoms in newborns and cord blood monoamine and prolactin concentrations. Arch Gen Psychiatry 60:720–726, 2003

Lam RW, Carter D, Misri S, et al: A controlled study of light therapy in women with late luteal phase dysphoric disorder. Psychiatry Res 86:185–192, 1999

Lee A, Minhas R, Matsuda N, et al: The safety of St. John's wort (*Hypericum perforatum*) in breastfeeding. J Clin Psychiatry 64:966–968, 2003

Llewellyn A, Stowe AN: Psychotropic medications in lactation. J Clin Psychiatry 59:41–52, 1998

Loprinzi CL, Kugler JW, Sloan JA, et al: Venlafaxine in management of hot flashes in survivors of breast cancer: a randomized controlled trial. Lancet 356:2059–2063, 2000

Loprinzi CL, Sloan JA, Perez EA, et al: Phase III evaluation of fluoxetine for treatment of hot flashes. J Clin Oncol 20:1578–1583, 2002

Mackenzie ER, Taylor L, Bloom BS, et al: Ethnic minority use of complementary and alternative medicine (CAM): a national probability survey of CAM utilizers. Altern Ther Health Med 9:50–56, 2003

McCann IL, Holmes DS: Influence of aerobic exercise on depression. J Pers Soc Psychol 46:1142–1147, 1984

McDonald SD, Ferguson S, Tam L, et al: The prevention of congenital anomalies with periconceptional folic acid supplementation. J Obstet Gynaecol Can 25:115–121, 2003

McLennan JD, Kotelchuck M: Parental prevention practices for young children in the context of maternal depression. Pediatrics 105:1090–1095, 2000

Min Y, Ghebremeskel K, Crawford MA, et al: Pregnancy reduces arachidonic and docosahexaenoic in plasma tricyglycerols of Korean women. Int J Vitam Nutr Res 70:70–75, 2000

Motl JM: Acupuncture, in Handbook of Complementary and Alternative Therapies in Mental Health. Edited by Shannon S. San Francisco, CA, Academic Press, 2002, pp 431–452

Neumeister A, Goessler R, Lucht M, et al: Bright light therapy stabilizes the antidepressant effect of partial sleep deprivation. Biol Psychiatry 39:16–21, 1996

Nonacs R, Cohen LS: Depression during pregnancy: diagnosis and treatment options. J Clin Psychiatry 63 (suppl 7):24–30, 2002

Nordeng H, Lindemann R, Perminov KV, et al: Neonatal withdrawal syndrome after in utero exposure to selective serotonin reuptake inhibitors. Acta Paediatr 90:288–289, 2001

Nulman I, Rovet J, Stewart DE, et al: Child development following exposure to tricyclic antidepressants or fluoxetine throughout fetal life: a prospective, controlled study. Am J Psychiatry 159:1889–1895, 2002

O'Hara MW: Depression during pregnancy, in Postpartum Depression Causes and Consequences. New York, Springer-Verlag, 1994, pp 110–120

O'Hara MW, Stuart S, Gorman LL, et al: Efficacy of interpersonal psychotherapy for postpartum depression. Arch Gen Psychiatry 57:1039–1045, 2000

Olsen SF, Sorensen JD, Secher NJ, et al: Randomized controlled trial of effect of fish oil supplementation on pregnancy duration. Lancet 339:1003–1004, 1992

Oren DA, Wisner KL, Spinelli M, et al: An open trial of morning light therapy for treatment of antepartum depression. Am J Psychiatry 159:666–669, 2002

Porzio G, Trapasso T, Martelli S, et al: Acupuncture in the treatment of menopause-related symptoms in women taking tamoxifen. Tumori 88:128–130, 2002

Rabl M, Ahner R, Bitschnau M, et al: Acupuncture for cervical ripening and induction of labor at term: a randomized controlled trial. Wien Klin Wochenschr 113:942–946, 2001

Roby CA, Anderson GD, Kantor E, et al: St. John's wort: effect on CYP3A4 activity. Clin Pharmacol Ther 67:451–457, 2000

Rodriguez-Palmero M, Koletzko B, Kunz C, et al: Nutritional and biochemical properties of human milk, II: lipids, micronutrients, and bioactive factors. Clin Perinatol 26:335–359, 1999

Rossouw JE, Anderson GL, Prentice RL, et al: Risks and benefits of estrogen plus progestin in healthy postmenopausal women: principal results from the Women's Health Initiative randomized controlled trial. JAMA 288:321–333, 2002

Salmaggi P, Bressa GM, Nicchia G, et al: Double-blind, placebo-controlled study of S-adenosyl-L-methionine in depressed postmenopausal women. Psychother Psychosom 59:34–40, 1993

Schmidt K, Olsen OV, Jensen PN: Citalopram and breast-feeding: serum concentration and side effects in the infant. Biol Psychiatry 47:164–165, 2000

Schmidt PJ, Rubinow DR: Menopause-related affective disorders: a justification for further study. Am J Psychiatry 148:844–852, 1991

Simon GE, Cunningham ML, Davis RL: Outcomes of prenatal antidepressant exposure. Am J Psychiatry 159:2055–2061, 2002

Slaven L, Lee C: Mood and symptom reporting among middle-aged women: the relationship between menopausal status, hormone replacement therapy, and exercise participation. Health Psychol 16:203–208, 1997

Smith RN, Studd JW, Zamblera D, et al: A randomized comparison over 8 months of 100 micrograms and 200 micrograms twice weekly doses of transdermal oestradiol in the treatment of severe premenstrual syndrome. Br J Obstet Gynaecol 102:475–484, 1995

Soares CN, Cohen LS: Perimenopause and mood disturbance: an update. CNS Spectr 6:167–174, 2001

Soares CN, Poitras JR, Prouty J, et al: Efficacy of citalopram as a monotherapy or as an adjunctive treatment to estrogen therapy for perimenopausal and postmenopausal women with depression and vasomotor symptoms. J Clin Psychiatry 64:473–479, 2003

Stahl SM: Essential Psychopharmacology: Neuroscientific Basis and Practical Applications. New York, Cambridge University Press, 2000

Stearns V, Beebe KL, Iyengar M, et al: Paroxetine controlled release in the treatment of menopausal hot flashes: a randomized controlled trial. JAMA 289:2827–2834, 2003

Steiner M, Dunn E, Born L: Hormones and mood: from menarche to menopause and beyond. J Affect Disord 74:67–83, 2003

Sumaya IC, Rienzi BM, Deegan JF II, et al: Bright light treatment decreases depression in institutionalized older adults: a placebo-controlled crossover study. J Gerontol A Biol Sci Med Sci 56:M356–M360, 2001

Terman M, Terman JS, Quitkin FM, et al: Light therapy for seasonal affective disorder: a review of efficacy. Neuropsychopharmacology 2:1–22, 1989

Thomas CS, Bottiglieri T, Edeh J, et al: The influence of S-adenosylmethionine (SAMe) on prolactin in depressed patients. Int Clin Psychopharmacol 2:97–102, 1987

Tiemstra JD, Patel K: Hormonal therapy in the management of premenstrual syndrome. J Am Board Fam Pract 11:378–381, 1998

Wadhwa PD, Sandman CA, Porto M, et al: The association between prenatal stress and infant birth weight and gestational age at birth: a prospective investigation. Am J Obstet Gynecol 169:858–865, 1993

Weinberg M, Tronick E: The impact of maternal psychiatric illness on infant development. J Clin Psychiatry 59 (suppl 2):53–61, 1998

Weissman MM, Leaf PJ, Holzer CE 3rd, et al: The epidemiology of depression: an update of sex differences in rates. J Affect Disord 7:179–188, 1984

Weissman AM, Levy BT, Hartz AJ, et al: Pooled analysis of antidepressant levels in lactating mothers, breast milk, and nursing infants. Am J Psychiatry 161:1066–1078, 2004

Wisner KL, Perel JM, Finding RL: Antidepressant treatment during breast-feeding. Am J Psychiatry 153:1132–1137, 1996

Wisner KL, Zarin DA, Holmboe ES, et al: Risk-benefit decision making for treatment of depression during pregnancy. Am J Psychiatry 157:1933–1940, 2000

Yamada N, Martin-Iverson MT, Daimon K, et al: Clinical and chronobiological effects of light therapy on nonseasonal affective disorders. Biol Psychiatry 37:866–873, 1995

Zeskind PS, Stephens LE: Maternal selective serotonin reuptake inhibitor use during pregnancy and newborn neurobehavior. Pediatrics 113:368–375, 2004

Zuckerman B, Amaro H, Bauchner H, et al: Depressive symptoms during pregnancy: relationship to poor health behaviors. Am J Obstet Gynecol 160:1107–1111, 1989

Spirituality, Mindfulness, and Mind–Body Practices

14

Mindfulness Training and Meditation

Jeffrey D. Rediger, M.D., M.Div.
Lauren Summers, M.Div. Candidate

In recent years, as society develops a fuller understanding of the human mind through advances in physics and neurophysiology and experiences a burgeoning interest in spirituality, Western scientists are slowly moving into realms that were previously considered outside the purview of traditional science. One of the most compelling areas of new inquiry is the study of the nature and capacity of human consciousness. The exploration of consciousness has enormous implications for all of the humanities and sciences, and especially psychiatry, because a deeper understanding of consciousness is the key to both self-understanding and cultural understanding. Because Westerners are conditioned by a pervasive materialist worldview, it is difficult for the Western mind to accept the claim that objective knowledge about ourselves and the world can arise independently of the five senses.

Meditation provides a particularly interesting window into the nature and capacities of human consciousness. Believed to enhance the success and improve the quality of life for many ordinary and extraordinary people—housewives, attorneys, adolescents studying martial arts, and even championship players on professional basketball teams like the Chicago Bulls and Los Angeles Lakers—meditation is a practice whose time has come. According to Salmon et al. (1998), by 1997, more than 240 hospitals and clinics in the United States and abroad were offering their medical patients stress-reduction programs based on mindfulness meditation, a particular type of meditation examined below.

As the interest in meditation grows, meditation is increasingly becoming the object of scientific investigation. The meeting of Eastern contemplative traditions with Western science is a meeting of great import and meaning. In a sense, it is a union of Western post–Enlightenment period rationalism with Eastern concepts of enlightenment.

Psychiatry stands to reap important insights from the scientific study of meditation. This chapter summarizes progress that has been made to date. The published research literature on mindfulness meditation as an intervention for psychiatric disorders is critically reviewed, clinical guidelines are presented, and future research goals are suggested.

MINDFULNESS MEDITATION

Mindfulness training is a form of meditation that has been investigated as a treatment for particular psychiatric disorders. Research into the relative advantages and disadvantages of mindfulness training with respect to other styles of meditation has been coordinated by the mindfulness-based stress reduction (MBSR) program, led by Jon Kabat-Zinn at the University of Massachusetts Medical School. Kabat-Zinn's initial focus was on the treatment of cancer, chronic pain, and other medical illnesses in which stress and anxiety are frequent comorbid complaints. The MBSR program began examining the efficacy of mindfulness training as an intervention for psychiatric disorders during the early 1990s, and many studies have subsequently been undertaken by independent researchers.

Kabat-Zinn's work came from his long-standing practice of Buddhist meditation, from which he developed an interest in exploring the beneficial health implications of vipassanâ meditation. *Vipassanâ* is a Buddhist meditation practice in which the objective is to seek insight into the nature of one's own thoughts. Vipassanâ can be translated as "insight meditation" or "seeing clearly." Kabat-Zinn was a pioneer in translating subtle Eastern concepts about the nature of consciousness and meditation into descriptions of mindfulness practices that are comprehensible to Western patients and health care providers. The neutral term *mindfulness* is a term used to describe a meditative approach that entails nonjudgmental, detached awareness of thoughts and feelings. Kabat-Zinn has described some of the reasons for his approach as follows:

> The choice of mindfulness as the primary meditative approach was due to its immediate applicability to a great variety of present-moment experiences. This orientation lends a quality of "ordinariness" to the intervention that makes it more acceptable and accessible to a wide range of people with different life stressors and different medical disorders. (Kabat-Zinn et al. 1992, p. 937)

Mindfulness meditation differs from TM in that the meditator may attend to a wide range of mental objects while maintaining moment-to-moment awareness rather than restricting his or her focus to a single mental task or object such as a mantra (Kabat-Zinn et al. 1992).

Kabat-Zinn and colleagues have explained this approach in light of the fight-

or-flight response: "The approach to present-moment experience characterized by mindfulness can abate or short-circuit the fight or flight reaction characteristic of the sympathetic nervous system, particularly in stressful or anxiety-producing social situations where it is nonadaptive" (Miller et al. 1995, p. 197). They believe that mindfulness increases the capacity of humans to bear physical pain and emotional stress by encouraging meditators to experience strong associated feelings through a detached self-observing stance that facilitates acceptance and release. This occurs as the meditator gains increasing experience and begins to realize the transient nature of feelings and thoughts. Subjective mental and emotional experiences come and go "like waves in the sea" and the meditator eventually realizes that he or she is not defined or limited by them. In contrast to other meditation practices that are more didactic or abstract, in mindfulness training, the meditator actually experiences having a body or mind rather than simply being a body and mind. In other words, the meditator realizes that he or she is more than the pain or stress. The pain and stress do not define the person or his or her choices, as is often assumed. Kabat-Zinn and colleagues have commented that mindfulness training permits the practitioner to meditate in both a group setting or solitude.

RESEARCH ON MEDITATION

Early Studies

The Western medical literature contains more than 30 years of published studies on meditation. One important general observation is that different types of meditation cannot be easily compared, either in terms of their therapeutic benefits or in terms of empirical measures of their cognitive, emotional, and bodily effects. Some forms of meditation are ecstatic or cathartic, whereas others promote calmness and relaxation. Some approaches attend to the fluctuation of internal experience (e.g., thoughts, emotions, bodily sensations), whereas others train the mind to pay attention to particular external auditory or visual cues. Physiological changes associated with meditation, including electrical brain activity, vary widely, depending on the style of meditation, the duration of practice, and many factors that are difficult to quantify. Claims of remarkable emotional and physiological benefits achieved by advanced meditators have attracted considerable attention from Western scientists. However, current research methods used to investigate these claims are limited by our incomplete understanding of consciousness in general and the absence of standardized protocols for measuring changes in functional brain activity during meditation.

Transcendental meditation (TM), an approach in which the meditator achieves a meditative state by repeating a word or phrase called a *mantra*, is a form of meditation that received considerable research attention during the 1970s and 1980s. During this period, the relaxation response of Dr. Herbert Benson (1975) was rigorously tested as an intervention for physical and psychological problems.

Most research into the effects of TM has been carried out at the Maharishi University of Management in Iowa, but other centers and individuals are engaged in TM research as well (Taylor 1999–2004). To date, most formal research studies on meditation have focused on physical problems and the general anxiety or stress associated with them. Fewer studies have examined claims of beneficial psychological changes, including an increased sense of general well-being and life satisfaction, and only a very few studies have examined particular psychiatric disorders.

Evidence-Based Studies

Although there has been a recent surge of interest in meditation as a treatment for psychiatric disorders, few evidence-based studies on this application have been completed. The studies reviewed in this chapter were identified through a literature search of the *Medline, PsychInfo, Cochrane,* and *PubMed* databases as well as an online bibliography of more than 1,700 meditation studies (Murphy and Donovan 1999–2004a). Search terms included "mindfulness," "meditation," "mind–body medicine," and "Buddhism." Books on meditation and psychology were consulted for bibliographical references. Only those studies that focused on mindfulness as the primary intervention were reviewed. All studies reviewed used empirical measurement of outcomes, were conducted in psychiatric patient populations, and were published in English-language peer-reviewed journals. Studies of medical patients that investigated the benefits of meditation for psychological health or for general stress and anxiety symptoms in the context of a primary medical disorder were excluded. (See Appendix 14–A for a brief summary of non-evidence-based research on transcendental meditation.)

Two controlled studies and one open study were found that applied TM to patients with anxiety neurosis, as defined by DSM-II criteria (American Psychiatric Association 1968; Benson et al. 1978; Ghoda 1974; Keshu et al. 1980). However, these studies are not included in this review, because the psychiatric diagnoses were not based on a structured clinical interview and the criteria used to diagnose anxiety neuroses in DSM-II vary significantly from criteria used in later DSM editions. The current review relied on diagnostic criteria established in DSM-III-R (American Psychiatric Association 1987) or later versions of the diagnostic manual. The parameters of study design, including sample size and randomization, were not taken into account in study selection, because doing so would have excluded most of the remaining studies from the review.

EVIDENCE FOR EFFICACY OF MEDITATION IN PSYCHIATRIC DISORDERS

At the time of this writing, only six studies met inclusion criteria for this review. Two studies investigated the effectiveness of the MBSR program as an intervention for anxiety disorders (Kabat-Zinn et al. 1992; Miller et al. 1995), one examined a mindfulness-based intervention for binge-eating disorder (Kristeller and Hallett 1999), and three explored the potential of meditation to change the course of major depressive disorder (Ma and Teasdale 2004; Teasdale et al. 2000; Williams et al. 2000). Several articles did not meet the selection criteria for this review but suggested beneficial effects of mindfulness training as a treatment for borderline personality disorder and obsessive-compulsive disorder. These studies will be briefly reviewed.

Generalized Anxiety Disorder and Panic Disorder

The first major study on mindfulness meditation as a treatment for psychiatric disorders was completed by Kabat-Zinn et al. (1992), who investigated the application of mindfulness meditation in the treatment of generalized anxiety disorder, panic disorder, and panic disorder with agoraphobia. The project was a prospective outcome study of group stress reduction with a repeated measures design. In all, 22 (92%) of the 24 enrolled participants (ages 24–64 years) completed the trial. The participants were screened by psychologists and psychiatrists trained in administering the Structured Clinical Interview for DSM-III-R and met criteria for generalized anxiety disorder or panic disorder with or without agoraphobia. A score in the 70th percentile on the anxiety subscale of the Symptom Checklist–90—Revised and 10 or more anxiety-related symptoms on the Medical Symptom Checklist were required for inclusion in the study. Patients with other primary psychiatric diagnoses, any psychotic or endocrine disorder, or significant alcohol or substance abuse were excluded. Individuals taking anxiolytics or other psychiatric medications were allowed to participate, with their medications being closely monitored throughout the study. All subjects were assessed in person at recruitment, weekly throughout the study period, and at 3-month follow-up. Study participants were also evaluated by telephone every month up to 3 months after the study ended using the Beck Anxiety Inventory, Beck Depression Inventory, and ratings of the frequency and severity of panic attacks. Subjects functioned as their own pretreatment and posttreatment controls.

All subjects participated in an 8-week treatment course at the stress reduction and relaxation program (SR&RP) clinic and were assigned to meditation classes with other students who had a range of medical and psychological disorders, some of whom were not enrolled in the study. The course involved weekly 2-hour classes and a 7.5-hour intensive silent "meditation retreat" held 2 weeks before the end of the program. Formal meditation techniques such as body scan, sitting meditation, and mindful hatha yoga were taught as well as informal mindfulness techniques that could be practiced independently. Participants kept daily journals, used audiotapes, and practiced formal and informal meditation techniques. The program was designed to increase the duration of time spent in meditation over the course of treatment until patients were meditating up to 45 minutes at a time. Instructors encouraged participants to silently observe anxious thoughts as they arose rather than respond to them. The same instructor remained with each class for the duration of the program. Instructors did not know which students were in the study, nor were they told about their students' DSM-III-R diagnoses.

The Beck Anxiety Inventory, the Beck Depression Inventory, the Hamilton Anxiety Scale, the Hamilton Rating Scale for Depression, the Fear Survey Schedule, and the Mobility Inventory for Agoraphobia were administered on a weekly basis, and a compliance questionnaire was used at the end of treatment and at follow-up.

The 22 subjects who completed the intervention (92%) achieved clinically and statistically significant reductions in both self-rated and clinician-administered measures of anxiety during the intervention, gains that were maintained at 3-month follow-up. Repeated measures analysis of variance indicated that the Hamilton and Beck anxiety and depression scale scores showed significant decreases over the course of the study and that these improvements were maintained at 3-month follow-up. Clinical improvements were unrelated to the type or dosing of conventional medications. Of the 13 participants who reported at least one panic attack during the week before the study began, only 5 reported a panic attack in the week before the posttreatment assessment (mean Hamilton panic score: 18 ± 8.40 [SD]; range: 13–34). This trend continued at follow-up. The comorbid depression reported by 8 participants was not associated with significant differences in outcome. An independent effect of mindfulness training on depressive symptoms was not investigated.

This study was significant because it was the first formal demonstration of the clinical benefits of regular mindfulness meditation in the treatment of anxiety disorders. However, the small study size and the absence of a randomly selected comparison group preclude general conclusions being drawn from it. Furthermore, the groups were too small to determine whether a mindfulness training program is equally effective for individuals who take psychiatric medications compared with those who do not.

In a second study, a 3-year follow-up of the same cohort showed maintenance of the gains and good compliance with regular meditation practice (Miller et al. 1995). Of the original 22 subjects, 1 declined to participate, 1 was unreachable, and 2 were noncompliant with several attempts to schedule interviews, leaving 10 subjects who were interviewed in person and 8 who were interviewed by telephone. As in the original study, repeated measures analysis demonstrated maintenance of gains obtained as demonstrated by scores on the Hamilton and Beck anxiety scales as well as on other standardized scales. Most respondents believed that mindfulness training had "lasting value." No differences in outcomes were noted between subjects who entered the study taking benzodiazepines or antidepressants and subjects who were taking no medications.

To determine whether these results could be generalized, Miller et al. (1995) also examined 58 of the "nonstudy" subjects reported on in the original study. All subjects had met the screening criteria, received identical treatment in the SR&RP, and showed reductions in anxiety comparable with those of the study subjects, as measured with a standardized symptom rating scale. All subjects were retested on this measure and on compliance measures. Data were available for 39 of these 58 nonstudy subjects at pretreatment, posttreatment, and 3-year follow-up. Significant reduction in anxiety was sustained for most of those who responded to the treatment, and Miller et al. (1995) concluded that the finding of significant clinical improvement in anxiety found in the intensively studied cohort could be generalized to the larger group of participants who also had high anxiety.

Miller et al.'s findings suggest that individuals with chronic anxiety, whether they are undergoing other forms of treatment for anxiety or not, can make substantial and enduring positive change in their lives by reducing their anxiety and panic through participation in a weekly outpatient group MBSR program (Miller et al. 1995). The researchers proposed that mindfulness training should be used as a short-term therapy with conventional medications and has the potential to serve as a long-term therapy in place of medications.

The appeal of mindfulness training lies in its orientation toward what is "right" with people rather than what is "wrong." This orientation originates from the goal of mindfulness training to nurture and strengthen a person's innate capacity for relaxation, self-awareness, insight, and positive behavioral change. Miller et al. (1995) noted that an important factor in the beneficial results that the group obtained from MBSR may have been related to the capacity of meditation to facilitate the development of latent human capacities. Self-improvement efforts are often overlooked in conventional psychiatry, which has a tendency to pathologize and medicalize symptoms. In contemporary Western psychiatry, symptoms are often viewed as problems to be removed rather than as opportunities for personal growth. The SR&RP clinic serves a heterogeneous population of medical patients referred by their physicians. The focus at the clinic is not on treating anxiety or panic but rather on learning to deal more effectively with stress, pain, and chronic illness by developing the capacity for self-observation and self-regulation of both psychological symptoms and maladaptive behaviors.

The value of mindfulness meditation lies in its capacity to cultivate and strengthen an individual's innate capacities for relaxation, awareness, insight, and behavior change. Miller et al. (1995) have theorized that this approach may interfere with the sympathetic nervous system's fight-or-flight reaction, particularly in anxiety-producing situations when this innate response is maladaptive. Mindfulness meditation encourages personal growth in many ways. It teaches an individual to respond to stressful situations with greater clarity and calmness rather than reacting with panic or fear. There may also be important additional benefits for patient populations, who gain a sense of community by establishing common bonds with other meditators who have different medical diagnoses.

The above findings (Kabat-Zinn 1992; Miller et al. 1995) are promising; however, their significance is limited by small study size and methodological flaws. Both studies lacked a randomized nontreatment control group for comparison. Small sample size is a problem for most studies reviewed in this chapter and is further discussed below. Both generalized anxiety disorder and panic disorder patients responded equally well to the SR&RP intervention; however, a larger sample size is needed to determine whether the SR&RP is equally effective in each case.

In view of the serious and pervasive economic pressures that affect the quality of conventional medical care, the effectiveness of mindfulness training as a group technique makes it attractive from a financial standpoint. The average duration of anxiety symptoms of individuals entering the Kabat-Zinn (1992) and Miller et al. (1995) studies was 6.5 years; 5 of the 22 individuals in the original study discontinued traditional treatment or sought it at reduced levels for at least 3 years after the studies ended. Further research is needed to determine whether meditators eventually require less psychotherapy, fewer emergency room visits, and lower levels of medication or whether their productivity losses are lower than those who do not meditate. A large, controlled study (Johnson 1987) found decreased hospital admissions, fewer inpatient days, and a reduced number of outpatient visits over a 5-year period in a population of 2,000 TM practitioners compared with 600,000 matched individuals who did not practice meditation. But it remains to be seen whether beneficial psychological and medical effects can be sustained through regular mindfulness meditation.

Binge-Eating Disorder

In a 6-week study, Kristeller and Hallet (1999) evaluated the efficacy of group mindfulness meditation for binge-eating disorder. Binge eating is believed to be related to anxiety, dysphoria, reactive thought patterns, and distorted awareness of normal physiological cues with regard to food intake. The researchers wanted to determine whether meditation-induced awareness of cognitive and affective states and bodily cues that reinforce binge-eating behaviors had therapeutic effects. Of the 21 women who began the program, 18 (86%) completed it. Women were accepted into the study if they met diagnostic criteria for binge-eating disorder, were obese (body mass index greater than 27), were not participating in a weight-loss program or psychotherapy, and did not have a comorbid personality or psychotic disorder. Individuals taking weight-loss medications either discontinued them or continued using them at the same dosage during the study period. The study used a single-group design with an extended baseline and a follow-up of 3 weeks. Standardized instruments were used to assess eating behavior and mood symptoms. All subjects reported the number of binge-eating episodes and the proportion of episodes considered "large" or "small" on a weekly basis and rated feelings of self-control and mindfulness when eating, as well as self-awareness of hunger and satiety cues. The women were divided into three groups and attended seven sessions over the 6-week period. All participants learned and practiced three forms of mindfulness: general mindfulness, eating meditation, and mini-meditations. General mindfulness was used to develop detached awareness of thought patterns and bodily sensations, eating meditation focused on cultivating awareness while consuming food, and mini-meditations were used at meal times and in an effort to help subjects resist urges to binge. All participants were instructed to meditate at home.

The three women who dropped out of the study early were not included in the analyses. None of the women achieved complete abstinence from binge eating during the study period, and individual weights remained unchanged. However, nine (50%) of the participants reported an average of one or fewer binges per week at the completion of treatment, and their scores on several measures of eating and mood showed significant improvements. Scores on the Binge Eating Scale decreased significantly, as did measures of depression, which dropped from 17.8 to 10.2 on the Beck Depression Inventory. Scores on the Beck Anxiety Inventory showed a decline in anxiety from 16.3 to 10.5. Important factors in the success of this intervention were the participants' increased ability to control eating, increased overall sense of mindfulness, and greater awareness of hunger and satiety cues and binge triggers. Helping participants achieve a detached noncritical attitude toward their eating behaviors was regarded as a unique advantage of mindfulness meditation.

Like the two studies reviewed above, the significance of this study was limited by the lack of randomization and the small number of subjects. In addition, follow-up was limited to 3 weeks, which did not permit observations about the duration of improvement.

Major Depressive Disorder

A fourth study examined ways of combining mindfulness training with cognitive therapies in the treatment of major depressive disorder. A group of researchers collaborated to develop a protocol that evaluated a mindfulness-based cognitive therapy (MBCT) intervention (Teasdale et al. 2000). The goal of the research was to identify an alternative treatment to conventional therapies, including medications, supportive psychotherapy, and cognitive-behavioral therapy (CBT). Because cognitive therapy has been shown to be as effective as conventional drugs for major depression (Jacobs 2001), the researchers theorized that mindfulness training would further improve outcomes, because it uses "intentional control of attention to establish a type of alternative information processing configuration (or cognitive model) that is incompatible with the depressive interlock configuration" (Teasdale 1999, p. 154). However, there are significant differences between the two approaches:

> Unlike CBT, there is little emphasis in MBCT on changing the content of thoughts; rather, the emphasis is on changing awareness of and relationship to thoughts. Aspects of CBT included in MBCT are primarily those designed to facilitate "decentered" views, such as "Thoughts are not facts" and "I am not my thoughts." (Teasdale et al. 2000, p. 617; Baer 2003, p. 129)

This study was the first randomized clinical trial to present evidence in favor of a mindfulness-based clinical intervention for major depressive disorder. The trial consisted of a group skills-training program based on the strategy of pharmacological withdrawal and psychological prophylaxis in the form of MBCT. Individuals considered most vulnerable to recurrent relapse were the focus of the study; they were chosen because the information-processing theory of depressive relapse suggests that people with a history of severe recurrent depressive episodes are susceptible to biological and cognitive triggers. The 145 study subjects (ages 18–65 years) participated in an 8-week treatment program and a 52-week follow-up period. They were all free of symptoms when they entered the trial, were not taking any medication, met DSM-III-R criteria for recurrent major depressive disorder, and had experienced at least two episodes of major depressive disorder in the previous 5 years, one of which had occurred in the previous 2 years. Exclusionary criteria included current or frequent practice of meditation or yoga, attendance at psychotherapy or counseling sessions more frequently than monthly, more than four previous sessions of CBT, current substance abuse, and the presence of a comorbid psychiatric disorder.

Patients were randomly assigned to continue with ongoing treatment or to add a component of eight MBCT classes (2-hour/week manualized group treatment sessions for 8 weeks with up to 12 participants in each group) to their current treatment. All participants completed homework assignments covering guided and unguided exercises on awareness. A primary goal of the MBCT therapy was to cultivate "an aware mode of being, characterized by freedom and choice." All participants were followed for 1 year, with follow-up at 1-, 2-, 3-, and 4-month intervals.

The results demonstrated that MBCT helped those who had the most frequent episodes of depression. For MBCT participants with three or more previous depressive episodes, relapse rates were close to half of those for participants who continued their previous treatment during the 1-year follow-up period. This treatment effect was both statistically and clinically significant. However, the intervention had little or no effect on subjects who reported only two previous episodes of depression. Teasdale et al. (2000) speculated that patterns of thinking become more autonomous after three episodes, thus creating a habitual cycle of vulnerability. Because MBCT works directly on this cycle, it is not effective until a patient has reached a certain threshold of "depressogenic" thinking.

The advantages of this study include its large sample size, the inclusion of a control group, and its randomized, double-blind design. However, the study design did not allow the beneficial effects of specific components of MBCT to be distinguished from other factors, such as therapeutic attention or group participation. The most significant finding of this study was the demonstration of the effectiveness of MBCT training in preventing a future event rather than the therapy's effectiveness in reducing baseline symptoms of depressed mood. Because the researchers assumed that depression-related difficulties in concentration interfere with the implementation of MBCT, selection criteria for the trial excluded patients whose illness had not already significantly improved or remitted (Teasdale et al. 2000). The researchers concluded that MBCT could not be recommended as a treatment for acute depression but was appropriate as a preventive maintenance intervention for patients who had been depressed but were currently in remission. It is important to remember that MBCT is not mindfulness meditation alone but a combination of mindfulness meditation and CBT.

Autobiographical Memory

Williams et al. (2000) used a subset of the study population from the Teasdale et al. (2000) study to investigate whether autobiographical memory could be affected by MBCT. Williams and colleagues cited evidence that showed correlations between "over-general memory" (i.e., retrieving generic summaries of past events rather than specific events) and depression, posttraumatic stress disorder, and suicidal ideation. The study drew on evidence suggesting that over-general memory processing impairs an individual's ability to find solutions to personal problems. Theorizing that reducing over-generality in autobiographical memory might also diminish a person's vulnerability to depression, the researchers examined whether a tendency to encode and retrieve general memories could be modified.

In this study, 41 of the original 45 patients recruited completed the program. The inclusionary and exclusionary criteria were essentially the same as those selected for the Teasdale et al. (2000) major depressive disorder relapse-prevention trial. The Hamilton Rating Scale for Depression and the standard Autobiographical Memory Test were administered to measure the severity of depression both at the outset and four times during the 12-month follow-up period. Participants were randomized to receive ongoing conventional treatment with or without MBCT. The control patients showed no change in specificity of memories recalled in response to cue words; however, the MBCT group demonstrated significantly fewer general and specific memories when asked to recall events from their past in response to cue words. The study concluded that MBCT may be an effective preventive intervention for major depressive disorder because it helps patients practice observing elements of their subjective experience in a nonjudgmental way. This improved perspective encourages a more specific encoding of events and a more specific retrieval of memories.

Although autobiographical memory is believed to be associated with depression, and Williams et al. (2000) demonstrated the benefits of MBCT in reducing overgeneral autobiographical memory in formerly depressed patients, this does not necessarily mean that MBCT is effective in treating depressive episodes or preventing their reoccurrence. The small sample size and absence of a control group did not support the inference that all observed memory changes were attributable to MBCT alone. Finally, no independent measure was varied during the treatment to evaluate whether or not participants were changing their cognitive style as predicted.

Ma and Teasdale (2004), in an attempt to replicate the results of the Teasdale et al. (2000) study, conducted a randomized trial in which 73 participants received MBCT and 68 continued their conventional therapy. They found the same pattern of results as Teasdale and colleagues, with MBCT leading to a reduction in the rate of depression relapse from 78% to 36% among participants with three depressive episodes or more. Once again, no effect was found for those who had previously experienced two or fewer episodes of depression. Ma and Teasdale (2004) concluded that MBCT is "probably efficacious." This trial successfully replicated the findings of the Teasdale et al. (2000) study. It also provided a more in-depth analysis of the results and answered several of the questions that were raised in the earlier study about patients with two versus three prior depressive episodes. MBCT decreased rates of depression by 54% among participants with three or more past episodes; however, as in the earlier study, MBCT was ineffective for participants with two or fewer episodes. It is possible that this latter group of patients, all of whom had experienced their first depressive episode later in life, represented a different subset compared with those in the three-episode category who first experienced depression earlier in life. The researchers proposed that patients who develop late-onset depression prompted by difficult life events do not benefit from MBCT and may in fact be adversely affected by it. These findings are consistent with those from studies on conventional cognitive therapies for late-onset depression that suggest that different strategies may be required for this population. Teasdale and colleagues have published additional discussions on issues connected with major depressive disorder and the theoretical framework supporting MBCT and have compared mindfulness and cognitive therapies in the treatment of major depressive disorder (Teasdale 1999; Teasdale et al. 1995).

INTERVENTIONS IN WHICH MINDFULNESS IS A SECONDARY GOAL

Two other approaches in conventional psychiatry have formally incorporated mindfulness training. However, these approaches are centered on individual psychotherapy and are thus only briefly mentioned in this review.

Dialectical Behavioral Therapy

One approach that has incorporated mindfulness training is dialectical behavioral therapy (DBT), as developed by Marsha Linehan (1993a, 1993b). DBT is a treatment for borderline personality disorder that combines cognitive and behavioral approaches to help patients internalize the dialectical qualities of acceptance and change. DBT teaches four core skills: mindfulness, interpersonal effectiveness, emotional regulation, and distress tolerance in combination with a comprehensive treatment program based on individual psychotherapy. To date, no studies have isolated mindfulness training from the other core skills to examine its relative efficacy. Mindfulness training may facilitate increased awareness and tolerance of affect that would otherwise be suppressed or invalidated.

Meditation-Based Treatment for Obsessive-Compulsive Disorder

Jeffrey Schwartz's (1997) treatment for obsessive-compulsive disorder is another approach that relies on mindfulness as part of an overall intervention. The four-step treatment strategy is designed to help patients develop mindful awareness of their thoughts. It combines meditative mindfulness training with cognitive-behavioral strategies with the goal of diminishing the severity of obsessions and compulsions. Schwartz has argued that mindfulness is an effective adjunct to more conventional cognitive-behavioral approaches because it allows patients to observe their own internal sensations with the calm clarity of an external witness. As with DBT, no trials have been designed that isolate mindfulness meditation as an independent intervention or primary treatment component.

Mindfulness and Cognitive-Behavioral Therapies

As has been seen, meditation is entering the discourse around evidence-based psychiatry largely under the umbrella of one particular type of practice—mindfulness training. Meditation is also used in conjunction with CBT in several studies described in this review. Mindfulness and CBT share many common qualities. The goal of cognitive restructuring and other CBT techniques is to recognize maladaptive thoughts as they arise and counteract or replace them with consciously chosen thoughts. This practice is highly compatible with mindfulness training, which teaches patients to monitor their thoughts not only while sitting in meditation but also while going about their daily activities. However, one important difference is that CBT attempts to replace maladaptive thought patterns, whereas mindfulness meditation facilitates enhanced awareness of them while emphasizing their transience. "Change appears to result from viewing one's thoughts as temporary phenomena without inherent worth or meaning, rather than as necessarily accurate reflections of reality, health, adjustment or worthiness" (Baer 2003, p. 130). Kabat-Zinn et al. (1992) have observed that both the mindfulness and the CBT approaches encourage patients to cultivate detached, nonjudgmental observation of thoughts and feelings and that both techniques rely on homework and the use of cues to reinforce new behaviors. One important difference between mindfulness and CBT is the cost of the intervention. As mentioned above, mindfulness meditation can be administered to diverse patient populations in group programs and does not require a formal clinical setting. Thus mindfulness training offers significant cost savings over the traditional model of individual care used in CBT. The isolation of mindfulness meditation and other forms of meditation from conventional therapies will be necessary to establish meditation as an effective intervention in mental health care. Larger, more rigorous studies are needed to expand on the preliminary findings of studies reviewed in this chapter.

CLINICAL GUIDELINES
Implications of Research

Several provisional guidelines on the use of mindfulness training can be outlined based on the above review. With regard to generalized anxiety disorder, panic disorder, and panic disorder with agoraphobia, the findings of Kabat-Zinn et al. (1992) suggested that a group stress–reduction intervention based on mindfulness meditation may have beneficial effects and that the positive changes persist over months or longer. This group approach holds promise as a cost-effective treatment for anxiety. However, group mindfulness training requires a high level of commitment from participants in terms of daily practice and homework. Thus group participants need to be highly motivated to achieve significant benefits from the therapy.

The findings of the pilot study of Kristeller and Hallet (1999) on binge eating suggest that mindfulness training results in modest reductions in anxiety and the number of weekly binges and contributes toward increased capacity for control over eating behavior. These results must be cautiously interpreted because of the small study size and absence of a control condition. Also, because follow-up was limited to 3 weeks in that study, it is unclear whether the beneficial changes persisted.

The findings of the other studies suggest that MBCT helps prevent relapse in patients who have a history of three or more episodes of depression and whose disorder is currently in remission (Teasdale et al. 2000). This conclusion can be made with greater confidence because the researchers used a large sample size and a randomized, double-blind design, and the results were replicated in other studies (Ma and Teasdale 2004). The latter group concluded that MBCT is "probably efficacious" for the prevention of depressive relapse for individuals with a history of three or more major depressive episodes. The specific, essential components of mindfulness meditation that are effective in treating this disorder have not been studied apart from the CBT cognitive components. There is no evidence to suggest that MBCT is helpful in the treatment of acute depression, and findings to date suggest that MBCT does not benefit patients who have a history of fewer than three depressive episodes.

In citing evidence that correlates over-general memory with depression, posttraumatic stress disorder, and suicidal ideation, Williams et al. (2000), using a subset of the Teasdale et al. (2000) study population, found modest evidence for MBCT's efficacy in improving the specificity of autobiographical memory in patients with major depression. Many studies have demonstrated that patients who have difficulty recalling specific memories also have problems solving interpersonal problems (Evans et al. 1992; Goddard et al. 1996). However, the theory that reducing over-generality in autobiographical memory may diminish a patient's vulnerability to depression requires further research; future studies are needed to characterize a putative link between over-general memory and depressed mood. Thus the clinical application of MBCT as a technique for enhancing autobiographical memory is based on limited evidence.

Therapeutic Effects of Meditation

Regular meditation can improve one's capacity to make contact with oneself and with internal resources that change the experience of affective and bodily states during times of stress. The development of this capacity is especially helpful during times of increased anxiety or depression. Meditation shifts the user's relationship with anxiety and depression by cultivating the user's capacity for nonjudgmental awareness and nonattachment to any particular feeling or thought. Over time, feelings and thoughts are regarded as being interim rather than accurate reflections of objective reality. The meditator develops a growing sense that reality is linked to something deeper. This altered approach can be of tremendous therapeutic benefit because many people who experience anxiety or depression believe that their self-deprecating thoughts and feelings reflect reality. In contrast to cognitive therapies, which are directed toward changing maladaptive thought patterns by substituting healthier thoughts, mindfulness meditation depends on the meditator's direct experience of the inaccuracy and limited nature of all thoughts in general and anxiety-related thoughts in particular (Miller et al. 1995).

As mentioned above, meditation is attractive in part because of its nonpathological orientation toward the range of human experience and its effectiveness in facilitating the development of latent capacities for self-observation and emotional self-regulation. Not only does this perspective highlight the limitations of traditional psychotherapy, which may allow patients to talk about change rather than actually experience it, but it also emphasizes self-development over clinical improvement. In view of the strong emphasis placed on external "fixes" in Western medicine, this approach has been welcomed and is moving medicine in a direction that will probably become increasingly important. Western medical practitioners and managed care companies are increasingly aware of the role that lifestyle choices and personal attitudes play in determining physical, psychological, and spiritual health. An approach that cultivates the capacity to experience oneself and one's choices in response to stress and promotes personal growth is very appealing.

A Caution About Meditation

It is important to be aware of the dangers of meditation. Different kinds of meditation vary significantly in terms of the goals and methodological orientation. Some approaches are activating whereas others are calming. Some have a clear cathartic effect whereas others aim to facilitate the tolerance of intense affect. Although meditators often report important salutary effects, meditation practice should be supervised by an instructor who is psychologically aware and able to assist participants in remaining grounded and in touch with themselves. Participants who are unusually sensitive or who have a fragile personality structure may experience significant deleterious effects if the contents of the unconscious press to the fore too quickly or are allowed to erupt in too reckless a manner. Manic episodes are occasionally precipitated by some of the more activating meditations, and, in extreme situations, a hidden psychosis may be unmasked. Finally, individuals with personality disorders should be screened carefully before undergoing meditation, because their involvement in a meditation group can cause havoc for the other participants and the instructor.

SELF VERSUS NO-SELF

Different understandings of the self distinguish Eastern and Western psychologies. Western psychology emphasizes strengthening the ego and the core self, whereas the Buddhist meditative tradition asserts that there is no core self. On the surface, these disparate orientations might appear to be working from opposite points of view; however, further examination of these two philosophies reveals a shared vision of optimal mental health.

Descartes' *Cogito ergo sum* ("I think, therefore I am") and Freud's "Where id was, there ego shall be" have resulted in psychotherapies that are usually directed toward strengthening the ego and correcting low self-esteem, with the goal of improving an individual's functioning in society. In contrast, most schools of Eastern thought acknowledge a model of self that emphasizes one's relationship to family, community, and society as the primary source of identity. Some Eastern meditative practices are based on the premise that the "I" is doomed to seek happiness by searching for positive experiences that ultimately will prove disappointing and unfulfilling. An important general goal in many Eastern traditions is to let go of concepts that are believed to be illusions about the self. This perspective may be difficult for Westerners to understand because they have been trained and socialized by a culture that is more oriented toward acquisitiveness than letting go. From an Eastern perspective, building oneself up with self-esteem, self-confidence, or self-control is valued principally as a strategy for embracing the true interconnectedness of all things. This outlook suggests that bolstering the ego in an attempt to develop a powerful, individuated self will ultimately lead to greater suffering. Thus from an Eastern perspective, the therapeutic task is not to repair the "deficiencies" of childhood as much as to find the doorways to psychological freedom contained within them.

Disparate conceptions of the self and the treatment of "disorders" of the self raise questions about language, culture, worldview, and epistemology that are beyond the scope of this chapter. It is sufficient to comment that the West and the East have developed typologies for different parts of the human life cycle. The West has focused on the developmental needs of a self in the process of individuation, and the East has emphasized cultivating a self that has wider, more interdependent ego boundaries, as was summarized by the psychotherapist and meditation teacher Jack Engler:

> It seems that our Western traditions have mapped out the early stages of that development and that the Buddhist traditions have mapped out the later or more advanced stages in which "de-centering" from the egocentrism of early development culminates in self altruism. And neither tradition knows much about the other. They are talking about the same continuum of development, but about different segments of it. (Engler 1999, p. 112)

Engler affirmed the same point in a phrase that has become a mantra among those who intermingle the two disciplines: "You have to be somebody before you can be nobody" (Engler 1999, p. 117). Engler further explained, "The farther reaches of meditation practice require a strong ego in the psychoanalytic sense of the capacity to assimilate, organize, and integrate experience; and a relatively well-integrated sense of self" (Engler 1999, p. 117). The story has been told of how the Dalai Lama has had difficulty grasping the notion of low self-esteem and was saddened to learn that so many people in the United States have deep feelings of self-loathing and inadequacy (Michalon 2001, p. 211). One can debate whether the causes of impoverished self-esteem in the West are due to a strong emphasis on achievement, acquisitiveness, accumulation, and individuality at the expense of family, community, connection, and wisdom. However, it is clear that even in the East, it is important to have a capable and well-integrated self before one can give it up.

EPISTEMOLOGICAL LIMITATIONS IN RESEARCHING THE EFFECTS OF MEDITATION

If physicians have an untiring proclivity to diagnose illnesses wherever they exist, that tendency probably also extends to problems of culture and other ideas. One could argue that the scientific study of meditation is plagued by certain epistemological limitations. In other words, the methods with which we attempt to evaluate and understand meditation are incapable of capturing its essential significance. It is important to remember that the scientific method as it is traditionally characterized measures quantitative change in variables that can be clearly defined and operationalized; however, this method is less effective at identifying changes that are difficult to quantify. When meditation approaches are unambiguously defined and empirically evaluated, there is a risk that contextual elements from the Buddhist tradition on which they are based will be overlooked. "The cultivation of awareness, insight, wisdom and compassion, [are] concepts that may be appreciated and valued by many people yet are difficult to evaluate empirically" (Baer 2003, p. 140). Appreciating the full significance of subjective experiences that cannot be empirically evaluated is challenging in a culture where the intellectual basis for comprehending such experiences has eroded.

Although more studies on meditation are needed, researchers must also develop more sophisticated study designs that examine different kinds of phenomena. Novel research methods will address the nonempirical but valid qualities of meditation interventions. Future understandings of meditation may best advance if researchers pay attention to the results of evidence-based research and the stories of advanced meditators. More than 1,000 studies of meditation have been published since the early 1970s, but most of them have concentrated on beginning users of meditation and typically fail to reflect the richness of experience described in the classic contemplative teachings (Murphy 1999–2004).

Detailed case histories may also be very helpful in expanding our ability to understand and develop latent capacities of human consciousness. With that goal in mind, this review ends with a few case reports. While many reports have methodological problems, some are quite compelling and are reported so frequently in the literature that they are worthy of further research. Murphy and Donovan (1999–2004b) discussed meditators' reports of rapturous feelings that cause gooseflesh, tremor in the limbs, and feelings of ineffable bliss. In reviewing the Vedic literature of ancient India, which predates Buddhist practices and is the source of much of the information on the historical evolution of yoga, they described how feelings of sublime happiness sometimes suffuse the meditator's body. Here they quote the philosopher Sri Aurobindo, who has written at length about meditation and its different aspects:

> These reports by contemporary researchers echo many traditional accounts of meditation's delight. The Vedas, for example, claim that through spiritual discipline "Man rises beyond the two firmaments, Heaven and Earth, mind and body...to the divine Bliss. This is the 'great passage' discovered by the ancient Rishis." Elsewhere Aurobindo writes that "A Transcendent Bliss, unimaginable and inexpressible by the mind and speech, is the nature of the Ineffable. That broods immanent and secret in the whole universe. It is the purpose of yoga to know and become it."
>
>   And in the Taittiriya Upanishad it is said that "For truly, beings here are born from bliss, when born they live by bliss and into bliss, when departing, they enter." (Murphy and Donovan 1999–2004b, p. 3)

Many fascinating case reports about the experiences of advanced meditators have been published over the past decades, some in prestigious journals. Of course, publication of these reports does not verify their reliability. Yet such accounts merit review because they offer a contextual foundation from which to expand research on meditation. One such account follows:

> During a remarkable experiment reported by L. K. Kothari and associates, a yogi was buried for 8 days in an earthen pit and connected with leads to an [electrocardiogram (ECG)] in a nearby laboratory. After the pit was boarded up, the subject's heart rate sometimes went as high as 50 beats per minute, until a straight line appeared on the ECG tracing when the yogi had been in the pit for 29 hours. There had been no slowing of his heart immediately before the straight line appeared, nor any sign of electrical disturbance, but the experimenters proceeded with certainty that their subject had not died. Suspecting that their ECG leads had been deliberately or accidentally disconnected, they checked their machine and continued to monitor its tracings. To their astonishment, it started to register electrical activity some 7 days later, about a half-hour before the yogi's scheduled disinterment. "After some initial disturbance," they wrote, "a normal configuration appeared. The 'speeded heart rate' was again there, but there was no other abnormality." When the pit was opened, the yogi was found sitting in the same posture he had started in, but in a stuporous condition. In accounting for his remarkable ECG record, the experimenters argued that a disconnection of the ECG lead would have produced obvious markings on the tracing, as they found when they tried to simulate ways in which the yogi might have tinkered with it. Furthermore, the yogi was ignorant about such machines, and the pit was completely dark. If the machine had malfunctioned in some way they could not ascertain, it seemed an extraordinary coincidence that it started again just a half-hour before their subject's scheduled release. Apparently, the yogi was operating with some kind of internal clock that did not depend upon the daily cycles of light and darkness, for the most likely cause of the straight line on his ECG tracing was a dramatic decrease in the activity of his heart. Kothari and his colleagues finally could not account for this remarkable cardiac record (Kothari et al. 1973; quoted in Murphy 1999–2004).

Claims like this one of remarkable control of psychological and physiological functions have been made by Eastern meditation practitioners for millennia. Yet these impressive abilities are perceived by Eastern contemplative traditions as mere by-products on a path to self-realization, which is believed to be the realization of one's ultimate interconnectedness with all things. Although some advanced meditators will support Western empirical study of "meditative by-products," they are quick to emphasize that when isolated from the tradition and culture of Eastern meditation, these impressive abilities are virtually meaningless. The study of extraordinary experiences is an appropriate starting point for revising Western scientific investigations of meditation that takes its cultural context into account.

CONCLUSION

Epstein (1988) noted that there is remarkable similarity between mindfulness as described by meditation teachers and Freud's characterization of the ideal mind state of the clinician during therapy. Freud described the latter as one of "evenly suspended attention," which he defined as suspending judgment and giving impartial attention to everything there is to observe. "Thus, Freud proposed an optimal attentional stance or state of mind characterized by two fundamental properties: the absence of critical judgment, or the presence of deliberate attempts to direct equal and impartial attention to all that occurs within the field of awareness" (Epstein 1988). As Miller et al. (1995) noted, this attentional stance is remarkably similar to the quality of mind that is the central aim of mindfulness meditation.

The meeting of East and West is a meeting of profound importance. The degree to which contemporary Western science is capable of uncovering objective truths independent of culture remains unclear. Because science presupposes the validity of its worldview, it is arguable that science has become a favored method for translating knowledge of other cultures into an idiom that is more comprehensible to Westerners (Taylor 1999–2004). Irrespective of this philosophical problem, Eastern approaches to consciousness and meditation promise to be fertile sources of novel insights into how healing occurs and the healing capacities that human beings possess.

REFERENCES

American Psychiatric Association: Diagnostic and Statistical Manual of Mental Disorders, 2nd Edition. Washington, DC, American Psychiatric Association, 1968

American Psychiatric Association: Diagnostic and Statistical Manual of Mental Disorders, 3rd Edition, Revised. Washington, DC, American Psychiatric Association, 1987

American Psychological Association: Template for Developing Guidelines: Interventions for Mental Disorder and Psychological Aspects of Physical Disorders. Washington, DC, American Psychological Association, 1995

Baer RA: Mindfulness training as a clinical intervention: a conceptual and empirical review. Clinical Psychology: Science and Practice 10:125–143, 2003

Benson H: The Relaxation Response. New York, William Morrow, 1975

Benson H, Frankel P, Apfel R, et al: Treatment of anxiety: a comparison of the usefulness of self-hypnosis and a meditational relaxation technique: an overview. Psychother Psychosom 30:229–242, 1978

Engler J: Buddhist psychology: contributions to Western psychological theory, in The Couch and the Tree: Dialogues in Psychoanalysis and Buddhism. Edited by Molino A. New York, North Point Press, 1999, pp 111–118

Epstein M: Attention in analysis. Psychoanalysis and Contemporary Thought 11:171–189, 1988

Epstein M: Thoughts Without a Thinker. New York, HarperCollins, 1995

Evans J, Williams JM, O'Loughlin S, et al: Autobiographical memory and problem-solving strategies of parasuicide patients. Psychol Med 22:399–405, 1992

Goddard L, Dritschel B, Burton A: Role of autobiographical memory in social problem solving and depression. J Abnorm Psychol 105:609–616, 1996

Ghoda M: Yoga, meditation and flooding in the treatment of anxiety neurosis. J Behav Ther Exp Psychiatry 5:157–160, 1974

Jacobs GD: Clinical applications of the relaxation response and mind-body interventions. J Altern Complement Med 7 (suppl 1):S93–S101, 2001

Johnson O: Medical care utilization and the transcendental meditation program. Psychosom Med 49:493–509, 1987

Kabat-Zinn J, Massion AO, Kristeller J, et al: Effectiveness of a meditation-based stress reduction program in the treatment of anxiety disorders. Am J Psychiatry 149:936–943, 1992

Keshu M, Bali J, Peeke H: Muscle biofeedback and transcendental meditation. Arch Gen Psychiatry 37:93–97, 1980

Kothari LK, Bordia A, Gupta OP: The yogic claim of voluntary control over the heart beat: an unusual demonstration. Am Heart J 86:282–284, 1973

Kristeller JL, Hallet CB: An exploratory study of a meditation-based intervention for binge eating disorder. J Health Psychol 4:357–363, 1999

Linehan MM: Cognitive-Behavioral Treatment of Borderline Personality Disorder. New York, Guilford, 1993a

Linehan MM: Skills Training Manual for Treating Borderline Personality Disorder. New York, Guilford, 1993b

Ma SH, Teasdale JD: Mindfulness-based cognitive therapy for depression replication and exploration of differential relapse prevention effects. J Consult Clin Psychol 72:31–40, 2004

Michalon M: "Selflessness" in the service of the ego: contributions, limitations and dangers of Buddhist psychology for Western psychotherapy. Am J Psychother 55:202–218, 2001

Miller JJ, Fletcher K, Kabat-Zinn J: Three-year follow-up and clinical implications of a mindfulness meditation-based stress reduction intervention in the treatment of anxiety disorders. Gen Hosp Psychiatry 17:192–200, 1995

Murphy M: Scientific studies of contemplative experience: an overview, in The Physical and Psychological Effects of Meditation. Edited by Murphy M, Donovan S. 1999–2004. Available at: www.noetic.org/research/medbiblio/ch1.htm. Accessed November 28, 2004.

Murphy M, Donovan S (eds): The Physical and Psychological Effects of Meditation. 1999–2004a. Available at: www.noetic.org/research/medbiblio/index.htm. Accessed October 11, 2004.

Murphy M, Donovan S: Subjective reports, in The Physical and Psychological Effects of Meditation. Edited by Murphy M, Donovan S. 1999–2004b. Available at: www.noetic.org/research/medbiblio/ch4.htm. Accessed November 28, 2004.

Salmon PG, Santorelli SF, Kabat-Zinn J: Intervention elements promoting adherence of mindfulness-based stress reduction programs in the clinical behavioral medicine setting, in Handbook of Health Behavior Change, 2nd Edition. Edited by Shumaker SA, Schron EB, Ockene JK, et al. New York, Springer, 1998, pp 239–268

Schwartz JM: Brain Lock: Free Yourself From Obsessive Compulsive Behavior (with Beyette B). New York, HarperCollins, 1997

Taylor E: Introduction, in The Physical and Psychological Effects of Meditation. Edited by Murphy M, Donovan S. 1999–2004. Available at: www.noetic.org/research/medbiblio/ch_intro1.htm. Accessed November 28, 2004

Teasdale JD: Metacognition, mindfulness and the modification of mood disorders. Clin Psychol Psychother 6:146–155, 1999

Teasdale JD, Segal ZV, Williams JMG: How does cognitive therapy prevent depressive relapse and why should attentional control (mindfulness) training help? Behav Res Ther 33:25–39, 1995

Teasdale JD, Segal ZV, Williams JMG: Prevention of relapse/recurrence in major depression by mindfulness-based cognitive therapy. J Consult Clin Psychol 68:615–623, 2000

Williams JMG, Teasdale JD, Segal ZV, et al: Mindfulness-based cognitive therapy reduces overgeneral autobiographical memory in formerly depressed patients. J Abnorm Psychol 109:150–155, 2000

APPENDIX 14-A

Non-Evidence-Based Research on Transcendental Meditation

Transcendental Meditation in Depression

The following is a summary of four published studies on the effects of the transcendental meditation (TM) technique on depression. The subjects in studies of drug users and Vietnam veterans are most likely to be clinically depressed, although this was not the criterion for subject inclusion in these studies, and it is not clear whether they were clinically depressed.

A 6.5-week longitudinal study of psychiatrically healthy university student volunteers compared ratings of depression, anxiety, and self-actualization in 33 subjects practicing TM and 19 control subjects who did not meditate. In addition, at posttest, a third group of 16 long-term (43 months) meditators was measured. The ratings for depression ($P<0.005$) and anxiety ($P<0.001$) decreased more in the TM than in the control group, and ratings in self-actualization increased more in the TM group ($P<0.025$). The long-term meditators showed even further significant reductions of depression and anxiety and increased self-actualization (Ferguson and Gowan 1976).

A randomized trial of 99 psychiatrically healthy university students compared TM, autogenic training (AT), and a delayed no-treatment control condition. Expectation levels at pretest were not different between the TM and AT groups. At 8 weeks, the TM group decreased significantly on depression ($P<0.01$) and anxiety ($P<0.01$) ratings, whereas the AT group did not change significantly on these measures and the control group increased significantly. At 16 weeks, the TM but not the AT group showed further significant decreases in depression and anxiety. Correlation analysis showed that the regularity of TM practice and close adherence to instructions for the duration of TM practice were both significant predictors of positive change (Kniffki 1979).

A 2-year longitudinal study of 146 young drug abusers (ages 14–25 years) found significant reductions in drug use and improved psychological health, including decreased depression and nervousness, with TM, especially in regular practitioners (Geisler 1978).

A 3-month randomized clinical trial of 18 Vietnam veterans seeking treatment for posttraumatic stress syndrome found significant reductions in their symptoms, including decreased anxiety ($P<0.005$) and depression ($P<0.025$) compared with a group receiving traditional psychotherapy (Brooks and Scarano 1985).

Transcendental Meditation in Posttraumatic Stress Syndrome

A study of war veterans suffering from posttraumatic stress syndrome randomly assigned subjects to a TM program or psychotherapy. The comparison subjects receiving psychotherapy were of similar age and background and were undergoing similar life problems as those who received the TM program. The TM group showed significant improvements compared with control subjects on all measures—decreased anxiety, decreased alcohol use, decreased marital problems, decreased startle response, decreased emotional numbness, and improved employment status (Brooks and Scarano 1985).

References

Brooks JS, Scarano T: Transcendental meditation in the treatment of post-Vietnam adjustment. J Couns Dev 64:212–215, 1985

Ferguson PC, Gowan JC: Psychological findings on transcendental meditation. Journal of Humanistic Psychology 16:483–488, 1976

Geisler M: Therapeutiche Wirkungen der Transzendentalen Meditation auf drogenkonsumenten [Therapeutic effects of transcendental meditation on drug use]. Zeitschrift für Klinische Psychologie 7:235–255, 1978

Kniffki C: Tranzendentale Meditation und Autogenes Training—Ein Vergleich [Transcendental Meditation and Autogenic Training: A Comparison]. Munich, Germany, Kindler Verlag, 1979

15

Religious Beliefs, Spirituality, and Intention

Andrew Freinkel, M.D.
James Lake, M.D.

An existential "divide" separates many patients and physicians, a divide that probably interferes with the quality of care that patients receive. According to patient surveys, as many as 77% of individuals who seek medical care feel that their religious or spiritual beliefs are directly related to their health concerns, whereas only 16% of conventionally trained physicians or nurses ever inquire about these important matters (Anderson et al. 1993; King and Bushwick 1994). An older study of 203 family practice adult inpatients found that 77% of patients wanted physicians to consider their spiritual needs, 37% wanted physicians to discuss these needs with them more frequently, and 48% wanted their physicians to pray with them if they could (King and Bushwick 1994). In a large multi-center trial, 67% of the patients felt that physicians should be aware of their spiritual beliefs, 33% wanted to be asked about these beliefs, and 10% said they would be willing to give up time discussing medical issues to address spiritual beliefs (MacLean et al. 2003). In contrast, although some studies have demonstrated that physicians are generally unwilling to pray with patients, physicians are open to doing so at the patient's request (Monroe et al. 2003). One important contribution to the literature on spirituality and health care comes from focus group work done at Johns Hopkins University (Hebert et al. 2001), where researchers found that patients want to share their spiritual beliefs, but only if they believe that their physician respects their values.

An important and understudied area of this research is the extent to which physicians themselves believe in God and the healing power of prayer. Clear regional and specialty differences exist with respect to this question. For example, in Kansas the percentage of family practitioners who disclose their religious beliefs is similar to the prevalence of patients who believe in the power of prayer (80%). This suggests that there is little difference between beliefs of patients and their physicians (Daaleman and Frey 1999). In the only survey of psychiatrists' religious beliefs, only 23% expressed a belief in God; however, 92% stated that it is appropriate to concern themselves with their patients' religious or spiritual beliefs (Neeleman and King 1993). Given the above findings, it is reasonable to imagine that however open-minded psychiatrists are, it may be difficult for their patients to relate to them on issues of spirituality. Although newer data might provide a more accurate picture of current attitudes, the most recent data (1978–1982) suggest that psychiatrists have little interest in spirituality. In fact, only about 2% of studies in the peer-reviewed psychiatric literature include a religious variable, even in studies of substance abuse treatment, where 12-Step programs based on shared spiritual beliefs can be a component (Larson et al. 1986).

The above findings suggest that patients and physicians have shared beliefs about the role of religion, spirituality, and prayer in illness and health. However, for reasons that remain unclear, these shared beliefs seldom influence the day-to-day practice of medicine. Despite the apparent significant role religion and prayer play in health care from the perspective of both patients and physicians, discussions of the evidence supporting religious and spiritual beliefs and practices in physical and mental health are seldom included in conventional medical training programs in Western countries (Puchalski and Larson 1998). Strong historical associations between religious beliefs and health stand in stark contrast to the failure of contemporary medicine to address these important issues. Recent studies have brought a renewed sense of legitimacy to the role of prayer in maintaining health and treating illness and have opened the door to novel understandings of the role of human intention in healing. Two central themes are addressed in this chapter: associations between religious beliefs and mental health and evidence for the efficacy of prayer and other spiritual practices as treatments for mental illness.

RELIGION AND MENTAL HEALTH

Historical Overview

The roles of healers and priests have overlapped since the beginning of recorded history. As recently as four centuries ago, the major world systems of medicine attributed mental illness to supernatural forces or presumed energetic or humoral imbalances, and typical treatments included magical incantations or prayers. Priests and other spiritual adepts were healers, and gifted healers were elevated to the status of priest or shaman. A dramatic conceptual leap took place in the early sixteenth century with the publication in 1563 of *De Praestigiis Daemonum* ("The Illusions of the Demons"), the first scholarly work to distinguish madness from demonic possession. Further progress was made a century later with the publication in 1621 of Robert Burton's seminal work *The Anatomy of Melancholy*, which invoked natural and supernatural causes of madness and other serious mental illnesses. From the early eighteenth century through much of the nineteenth century, the Quakers and other radical religious movements spearheaded humanitarian reforms in standards of care for incurably insane individuals, who had previously been condemned to the dungeons and asylums of England, continental Europe, and the American colonies. The nineteenth century reform efforts of Benjamin Rush, considered by many to be the father of American psychiatry, were motivated by strong Christian beliefs and a spiritual upbringing.

By the early twentieth century, Freud had dismissed religious beliefs as signs of pathology or shared delusions. Despite an antagonistic cultural background, some Christian groups, including the Emmanuel movement, advanced early forms of spiritual psychotherapy that combined spiritual self-development with stress-reduction methods. Psychoanalysis, which pathologized or dismissed the psychological dimensions of religious experience, was the dominant intellectual framework in which psychiatry evolved during the first half of the twentieth century.

Today, biological models are widely accepted as correct and sufficient explanations of the causes and characteristics of mental illness. In these first years of the twenty-first century, psychiatrists are being trained to view spiritual or religious beliefs and practices as ancillary data that provide useful information about the patient's social or cultural background. As is clear to many researchers in this area, societal views toward the role of religious beliefs shift with regularity, but often in the absence of convincing data.

Influence of Religious or Spiritual Beliefs on Mental Health

The relation of religious or spiritual beliefs to mental health is complex and multileveled and involves social, psychological, and biological factors. To date most studies have examined the relation between participation in group religious practices and health in general. In contrast to the shared experiences of religious affiliation and practice, spirituality refers to individual experiences or beliefs that typically take place outside of organized social settings. The association between health and spirituality has eluded analysis because of the intrinsically subjective nature of spiritual beliefs and experiences, and few studies have been done on spirituality and health (Thoresen and Harris 2002). This section reviews what is known about the role of religiosity in mental health.

Religious practices probably have indirect and direct effects on mental health and general well-being that are both protective and health promoting. Epidemiological studies suggest that religious beliefs have a primary protective effect on mental health (Levin 1996). Numerous social, behavioral, and psychological models have been advanced in efforts to explain the observed relation between religious or spiritual practices and mental health. Religious involvement promotes optimism, which increases an individual's resilience for coping with stressful situations (Taylor 1989). Religious or spiritual values are correlated with mental health and health-promoting lifestyle choices, including exercise, diet, and moderate alcohol use (Hamburg et al. 1982). Regular involvement in religious activities has beneficial effects on general emotional well-being by providing a person access to a supportive network of like-minded believers during stressful periods, offering a sense of coherence or meaning that supports an individual's coping efforts, and enhancing self-confidence (Ellison 1994). The social and psychological benefits of religious involvement are achieved through regular contact with a supportive group in a safe and encouraging environment.

In contrast to the positive findings of most studies, some evidence suggests that religious coping methods are sometimes maladaptive and that discouraging experiences can take place in the context of organized religious activity. In such cases, religious involvement is sometimes associated with an increased risk of mental health problems (Krause et al. 1998; Pargament 1997). The complex and poorly defined interaction between personal, intelligence, social, and economic variables and the dimensions of religious experience preclude inferences of a strict causal relation between specific mental health problems and religiosity. What is known about the association between specific psychiatric disorders and specific factors of religious or spiritual engagement is reviewed in the following section.

Influence of Religious Beliefs on Specific Psychiatric Disorders

Because most data on the relation between religious practices and mental health come from epidemiological surveys or retrospective analyses, it is difficult to form strong arguments for direct beneficial effects of a religious or spiritual practice on any particular psychiatric disorder. Furthermore, the prevalence of specific mental health problems is different in disparate religious groups (Koenig et al. 1994). Significant findings from published research studies are discussed in this section.

Most studies on religion and mental health provide limited clinical data because they examine the relation between general beliefs (*religiosity*) and broad measures of mental or emotional well-being. Recent studies have used factor analysis to attempt to deconstruct religiosity into discrete dimensions. A meta-analysis of 89 studies on religion and mental health showed that regular involvement in organized religious activity is associated with a relatively reduced risk of depressed mood (Koenig et al. 1995). A survey study of over 3,000 adolescent girls found that two dimensions of religiosity, personal devotion and participation in a religious community, were correlated with moderately reduced risk of depression in adolescent girls and highly reduced risk (up to 43%) in more mature girls (Miller and Gur 2002). Another survey study used in-person interviews with over 1,000 pairs of adult twins to clarify associations between specific factors of religiosity and specific psychiatric disorders (Kendler et al. 2003). Religiosity was deconstructed into seven specific factors: general religiosity, social religiosity, involved God, forgiveness, God as judge, unvengefulness, and thankfulness. Social religiosity and thankfulness were associated with reduced risk for alcohol and substance abuse, antisocial behavior, major depressive disorder, generalized anxiety disorder, panic disorder, and bulimia. Four different factors—general religiosity, involved God, forgiveness, and God as judge—predicted reduced risk for substance abuse and antisocial behavior, but not for other major psychiatric disorders. These findings were limited by the cross-sectional design of the study; thus it is not possible to infer a causal relation between discrete factors of religiosity and specific psychiatric disorders. In a similar fashion, McClain et al. (2003) demonstrated a relationship between spiritual well-being and alleviation of end-of-life despair.

Even in view of the strong evidence supporting the mental health benefits of religious involvement, psychiatrists hesitate to approach this dimension of human experience as a potentially useful adjunct to conventional care, even though they are willing to consider other nonconventional adjuncts to mental health treatment. For example, if a clinician learned about research findings showing a relation between an herb and improved mental health, he or she would probably feel comfortable accepting a causal inference.

The relation between religious beliefs or affiliation with organized religion and specific psychiatric disorders is complex and difficult to delineate. A review of 80 published and unpublished studies revealed that organized religious affiliation was generally associated with decreased risk of depressed mood; however, private religious activities and certain religious beliefs did not predict lower risk (McCullough and Larson 1999). The findings of a survey of elderly men ($N=832$) with medical problems suggested that cognitive, but not somatic, symptoms of depression are less severe in individuals who use religion to help them cope (Koenig et al. 1995). Elderly depressed patients who participate in an organized religious activity have fewer symptoms, less severe symptoms, and are less likely to commit suicide (Koenig et al. 1997). Depressed medically hospitalized elderly patients who have strong religious beliefs are significantly more likely to have complete remission of mood symptoms compared with those who do not hold strong religious or spiritual beliefs (Koenig et al. 1998). This effect was not found to be related to the frequency of participation in organized or private religious practices.

Findings of a large survey study suggest that religious beliefs are associated with improved self-management of symptoms in patients with bipolar disorder (Mitchell and Romans 2003). Results from the National Institute of Mental Health's Epidemiologic Catchment Area survey ($N=2,969$) support the view that regular weekly attendance at religious services is associated with significantly lower incidence of most anxiety disorders, including agoraphobia, generalized anxiety disorder, and social phobia in general, and a relatively higher incidence of obsessive-compulsive disorder in younger individuals with strong religious beliefs (Koenig et al. 1993). Religious beliefs and practices are an important source of encouragement, social support, and insight among individuals with chronic severe mental illness, including schizophrenia (Sullivan 1993). Support groups built around shared spiritual themes have beneficial effects on self-esteem, quality of life, and community involvement in schizophrenic patients (Sageman 2004).

Rates of alcohol and drug abuse are generally lower in groups that follow organized religious practices (Ndom and Adelekan 1996). Feelings of deep personal devotion and conservative religious values are correlated with a generally reduced risk of alcohol or substance abuse and dependence; this relation is somewhat stronger in adolescents than in adults (Miller et al. 2000). The 12-Step programs that incorporate religious and spiritual values have a strong record of success in prolonging abstinence in recovering alcoholic individuals and those who abuse narcotics (Carroll 1993). Death anxiety is lower among individuals who follow a religious or spiritual practice in which a belief in an afterlife plays a central role (Chibnall et al. 2002; Klenow and Bolin 1989). Although religious beliefs or practices do not cause schizophrenia or other psychotic disorders, deeply held religious beliefs can exacerbate delusions (Tateyama et al. 1993).

PRAYER IN MENTAL HEALTH

Recent theories have attempted to explain the indirect and direct effects of prayer or other spiritual practices on mental health, both in individuals who pray, and in a prayed-for person or group. This section reviews the evidence for beneficial effects of prayer on physical and mental health.

Overview

A joint survey by *USA Today,* Stanford Medical Center, and *ABC News* of more than 1,000 respondents found that nearly 80% of the U.S. population believes that prayer can help people recover from disease ("Too many Americans in pain," 2005). The results of another study (Samano et al. 2004) suggest that about 75% of cancer patients who use complementary medicine treatments believe in the efficacy of prayer in cancer treatment. A smaller study (McCaffrey et al. 2004) reported similar—though less robust—findings. However, only 11% of individuals who pray in efforts to improve their health disclose this fact to their physicians. Although many physicians consider that a patient's religious or spiritual issues are the domain of a chaplain or of religious clergy, a large national poll found that almost 50% of patients would like to share in prayer with their physicians (Yankelovich 1996). Physicians who have strong religious beliefs frequently pray alone for their patients (Olive 1995). Findings from surveys and meta-analyses of studies on prayer suggest that a significant percentage of severely depressed or anxious individuals engage in prayer in an effort to address their mental health concerns, and approximately 33% of these report that prayer is very helpful in improving their symptoms (Astin et al. 2000; Barnes et al. 2004). Furthermore, of individuals who indicated that they used prayer to self-treat any psychiatric symptom, only 10% reported having sought treatment from a psychiatrist or family physician during the previous year. Renewed scientific interest in prayer led to the establishment of an Office of Prayer Research by delegates to the 2004 meeting of the Parliament of the World's Religions; at this think-tank on prayer, "men and women of science and spirit will work toward a common goal: learning more about the power of prayer" (Levitin 2004).

Beneficial Effects of Prayer on the Mental Health of the Individual Who Prays

Studies on the neurophysiology of prayer comprise an important part of ongoing research on the role of consciousness in health and illness. A serotonin hypothesis has been proposed to explain individual differences in the capacity to achieve transcendent spiritual experiences (Borg et al. 2003). Findings of a small functional brain-imaging study using positron emission tomography indicated that high serotonin receptor binding correlates with a relatively greater capacity for experiences of "self-transcendence." On the basis of neurophysiological studies of brain function during ecstatic religious or mystical states, D'Aquili and Newberg (1993, 2000) proposed a spiritual continuum model to explain the range of reported mystical and religious experiences. The model postulates that the human capacity for spiritual experiences is embedded in complex neural connections between primitive brain areas (the limbic system) and association areas of the neocortex that confer significant evolutionary advantages on humans. According to the theory, individual or group prayer, meditation, and other forms of ritual contemplation are unitive experiences that share common experiential and neurophysiological features. The kind and intensity of a spiritual experience are determined by the particular brain regions involved in that experience and the degree of shared activity among the regions. (See Chapter 14, "Mindfulness Training and Meditation," for a review of research on the mental health benefits of meditation.)

Beneficial Effects of Prayer on the Person Being Prayed For

There has been confusion around terminology used to describe spiritual treatment approaches. Among researchers, the term *prayer* refers to a request made to a loved one or a traditional healer by a patient requesting that an intention be directed at the patient with the goal of "causing" clinical improvements in a specified health problem. In contrast, in *intercessory prayer,* the patient asks a loved one or traditional healer to pray for God to intercede on his or her behalf, with the goal of improving a specific medical problem. In monotheistic religions, this request is generally made of a supernatural entity. *Distant healing,* one spiritual practice that is well suited for examination in clinical trials, is typically performed by a designated healer at a distance from the patient, sometimes by telephone or other modern means, and often without the patient's awareness. The putative health benefits of prayer and directed intention have been examined in many studies funded by the National Institutes of Health (e.g., see NCT00079534 and NCT00067717 at www.clinicaltrials.gov).

Dossey (1993) provided a comprehensive review of theories explaining the apparent effects of prayer on illness. The nonlocal healing approaches reviewed included intercessory monotheistic prayer as well as less-prevalent prayer systems such as therapeutic touch, qigong (see Chapter 17), Johrei, and Reiki. Findings of individual studies and meta-analyses of controlled trials on prayer and other forms of distant healing intention are highly inconsistent, and basic issues pertaining to appropriate study methodologies continue to be debated in the research community.

A systematic review of 21 studies of distant healing identified 12 studies with adequate design and control conditions that reported significant beneficial effects of prayer on humans, animals, and microorganisms (Benor 2001). A systematic review of 23 controlled trials of different healing approaches concluded that beneficial outcomes are reported almost 60% of the time when distant healing intention alone is used to treat a particular medical or psychiatric disorder (Astin et al. 2000). However, findings of other reviews (Alpher and Blanton 1991; Aviles et al. 2001; Ernst 2003) suggest that distant healing intention does not result in beneficial effects on health.

An attempted meta-analysis (Astin et al. 2000) covered 59 randomized, controlled studies on healing intention in humans (including 10 dissertation abstracts and five pilot studies) up to the year 2000. Of the 22 fully reported trials, the results of 10 suggested significant beneficial effects of being prayed for; however, only 8 were rated as methodologically sound, 5 of which showed significant effects. The heterogeneity of the studies precluded a formal meta-analysis. The authors noted that the small sample sizes in the 15 dissertations and pilot studies may have contributed to the lack of significant effects in 11 of those studies, and that inclusion of abstracts and pilot studies weakened the strength of the meta-analysis.

In a meta-analysis of studies on intercessory prayer, Jonas and Crawford (2003) examined 13 randomized studies, of which 46% demonstrated beneficial health effects that were statistically significant compared with the control condition. In a review of 90 randomized, controlled studies (Crawford et al. 2003), positive outcomes were reported in 70%–80% of these clinical and laboratory studies. However, the authors noted,

Major methodological problems of these studies included adequacy of blinding, dropped data in laboratory studies, reliability of outcome measures, rare use of power estimations and confidence intervals, and lack of independent replication. Many studies of the effects of intention on healing contained major problems that must be addressed in any future research. (Crawford et al. 2003, p. A96)

The possibility of a clinically effective nonlocal intervention is, of course, the holy grail of distant healing research and, for that matter, an important touchstone for the entire issue of the efficacy of prayer and intention on health. The question of whether or not prayer or directed intention can positively impact a solid tumor is in some sense the paradigmatic question. In a just-concluded triple-blinded, multisite, 4-year study on distant healing intention as an adjunct therapy for glioblastoma in which one of the authors of this chapter was the principal investigator, patients were randomized to a control (not prayed for) or treatment (prayed for) group (A. Freinkel et al., "Efficacy of Distant Healing in Glioblastoma Treatment," in preparation). Photographs of patients were sent to healers who had little specific knowledge of them, and each healer was instructed to concentrate positive healing intention on the designated patient. Through this triple-blinded research model, the advantage of the "placebo effect" emanating from the knowledge of being prayed for was negated and the anonymous quality of the prayer eliminated any empathic or spiritual connection between the patient and healer. Some religious authorities have argued that prayers are unlikely to be effective when the intercessor and the designated recipient of the prayer or healing intention do not know one another. Preliminary results of this as-yet unpublished study do not support the hypothesis that prayer and other forms of distant healing intention have a beneficial health effect on patients diagnosed with glioblastoma. However, other studies have reported beneficial effects distant intention on different types of disorders and less serious illnesses. Many questions remain unanswered, such as whether certain forms of prayer or other forms of distant healing intention are more effective than others, what the putative role of empathy in healing is, whether the distance of the intercessor or duration of the intercession influences the outcome, whether the frequency or quality of the prayer or intention affects the outcome, how to interpret the highly inconsistent outcomes associated with disparate research methodologies and statistical methods, and what the possible influence of researchers' and patients' attitudes or beliefs are on outcomes.

Beneficial Effects of Intercessory Prayer on Specific Psychiatric Disorders

The caution with which one must view reports of beneficial effects of distant healing intention on physical illness, such as cancer or heart disease, may not apply to psychiatric disorders. Initial research on distant healing as an unspecified tonic almost certainly oversimplified the phenomenon. For example, many writers (E. Targ, personal communications) have felt that distant healing has only positive effects; that is, its valence is only positive when given with positive intention. Others (e.g., Dossey 2003) have often considered the possibility that distant healing could potentially have a negative effect on somatic illness, so that the distant intention paradoxically shortens the survival of the patient. In this scenario, it has been suggested that the patient was somehow "destined" to die of the illness and thus the effect of the "healing" was an earlier and less painful death. Such speculation very rapidly devolves into clinically unanswerable matters of personal theology.

The apparent limitations of beneficial effects of prayer on physical diseases, including cancer, heart disease, or diseases of the brain, could well be artifacts of experimental design. In research conducted by one of the authors of this chapter, for example, attempts to adequately "blind" the participants resulted in a lack of personal connection between the "healer" and the patient (A. Freinkel et al., "Efficacy of Distant Healing in Glioblastoma Treatment," in preparation). If the beneficial effects of prayer and intention do in fact depend on personal interaction and empathic connection, such research might inevitably demonstrate negative results. Thus the most important question—Does a person praying directly for someone who they know and intensely care about have a clinical effect?—remains unanswered. However, such limitations may have no impact with respect to illnesses that are not related to clear pathology at a macroscopic or organ level. Thus the possible beneficial clinical effects of prayer and distant healing intention on psychiatric symptoms continues to be a viable research area.

When approaching mental health problems, numerous effective "spiritual" treatments already exist. In many cases, there are probably few differences in outcomes between a cognitive-behavioral therapy protocol for depression and weekly hope-centered pastoral counseling. In one 12-week, randomized, controlled, double-blind investigation of intercessory prayer on depression, all subjects knew that they were enrolled in the study, but none were told whether they had been assigned to the group receiving prayer. Significant and equivalent improvements in mood were reported in individuals who were prayed for ($n=496$) and individuals who prayed ($n=90$). Positive outcomes were highly correlated with subjects' belief in the capacity of prayer to heal and that they were the recipients of prayer (O'Laoire 1997). The reliability of the findings from this study is limited by the fact that standardized rating scales were not used. However, the outcomes were consistent with a strong placebo or positive expectation effect of prayer in depressed mood.

A controlled, double-blind study on distant healing in patients who met DSM-IV (American Psychiatric Association 1994) criteria for major depressive disorder compared intercessory prayer and antidepressants with conventional antidepressants alone (Greyson 1996). The outcomes, measured using standardized mood rating scales, did not show differential benefits of intercessory prayer over conventional medications alone; however, the small number of individuals enrolled in the study precluded significant findings. A 6-week double-blind, sham-controlled trial on distant Reiki in depressed patients, some of whom met DSM-IV criteria for major depressive disorder, found significant beneficial effects of regular Reiki treatments using standardized mood rating scales (Shore 2004); patients assigned to the sham Reiki treatment group did not improve.

Intercessory prayer may have beneficial effects on anxiety. In a randomized, double-blind study, patients who complained of transient anxiety after pituitary surgery were randomly assigned to a prayer group or a wait-list condition. Patients who were prayed for reported less postoperative anxiety in general and requested fewer pain medications compared with patients in the wait-list group (Green 1993). The researchers attributed the beneficial effects of prayer to suggestion and shared expectations. No benefits of intercessory prayer as a treatment of alcohol abuse were found in a 6-month pilot study ($N=40$) (Walker et al. 1997), with no differences being found in alcohol use patterns between patients who were prayed for and patients who were placed on a wait list.

TAKING A PATIENT'S RELIGIOUS AND SPIRITUAL HISTORY

Surveys suggest that most medically ill patients would like physicians to ask them about their religious or spiritual beliefs, especially if they become gravely ill (Ehman et al. 1999). It is sometimes assumed that clinicians are easily able to remove their own cultural and, in this case, spiritual biases, but this neutrality is probably seldom achieved in the day-to-day clinical practice of psychiatry. Relatively few clinicians are able to recognize their own reactions to patients' beliefs and values. This is critically important in issues as controversial as religious beliefs. Belief structures are at the very center of what makes an individual unique. In view of these issues, we strongly recommend that every clinical interview cover the patient's religious or spiritual beliefs and practices. Responses to a few open-ended questions generally provide useful information about the relation between the patient's complaints and religious beliefs and practices. FICA, a simple screening tool for taking a religious-spiritual history, includes a few simple questions (Puchalski and Romer 2000):

- **F (Faith and Belief)**—Do you consider yourself spiritual or religious?
- **I (Importance)**—How important are these beliefs to you? Do they influence how you care for yourself?
- **C (Community)**—Do you belong to a spiritual community?
- **A (Address in Care)**—How might health care providers best address your needs in this area?

The mental health professional who solicits information about religious or spiritual issues should be careful to avoid making remarks that might be construed as critical or judgmental of patients' beliefs. Patients sometimes misconstrue such comments as the caregiver's arrogance, an assumption that would interfere with good care. It is always unethical and often detrimental to impose one's own religious or spiritual views on a patient. With this caveat in mind, a good clinical interview is always guided by tact and respect for the patient and his or her needs, as in the following case example.

Robert was age 38 years when he began to experience unexplained feelings of dread that became especially intense in the hours before going to bed. Chronically disturbed sleep had left him feeling depleted and "dull" at work. He had recently broken up with his fiancée and spent many evenings staring at reruns of old movies on cable television. He developed the habit of drinking a nightcap "to quiet the dreams."

Two years passed before Robert sought professional help because he was worried about losing his job. His psychiatrist took a complete medical and psychiatric history and concluded that Robert met DSM-IV criteria for a major depressive episode with prominent vegetative symptoms combined with moderate alcohol abuse. Robert denied a suicidal plan or thoughts. He had no significant psychiatric history and no identifiable medical problems. During the intake, the psychiatrist found that Robert lacked insight into the possible causes of his intense feelings of dread and encouraged him to explore those feelings in psychotherapy. Robert refused therapy, saying, "I just need the right medications to stop these thoughts and make me sleep." Treatment options were discussed, and Robert agreed to a trial of mirtazapine (Remeron) 15 mg at bedtime. He also agreed to monitor his use of alcohol and to work on improving his sleep hygiene, including listening to relaxing music while taking a hot bath in the hour before going to sleep.

At the 2-week follow-up appointment, Robert reported that his sleep had improved dramatically, but he complained of intense cravings for sweets at night. He stated that he had been listening to music at night, but said, "The feelings kept on coming into my head. I don't know what's going on." To explore the possible causes of Robert's feelings of dread, the psychiatrist asked Robert to describe the feelings and associated memories. Within a few minutes, Robert recalled that when he was age 12 years, his father, age 38 years at the time, had a massive heart attack but survived. Robert later became estranged from his father in late adolescence, but the times he did spend with his father were typically associated with feelings of "darkness, just waiting for death." Robert wondered, "How could I have forgotten all that?"

During the next three sessions, Robert became aware of the fact that he had no spiritual beliefs. He realized that he had "stopped thinking about that stuff when I...shut out my father....The fear of death was just too great....There was this dark space at night when [my father] would just lie there....Every night I thought it would be the last time I would see him....He never talked about it....I couldn't handle it." Robert realized that he had actively avoided exploring spiritual dimensions of his life, including a fear of his own mortality, because of his experience with his father and had in fact "sealed off the fear" until it hit him when he was the same age as his father was when he had the heart attack.

In the ensuing months, continued work on these insights in psychotherapy and through journaling brought progressively greater relief to Robert. His depressed mood gradually lifted, and he decided to stop taking mirtazapine, remarking, "Now that I've found out what the real problem is, I guess I don't need to take a medication to fix a deeper problem." His feelings of dread markedly diminished and Robert was eventually able to significantly reduce his drinking. After discontinuing the mirtazapine, Robert was able to sleep well using relaxing music and hot baths, his nighttime cravings for chocolate stopped, and he had no further complaints of significant daytime fatigue. Although Robert had originally described himself as "a devout agnostic," in an effort to "look at my own fears around death," he had begun to explore many possible religious and spiritual directions. He had read several books on Christian and Buddhist views on living and dying, had attended services at a Unitarian church, and was planning to attend a weekend Buddhist retreat in the near future. On reviewing his rapid progress after 3 months of therapy, Robert described his increasing insight into "the spiritual side of the problem" as "the big idea…that really took care of this thing."

REFERENCES

Alpher VS, Blanton RL: Motivational processes and behavioral inhibition in breath holding. J Psychol 125:71–81, 1991

American Psychiatric Association: Diagnostic and Statistical Manual of Mental Disorders, 4th Edition. Washington, DC, American Psychiatric Association, 1994

Anderson J, Anderson L, Felsenthal G: Pastoral needs for support within an inpatient rehabilitation unit. Arch Phys Med Rehabil 74:574–578, 1993

Astin JA, Harkness E, Ernst E: The efficacy of "distant healing": a systematic review of randomized trials. Ann Intern Med 132:903–910, 2000

Aviles JM, Whelan SE, Hernke DA, et al: Intercessory prayer and cardiovascular disease progression in a coronary care unit population: a randomized controlled trial. Mayo Clin Proc 76:1192–1198, 2001

Barnes PM, Powell-Griner E, McFann K, et al: Complementary and alternative medicine use among adults: United States, 2002. Adv Data (343):1–19, 2004

Benor DJ: Healing Research, Vol 1: Spiritual Healing: Scientific Validation of a Healing Revolution (Professional Supplement). Southfield, MI, Vision Publications, 2001

Borg J, Andree B, Soderstrom H, et al: The serotonin system and spiritual experiences. Am J Psychiatry 160:1965–1969, 2003

Carroll S: Spirituality and purpose in life in alcoholism recovery. J Stud Alcohol 54:297–301, 1993

Chibnall J, Videen S, Duckro P, et al: Psychosocial-spiritual correlates of death distress in patients with life-threatening medical conditions. Palliat Med 16:331–338, 2002

Crawford CC, Sparber AG, Jonas WB: A systematic review of the quality of research on hands-on and distance healing: clinical and laboratory studies. Altern Ther Health Med 9 (3 suppl):A96–A104, 2003

Daaleman TP, Frey B: Spiritual and religious beliefs and practices of family physicians: a national survey. J Fam Pract 48:98–104, 1999

D'Aquili E, Newberg A: Religious and mystical states: a neuropsychological substrate. Journal of Religion and Science 28:277–200, 1993

D'Aquili EG, Newberg AB: The neuropsychology of aesthetic, spiritual, and mystical states. Journal of Religion and Science 35:39–51, 2000

Dossey L: Healing Words: The Power of Prayer and the Practice of Medicine. New York, HarperCollins, 1993

Ehman J, Ott B, Short T, et al: Do patients want physicians to inquire about their spiritual or religious beliefs if they become gravely ill? Arch Intern Med 32:210–213, 1999

Ellison C: Religion, the life stress paradigm, and the study of depression, in Religion in Aging and Health: Theoretical Foundations and Methodological Frontiers. Edited by Levin JS. Thousand Oaks, CA, Sage, 1994, pp 78–121

Ernst E: Distant healing: an "update" of a systematic review. Wien Klin Wochenschr 115:241–245, 2003

Green W: The therapeutic effects of distant intercessory prayer and patients' enhanced positive expectations on recovery rates and anxiety levels of hospitalized neurosurgical pituitary patients: a double-blind study. Doctoral dissertation, California Institute of Integral Studies, San Francisco, CA, 1993

Greyson B: Distance healing of patients with major depression. Journal of Scientific Exploration 10:1–18, 1996

Hamburg D, Elliott G, Parron D (eds): Health and Behavior: Frontiers of Research in the Biobehavioral Sciences. Washington, DC, National Academy Press, 1982

Hebert RS, Jenckes MW, Ford DE, et al: Patient perspectives on spirituality and the patient-physician relationship. J Gen Intern Med 16:685–692, 2001

Jonas WB, Crawford CC: Science and spiritual healing: a critical review of spiritual healing, "energy" medicine, and intentionality. Altern Ther Health Med 9(2):56–61, 2003

Kendler K, Liu X, Gardner CO, et al: Dimensions of religiosity and their relationship to lifetime psychiatric and substance use disorders. Am J Psychiatry 160:496–503, 2003

King D, Bushwick B: Beliefs and attitudes of hospital inpatients about faith-healing and prayer. J Fam Pract 39:349–352, 1994

Klenow D, Bolin R: Belief in an afterlife: a national survey. Omega 20:63–74, 1989

Koenig H, Futterman A: Religion and health outcomes: a review and synthesis of the literature. Paper presented at the Conference on Methodological Advances in the Study of Religion, Health and Aging, Kalamazoo, MI, March 16–17, 1995

Koenig H, Ford S, George L, et al: Religion and anxiety disorder: an examination and comparison of associations in young, middle-aged and elderly adults. J Anxiety Disord 7:321–342, 1993

Koenig H, George L, Meador K, et al: Religious affiliation and psychiatric disorders among Protestant baby boomers. Hosp Community Psychiatry 45:586–596, 1994

Koenig H, Cohen H, Blazer D, et al: Cognitive symptoms of depression and religious coping in elderly medical patients. Psychosomatics 36:369–375, 1995

Koenig H, Hays J, George L, et al: Modeling the cross-sectional relationships between religion, physical health, social support, and depressive symptoms. Am J Geriatr Psychiatry 5:131–143, 1997

Koenig H, George L, Peterson B: Religiosity and remission of depression in medically ill older patients. Am J Psychiatry 155:536–542, 1998

Krause N, Ellison C, Wulff K: Church-based emotional support, negative interaction, and psychological well-being: findings from a national sample of Presbyterians. J Sci Study Relig 37:726–742, 1998

Larson DB, Pattison EM, Blazer DG, et al: Systematic analysis of research on religious variables in four major psychiatric journals, 1978–1982. Am J Psychiatry 143:329–334, 1986

Levin J: How religion influences morbidity and health: reflections on natural history, salutogenesis and host resistance. Soc Sci Med 43:849–864, 1996

Levitin M: International prayer research office announced. Science and Theology News, September 1, 2004. Available at: www.stnews.org/News-656.htm

MacLean CD, Susi B, Phifer N, et al: Patient preference for physician discussion and practice of spirituality: results from a multicenter patient survey. J Gen Intern Med 18:38–43, 2003

McCaffrey A, Eisenberg D, Legedza A, et al: Prayer for health concerns: results of a national survey on prevalence and patterns of use. Arch Intern Med 64:858–862, 2004

McClain CS, Rosenfeld B, Breitbart W: Effect of spiritual well-being on end-of-life despair in terminally ill cancer patients. Lancet 361:1603–1607, 2003

McCullough M, Larson D: Religion and depression: a review of the literature. Twin Res 2:126–136, 1999

Miller L, Gur M: Religiosity, depression and physical maturation in adolescent girls. J Am Acad Child Adolesc Psychiatry 41:206–214, 2002

Miller L, Davies M, Greenweald S: Religiosity and substance use and abuse among adolescents in the National Comorbidity Survey. J Am Acad Child Adolesc Psychiatry 39:1190–1197, 2000

Mitchell L, Romans S: Spiritual beliefs in bipolar affective disorder: their relevance for illness management. J Affect Disord 75:247–257, 2003

Monroe MH, Bynum D, Susi B, et al: Primary care physician preferences regarding spiritual behavior in medical practice. Arch Intern Med 163:2751–2756, 2003

Ndom RJ, Adelekan ML: Psychosocial correlates of substance use among undergraduates in Ilorin University, Nigeria. East Afr Med J 73:541–547, 1996

Neeleman J, King MB: Psychiatrists' religious attitudes in relation to their clinical practice: a survey of 231 psychiatrists. Acta Psychiatr Scand 88:420–424, 1993

O'Laoire S: An experimental study of the effects of distant, intercessory prayer on self-esteem, anxiety and depression. Altern Ther Health Med 3:38–53, 1997

Olive K: Physician religious beliefs and the physician-patient relationship: a study of devout physicians. South Med J 6:274–279, 1995

Pargament K: The Psychology of Religion and Coping: Theory, Research and Practice. New York, Guilford, 1997

Puchalski CM, Larson DB: Developing curricula in spirituality and medicine. Acad Med 73:970–974, 1998

Puchalski CM, Romer AL: Taking a spiritual history (FICA) allows clinicians to understand patients more fully. J Palliat Med 3:129–137, 2000

Sageman S: Breaking through the despair: spiritually oriented group therapy as a means of healing women with severe mental illness. J Am Acad Psychoanal Dyn Psychiatry 32:125–141, 2004

Samano ES, Goldenstein PT, Ribeiro Lde M, et al: Praying correlates with higher quality of life: results from a survey on complementary/alternative medicine use among a group of Brazilian cancer patients. Sao Paulo Med J 122:60–63, 2004

Shore A: Long-term effects of energetic healing on symptoms of psychological depression and self-perceived stress. Altern Ther Health Med 10:42–48, 2004

Sullivan WP: "It helps me to be a whole person": the role of spirituality among the mentally challenged. Psychosocial Rehabilitation Journal 16:125–134, 1993

Tateyama J, Asai M, Kamisada M, et al: Comparison of schizophrenic delusions between Japan and Germany. Psychopathology 26:151–158, 1993

Taylor S: Positive Illusions: Creative Self-Deception and the Healthy Mind. New York, Basic Books, 1989

Thoresen C, Harris A: Spirituality and health: what's the evidence and what's needed? Ann Behav Med 24:3–13, 2002

Too many Americans in pain; too few taking appropriate steps to resolve it. Dynamic Chiropractic 23(15), July 16, 2005

Walker S, Tonigan J, Miller W, et al: Intercessory prayer in the treatment of alcohol abuse and dependence: a pilot investigation. Altern Ther Health Med 3:79–86, 1997

Yankelovich Partners, Inc: Time/CNN poll on religion and health, June 12–13, 1996

16

Yoga

Patricia L. Gerbarg, M.D.
Richard P. Brown, M.D.

Yoga is an experiential psychophilosophical system that can enhance physical and mental health. Yoga means "to unite" the individual life energy, *prâna*, with the universal energy, *Brahman*. The methods for achieving this union increase awareness of the mind and body through self-observation, enhance the capacity to control the mind (fluctuations of consciousness) and physiological processes, increase energy, reduce the influence of negative emotions and experiences, uncover the true self, and free the individual to improve his or her quality of life.

The history, philosophy, and practices of the many schools of yoga have been reviewed elsewhere (Becker 2000; Cummins 2002; Feuerstein 1998). Variations of the basic yogic techniques—*asanas* (postures and stretching), *pranayama* (yoga breathing), meditation, and relaxation—are used by most yoga practitioners. The ancient *rishis* (Hindu sages) knew that each practice enhances the others. This chapter focuses on pranayama and asanas.

Derived from wisdom as ancient as 5000 B.C.E., yogic ideas and practices were systematized by Patanjali in the *Patanjali Sutras* (200 C.E.) as "the eight limbs of yoga." These are briefly summarized below.

1. *Yama and Niyama:* Ethical and moral standards such as honesty, nonviolence, patience, compassion, and contentment with what one has (not being greedy), study of ancient wisdom to overcome dysfunctional habits, and devotion
2. *Svadhyaya:* The study of ancient yoga scriptures and knowledge
3. *Asanas:* Physical yoga postures, meditation on the body to experience the self
4. *Pranayama:* Yoga breathing techniques
5. *Pratyahara:* Turning the attention away from the senses toward the inner world of self-experience
6. *Dharana:* Concentration to focus attention

7. *Dyana:* Meditation with mental clarity and total calmness
8. *Samadhi:* Ecstasy or bliss that occurs when one is reunited with the true self, which is one and the same as universal energy or the divine

Western psychiatry has struggled to comprehend yoga science since Freud admitted his discomfort with the subject in *Civilization and Its Discontents:*

> It is very difficult for me to work with these almost intangible qualities. Another friend of mine…has assured me that through the practices of yoga, by withdrawing from the world, by fixing the attention on bodily functions and by peculiar methods of breathing, one can in fact evoke new sensations…which he regards as regressions to primordial states of mind which have long ago been overlaid. He sees in them a physiological basis, as it were, of much of the wisdom of mysticism…. (Freud 1930/1968, pp. 72–73)

Had Freud delved deeply into yoga science, he would have discovered that despite its exotic appearance, many principles of yoga are based on neuropsychological concepts corresponding to modern science. Little is known about the philosopher-yogin Patanjali, who is believed to have compiled the *Yoga-Sutras* that became the basis of Classical Yoga. This work, containing aphorisms on the practical and philosophical wisdom of Raja yoga, attributed the neuroses (depression, tremor, languor, doubt, heedlessness, sloth, dissipation, false vision, and instability) to "fluctuations in the state of consciousness." To restrict the fluctuations of consciousness, the *Yoga-Sutras* prescribed a list of remedies, including yoga breathing ("the expulsion and retention of breath [*prâna*] according to the yoga rules") and dream analysis ("[restriction is achieved when consciousness] rests on insights [arising from] dreams and sleep") (Feuerstein 1998, pp. 291–292).

Although yoga is steeped in tradition, it is remarkably innovative. Yoga masters who develop fresh insights, techniques, and approaches to the problems of modern life are deeply honored, particularly if their contributions benefit mankind. A love of creativity and adaptability to the changing world has kept yoga alive and relevant.

THE IMPORTANCE OF THE TEACHER

Just as health care practitioners bring a wide range of skills and personalities to their work, so also do teachers of yoga. They are subject to the same challenges: the effects of transference; their own needs for love, recognition, or power; and temptations to exploit trainees financially or sexually. In referring patients to yoga instructors, it is important for the referring clinician to obtain information about the teacher, the course, and the sponsoring organization. By speaking directly with local yoga teachers, clinicians can develop a better sense of the yoga teacher's training, experience, and ability to collaborate in patient care. Learning about yoga practice by taking yoga courses can be invaluable for clinicians.

A yoga teacher should be aware of a patient's vulnerabilities and how to help the patient deal with the challenges of yoga training. For example, patients with an anxiety disorder, posttraumatic stress disorder (PTSD), and social phobia may have difficulty dealing with the group situation at first. The teacher can provide more support, introduce the patient to other course participants, and assign the patient small tasks at first.

Only a competent yoga teacher can properly convey yogic techniques. These techniques should not be "learned" from a book; instead, skilled training is strongly advised. A good yoga teacher makes participants feel safe and relaxed and has the wisdom to explain how to apply basic yoga knowledge to problems of everyday life. An advanced teacher or yoga master can have a profound effect on the life of a serious student. In the presence of a yoga master, some people experience intense empathy, connectedness, awareness, peacefulness, and joy. The life work of a fully enlightened yoga master will reflect his or her dedication to uplifting mankind. A true master may be seen as a window to the infinite capacity for love contained in the self.

YOGA AND THE RESPONSE TO STRESS: NEUROPHYSIOLOGICAL MODEL

Until recently, research on stress focused on the sympathetic nervous system (SNS) and the hypothalamic-pituitary-adrenal axis. Yoga postures and breathing practices were seen as reducing sympathetic activity and thereby shifting the autonomic balance toward parasympathetic dominance (Malathi and Damodaran 1999). The possibility that yoga practices also stimulated the parasympathetic nervous system (PNS) through activation of vagal afferents was recognized in ancient yoga science (Rama et al. 1998) but has only recently been considered by Western science (Brown et al. 2003).

Vagal activity has been linked to emotional regulation, psychological adaptation (Beauchaine 2001; Sargunaraj et al. 1996), emotional reactivity, empathic response, and attachment (Porges 2001). Autonomic dysfunction plays a role in emotional disorders in infants and children (Bazhenova et al. 2001; Boyce et al. 2001; Mezzacappa et al. 1997; Monk et al. 2001), including attention-deficit/hyperactivity disorder (ADHD) (Beauchaine et al. 2001) and autism (Porges 2004). PNS underactivity has been found in adults with anxiety (Kawachi et al. 1995; Thayer et al. 1996), panic (B.H. Friedman and Thayer 1998), depression (Carney et al. 1995; Lehofer et al. 1997), PTSD (Sahar et al. 2001), hostility, and aggression, as well as in criminal offenders (Beauchaine et al. 2001; Mezzacappa et al. 1997).

Mind–body interventions, such as progressive relaxation, meditation, and many yoga techniques, calm the stress response system. Because breathing is under both voluntary and involuntary control, it provides a point of entry for controlling the autonomic nervous system (ANS). Experienced yogis have demonstrated the power of breathing techniques to control autonomic functions such as heart rate. Ancient yoga science described subtle energy channels, *nadis,* and vital energies, *prânas,* that can be viewed as nonphysical counterparts of nerves and electrical impulses. The locations of spiritual centers, *chakras,* correspond to major nerve plexuses and glands. Yoga breathing brings autonomic functions under voluntary control, initially by controlling the vagus nerve and the heart rhythm (Rama 1998).

Yoga masters used pranayama to regulate the body and the mind and develop character. These effects can be understood in the context of modern neurophysiology and neuroendocrinology. The voluntary control of breathing impacts ANS functions, heart rate variability, and cardiac vagal tone (Fokkema 1999). Yoga breathing influences central nervous system excitation (Lehrer et al. 1999; Sovik 2000) as measured by electroencephalogram (EEG; Balzamo et al. 1991; Roldan and Dostalek 1983, 1985), magnetoencephalogram (Carbon et al. 2000), and magnetic resonance imaging (Posse et al. 1997a, 1997b). Neuroendocrine functions affected by yoga breathing include decreased release of cortisol, a stress hormone (Gangadhar et al. 2000); increased prolactin, an antistress, social-bonding hormone (Janakiramaiah et al. 1998); and possibly vasopressin and oxytocin. Although many studies have documented the effects of yoga on brain function and physiological parameters, the underlying mechanisms have not been well understood. In particular, the neuropsychological bases for the observed shifts in emotional tone, attention, cognitive function, relatedness, centeredness, and well-being have not been elucidated. An integrative model of the effects of yoga breathing on mental states (Brown et al. 2003) will be presented.

The simplest pranayama is slow breathing. Any form of meditation that includes a focus on the breath will tend to induce slow breathing. The forms of pranayama—slow breathing, abdominal breathing, unilateral nostril, alternate nostril, *ujjayi, bhastrika,* cyclical breathing, breath holding, chanting, prayer, and singing—can be modified by the use of different frequencies, tidal volumes, number of repetitions, physical postures (*asanas*), and the use of the mouth or nose. Many yoga traditions use pranayama, including Integral, Kripalu, Ashtanga, Iyengar, Viniyoga, Kundalini, Raja, Hatha, Zen, Buddhist, Tibetan, and Sudarshan Kriya yogas. This chapter focuses on unilateral forced nostril breathing, forced alternate nostril breathing, and Sudarshan Kriya yoga as they contribute to the development of an integrative neurophysiological model.

Unilateral Forced Nostril Breathing

Unilateral forced nostril breathing (UFNB) is achieved by gently compressing one side of the nasal ala with the tip of the thumb to occlude the nostril. Research suggests that UFNB activates the contralateral cerebral hemisphere and the ANS. UFNB results in a shift toward greater EEG activation in the contralateral cerebral hemisphere (Morris 1998; Schiff and Rump 1995; Werntz et al. 1987). A natural ultradian rhythm of alternating cerebral dominance linked to the nasal cycle (natural rhythmic shifts in airflow through the right and left nostrils) has been hypothetically attributed to a lateralized rhythm of relative sympathetic and parasympathetic dominance (Schiff and Rump 1995; Telles et al. 1994; Werntz et al. 1983). Stancak and Kuna (1994) determined that 10 minutes of forced alternate nostril breathing (FANB) in subjects with 2–20 years experience in yoga breathing increased power in the beta and partially in the alpha bands on EEG topography, reflecting cortical excitation. During the second 5 minutes of the FANB, beta 1 band asymmetry decreased, suggesting a balancing effect on the functional activity of the right and left hemispheres.

Ancient yogis called right-nostril breathing *surya anuloma viloma* (heat generating) and left-nostril breathing *chandra anuloma viloma* (heat dissipating). A study at the Vivekananda Kendra Yoga Research Foundation showed that slow right-nostril breathing accelerated metabolism (37% increased oxygen consumption), whereas slow left-nostril breathing increased oxygen consumption by 24% (Telles et al. 1994). The blocking of one nostril creates increased airway resistance, thereby requiring increased respiratory effort. The effects of slow breathing, breath holds, and airway resistance on vagal afferent stimulation would be considered when evaluating the influence of UFNB and FANB on the nervous system.

Small pilot studies have found emotional and cognitive correlates with UFNB. Although there have been contradictory results using different techniques, overall the research supports the concept that UFNB activates the contralateral cerebral hemisphere (Block et al. 1989; Klein et al. 1986). These studies need to be replicated in larger controlled trials that consider the effects of the specific parameters of each breath technique.

Sudarshan Kriya Yoga

Sudarshan Kriya yoga (SKY), developed by Sri Sri Ravi Shankar, combines ancient and modern pranayama with meditation, chanting, and yoga knowledge (Muskin 2004). SKY is a good example of a yoga program with mental health benefits for healthy individuals as well as those with a psychiatric disorder. SKY is taught in The Art of Living Foundation courses (www.artofliving.org). The benefits are enhanced by elements of supportive group therapy, cognitive therapy, and attitudinal change (e.g., accepting people, valuing human diversity, reducing guilt, letting go of negative thinking, being in the present moment, dealing with stress). SKY uses *ujjayi* (victorious breath), *bhastrika* (bellows breath), the "om" chant, and *Sudarshan Kriya* (SK) cyclical breathing. These breathing patterns are described below, as is a unifying neurophysiological model for the action of yoga breathing. Research studies, treatment programs, risks and benefits, and treatment guidelines are also discussed.

Ujjayi Breathing

Ujjayi is a form of slow breathing through the nose against airway resistance (created by a slight contraction of laryngeal muscles and partial closure of the glottis) performed with the eyes closed. In the basic SKY course, *ujjayi* is done at a rate of 2–5 breath cycles per minute (cpm). The breath is held at the end of inspiration and expiration. The expiratory phase is longer than the inspiratory phase. Slow breathing and prolonged expiration have been shown to increase vagal tone (Cappo and Holmes 1984; Lehrer et al. 1999; Sakakibara and Hayano 1996); decrease chemoreflex sensitivity, which is mediated by the vagus (Spicuzza et al. 2000); increase respiratory sinus arrhythmia (Sovik 2000); and improve arterial baroreflex sensitivity, oxygenation, and exercise tolerance (Bernardi et al. 1998; Bowman et al. 1997). Adaptation of chemoreceptors and pulmonary stretch receptors may increase vagal afferent activity in the brain stem center (nucleus tractus solitarius) with projections to the thalamus and limbic systems (Bernardi et al. 1998; E.H. Friedman and Coats 2000) (Figure 16–1). This vagal activity is both physically and emotionally calming.

Contraction of the laryngeal muscles increases airway resistance, making it possible to prolong inspiration and expiration. It also stimulates somatosensory nerves that activate vagal afferents. Breathing against airway resistance increases heart rate variability, respiratory sinus arrhythmia, and baroreceptor stimulation (increased intrathoracic pressure) (Calabrese et al. 2000). Inspiratory resistive loads increase signal intensity in the parabrachial nucleus (PBN) and locus coeruleus on magnetic resonance imaging (Gozal et al. 1995). The PBN and locus coeruleus receive vagal afferents from the lungs and chest wall. Holding breath at end-inspiration and end-expiration augments vagal output (Telles and Desiraju 1992).

In clinical studies, unilateral electrical vagal nerve stimulation has been shown to improve mood in patients with refractory depression (Sackeim et al. 2001), memory in humans and rats (Clark et al. 1998, 1999), and cognition in healthy individuals, patients with epilepsy, and patients with Alzheimer's disease (Sjogren et al. 2002). Positron emission tomography studies have demonstrated that vagal nerve stimulation activates the thalamus (Schachter and Saper 1998).

We therefore postulate that *ujjayi* breathing activates vagal afferents to the nucleus tractus solitarius in the brain stem and PBN (see Figure 16–1). Two paths diverge from the PBN: the first projects to the limbic system, activating hypothalamic vigilance areas (increasing attention), and the second activates the thalamic nuclei that project to the cerebral cortex (parietal areas in particular), prefrontal cortex, and limbic system. The hypothesis that slow *ujjayi* breathing activates vagal afferents that quiet parietal cortical activity and activate hypothalamic vigilance areas would help explain the mental state of calm alertness associated with this type of breathing. The vagal afferent stimulation of limbic structures (with the release of prolactin and possibly oxytocin) and forebrain reward areas would enhance feelings of joy, well-being, and bonding.

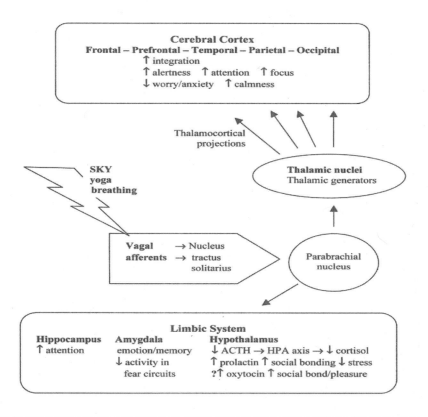

FIGURE 16–1. Proposed neurophysiological model of yoga breathing.

Yoga breathing stimulates somatosensory vagus afferents to the brain stem centers, the nucleus tractus solitarius and the parabrachial nucleus. Two paths diverge: one goes to the thalamus with projections to the cerebral cortex; the other goes to the limbic system. ACTH = adrenocorticotropic hormone; HPA = hypothalamic-pituitary-adrenal; SKY = Sudarshan Kriya Yoga; ↑ = increase; ↓ = decrease; ? = possible effect.

Variants of *ujjayi* breathing occur naturally. An *ujjayi*-like breathing that Fokkema (1999) called "strained breathing" has been observed in animals defeated in battle. It enables the animal to conserve energy while being alert and prepared for survival maneuvers. Mild forms of *ujjayi*-like breathing occur in toddlers playing with building blocks, children doing math problems, adults doing tasks that are mentally or physically stressful (D. Fokkema, personal communication, July 2004), and during sexual arousal, particularly in women (Fox and Fox 1969). Intense *ujjayi* breathing is used in martial arts to prepare for maximum exertion.

Bhastrika Breathing

The second breath technique used in SKY is *Bhastrika,* which is a strong, quick inhalation followed by a forceful exhalation at 30 cpm that stimulates the SNS and causes excitation on EEG (Roldan and Dostalek 1983, 1985) with temporo-parietal activation. Rhythms similar to gamma frequency bands associated with synchronization of neural assemblies have been observed (Kwon et al. 1999). *Bhastrika* provides mild SNS stimulation that over time could increase the capacity to respond to stressors without exhausting energy reserves. The subjective experience is one of stimulation followed by a sense of calmness. After *bhastrika,* "om" is chanted three times with a very long expiration.

Sudarshan Kriya Breathing

Sudarshan Kriya (SK) breathing is a unique form of cyclical breathing at three different rates through the nose with no airway resistance. Slow cycles of SK breathing are calming; medium and rapid cycles are analogous to very brief (<1 minute's duration), mild, controlled hyperventilation. Rapid cycles are followed by slow cycles for rest and recovery.

A 30-day pilot study using *Santhi Kriya* (a variation of cyclical breathing) for 10 minutes found a gradual, significant increase in alpha activity in the occipital and prefrontal areas before each day's practice, indicating a growing state of calmness (Satyanarayana et al. 1992). Hyperventilation for 100–300 seconds increased blood flow to and activation of the thalamus, leading to increased excitation of sensorimotor cortex and decreased excitation of the frontal and parietal cortex (Posse et al. 1997a, 1997b; Prevett et al. 1995). We hypothesize that, like hyperventilation, the medium and rapid SK cycles activate the thalamus and that thalamic projections excite sensorimotor cortex and quiet frontal and parietal cortical areas.

In one study, 19 experienced SKY practitioners showed increased beta activity (13–30 Hz) in the right and left parieto-occipital regions and increased alpha activity compared with that seen in control subjects (Bhatia 2002; Bhatia et al. 2002). This alpha and beta activity probably reflects calm relaxation with increased vigilance and attention (Bhatia 2002). Further studies are needed to better understand the vagal, thalamic, limbic, and cortical effects of SKY.

CLINICAL USES OF YOGA

Anxiety, Phobias, and Stress Overreactivity

Asanas, meditation, and pranayama—in particular, slow *ujjayi* breathing, UFNB, and FANB—increase PNS activity and reduce SNS activity, producing a state of physical and mental calmness. In 22 medical patients with an anxiety disorder, 8 weeks of mindfulness meditation, asanas, and relaxation techniques significantly improved the patients' anxiety and reduced panic attacks. At 3-year follow-up,

18 subjects maintained the practice and their improvements on depression and anxiety scales (Miller et al. 1995).

In a 3-month, randomized study of 50 first-year medical students, 25 were given three 1-hour sessions per week of yoga postures, pranayama, and meditation and the other 25 (the control group) used the time for reading. The yoga program significantly reduced anxiety levels on the day of examinations (Malathi and Damodaran 1999). In another study, six sessions of meditation, Hatha yoga, pranayama, and imagery significantly reduced anxiety and depression and improved self-efficacy in the caregivers of 12 patients with dementia (Waelde et al. 2004).

Individuals with severe anxiety or panic attacks may need extra preparation and reassurance before starting a yoga course. Sometimes when patients with a panic disorder attempt rapid breathing practices, they become worried about hyperventilating, and their anxiety can trigger a panic attack. This problem can be prevented by explaining to them the differences between controlled rapid breathing and uncontrolled hyperventilation. In addition, if they begin to feel anxious, patients with an anxiety disorder can be instructed to reduce the frequency of respirations until they become more comfortable.

Obsessive-Compulsive Disorder

In a pilot study (Shannahoff-Khalsa 2003) and a 12-month randomized trial (Shannahoff-Khalsa et al. 1999), Kundalini yoga using eight yoga practices (including asanas, meditation, and slow [1-cpm] left-nostril breathing with breath holds) improved symptoms of obsessive-compulsive disorder. Subjects in the Kundalini program showed significantly greater improvement than the control group, which was given relaxation and mindfulness training.

Posttraumatic Stress Disorder

SKY has been found to relieve symptoms of PTSD (Descilo et al. 2006). Dr. Sharon Sageman has noted SKY courses include aspects of cognitive-behavioral therapy and psychoeducation about human values of acceptance, social responsibility, and community service (Sageman 2002). SKY breathing sometimes evokes trauma-related sensations, movements, and affects in a safe, supportive setting. When this occurs, there is usually no conscious reexperiencing of the trauma. We (P.L. Gerberg and R.P. Brown) have observed that many patients with PTSD experience improvement in physical and psychological symptoms with SKY breathing. The overall effect is amelioration of feelings of fear, neglect, abuse, rejection, depression, isolation, and worthlessness. Patients with PTSD should be informed of the possibility of physical or emotional reactions. The therapist should monitor the patient during and after the course to help process intense emotions that may emerge.

Mood and Depression

A nonrandomized study of 87 "normal" college students found that both swimming and Hatha yoga (postures, stretches, and breathing) significantly improved depression scores and reduced indexes of stress (anger, confusion, and tension) compared with the control condition in which subjects only attended lectures (Berger and Owen 1992). In male students, yoga produced a greater mood elevation than swimming. In another study, compared with visualization and relaxation, 30 minutes of asanas and pranayama significantly improved perceptions of increased mental and physical energy, alertness, enthusiasm, and positive mood in a group of 71 "normal" adults (Wood 1993).

Three open studies found that SKY significantly improved depression (Janakiramaiah et al. 1998; Naga Venkatesha Murthy et al. 1997, 1998), and a randomized comparison study of 45 hospitalized patients with severe melancholic depression reported SKY to be as effective as imipramine (150–225 mg/day) and almost as effective as electroconvulsive therapy, but with no adverse side effects (Janakiramaiah et al. 2000). SKY has also been shown to normalize P300 event–related evoked potential amplitude in depressed patients (Bhatia et al. 2002; Naga Venkatesha Murthy et al. 1998).

In a randomized, wait-list control study of 28 mildly depressed young adults, two 1-hour Iyengar yoga classes per week for 5 weeks (using postures only) significantly reduced depression, fatigue, and trait anxiety scores (Woolery et al. 2004).

Bipolar Disorder

Yoga should be used with caution in bipolar I patients or those with an unstable rapid-cycling disorder, because rapid breathing can precipitate mania. Occasionally, bipolar patients may overuse the practices for self-stimulation, triggering manic symptoms. However, bipolar II patients whose hypomania is well controlled on antipsychotic medication and mood stabilizers other than lithium (yoga breathing can lower lithium levels by increasing excretion) have benefited from SKY. Patients taking lithium may be considered for yoga breathing if serum lithium levels are monitored and dosages are adjusted. Avoiding rapid-cycle breathing—and, in some cases, *bhastrika* breathing—will reduce the possibility of triggering a manic reaction. Bipolar patients with predominantly depressive symptoms often respond well to pranayama and asanas.

Schizophrenia and Psychoses

General yoga classes are not recommended for psychotic patients. However, one author reported that after 2 months of pranayama, 60 hospitalized schizophrenic patients became calmer and more relaxed (Higashi 1964). A study of nonverbal expressive group therapy compared four patient groups: psychotic, psychosomatic, heterogeneous, and control. The program included deep-breathing yoga and movement. All patients responded well with decreased anxiety, improved sociability, and reduced medication requirements (Jordan 1989).

Sageman (2004) introduced *ujjayi* breathing to a therapy group for women with severe chronic mental illness, predominantly schizophrenia. Most were Latino or African American women living below the poverty line who had a history of abuse, childhood trauma, and repeated psychiatric hospitalizations. The patients learned *ujjayi* quickly and responded with rapid improvement in mood, energy, and attention. Their affect and behavior shifted from sad, tense, or withdrawn to more cheerful, alert, and interactive (Sageman 2004).

Schizophrenic patients may benefit from modified nonstimulating yoga techniques in a supportive setting with skilled mental health professionals.

Stress-Related Medical Conditions

In a 2-month randomized study of 22 men with irritable bowel syndrome, those assigned to a yoga program consisting of 12 yoga postures and right nostril breathing (twice a day) had greater improvement in bowel symptoms and autonomic functions than those assigned to standard treatment with loperamide 2–6 mg/day (Taneja et al. 2004). Studies have also reported improvements in asthma (Nagendra and Nagarathna 1986; Singh et al. 1990), hypertension (Raub 2002), and cholesterol levels (Becker 2000).

We (P.L. Gerbarg and R.P. Brown) have found yoga asanas and pranayama to be helpful in patients with a wide range of medical disorders, including chronic fatigue, chronic pain, fibromyalgia, neck and back pain, temporomandibular joint pain, cancer, diabetes, asthma, and multiple sclerosis and other neurological disorders. Reducing stress and anxiety can ameliorate pain and other stress-related symptoms. Further research is needed to better understand how yogic techniques improve medical conditions beyond the basic reduction of stress reactivity.

Attention-Deficit/Hyperactivity Disorder

Because yoga breathing quiets the mind and heightens attention, it may prove helpful for ADHD and attention-deficit disorder. Studies of ADHD have demonstrated slower brain waves (Clark et al. 1998), deficits in cerebral lateralization (Heilman et al. 1991), and reduced oxygen consumption (Zametkin et al. 1990). Yoga breathing has been shown to improve brain wave activity, cerebral lateralization (Werntz et al. 1983), oxygen consumption (Telles and Desiraju 1991), and cognition (Jella and Shannahoff-Khalsa 1993; Naveen et al. 1997). Although meditation has been reported to be helpful in this population (Arnold 2001), patients with ADHD often have difficulty sitting still or concentrating enough to meditate, whereas they can benefit from asanas and pranayama.

A small controlled pilot study of the effects of yoga (breathing, postures, and relaxation) on attention and behavior in 19 boys diagnosed with ADHD (ages 8–13 years) found that the number of yoga sessions attended and the amount of home practice correlated with improvements on the Conners Parent Rating Scale, the Test of Variables of Attention response time variability scores, and the Global Emotional Lability subscale of the Conners Teacher Rating Scale (Jensen and Kenny 2004). A larger study is under way (D. T. Kenny, personal communication, September 5, 2004).

Addictions

In a 3-week study of hospitalized alcohol-dependent patients, those treated with SKY plus standard treatment had greater reductions in depression, anxiety, and cortisol levels than did patients given standard treatment and rehabilitation (Vedamurthachar 2002; Vedamurthachar et al. 2002). In a randomized study of 61 patients at a methadone maintenance program, traditional group therapy and Hatha yoga (asanas, pranayama, and relaxation) were equally effective in significantly reducing drug use and criminal activity (Shaffer et al. 1997).

Prison Programs

More than 100,000 prison inmates and staff in India, Europe, Africa, and the United States have been taught a modified SKY program. Prison authorities report that even in violent criminals and terrorists in maximum security prisons such as Delhi's Tihar Jail and Patna's Beur Model Jail, SKY significantly reduced violent behavior and improved the quality of life for prison staff and prisoners (Chaudhary 2004; Mukherjee 2004; Tang 2003). In a 4-month open pilot study, 86 juvenile offenders (ages 13–18 years) convicted of violent crimes with deadly weapons (gang members of Los Angeles County) were given SKY for 1 week (20–25 hours) in the Prison Smart Program, followed by 30 minutes of guided meditation and pranayama for 3 nights per week. Participants showed a significant overall reduction in anxiety, anger, reactive behavior, and fighting (Suarez 2002).

Public Health Programs: Emergency Response

Yoga breathing can be taught to large groups in just a few days. SKY has been used to relieve stress, anxiety, insomnia, depression, and PTSD after large-scale disasters, such as the wars in Kosovo, Bosnia, Iraq, and Sudan (Biswas 2004; Joseph 2004; Luedemann 2004); natural disasters, such as the Gujarat, India, earthquake in 2000 (Gupta 2001; "Restructuring Gujarat with human values" 2001) and Hurricane Katrina (Gerbarg and Brown 2005); and terrorism, such as the September 11, 2001, attack on the World Trade Center in New York City ("Helping New Yorkers take a deep breath" 2001). Scientific studies were not conducted during these mass disasters; however, many trauma survivors reported improvement in anxiety, mood, flashbacks, and daily functioning after learning yoga breathing (Gerbarg and Brown 2005).

In a controlled study of 180 survivors of the 2004 Southeast Asia tsunami living in refugee camps in Nagapattinam, Teresa Descilo and colleagues (2006) showed that a short 8-hour version of the SKY course rapidly and significantly reduced symptom scores of PTSD and depression on standardized tests. Improvements were sustained at the 3- and 6-month follow-ups. Yoga programs should be included in emergency response planning for disasters such as floods, earthquakes, war, and terrorism.

REFERRALS, RISKS, AND BENEFITS OF YOGA

SKY and other yoga programs can augment the psychotherapeutic and pharmacological treatment of patients with anxiety, depression, PTSD, ADHD, and stress-related physical illness. It can serve as an alternative treatment for those who prefer not to take medications. Patients with major depression may need a longer SKY course or several cycles of courses. Patients with psychotic disorders, severe borderline pathology, or difficulty maintaining a sense of reality should not undertake SKY training. High-functioning borderline patients can benefit from the course if they are able to attend sessions consistently and maintain appropriate boundaries.

During pregnancy, women are advised to avoid breath holding, straining, or *bhastrika*. Patients with high blood pressure, cerebral vascular disease, or a history of migraine headaches should also use caution, as they may not be able to tolerate breath holding, *bhastrika,* or head-down postures. Yoga breathing must be modified by a knowledgeable instructor for patients with epilepsy to reduce the risk of seizure. Yogic stretches should be initiated gradually in accord with each person's physical condition to avoid injuries.

The referring physician or health care professional is encouraged to take yoga courses before referring patients to them. By understanding the programs, health care providers will be better able to prepare patients for courses, support their daily practice, and integrate yoga lessons into patients' overall treatment. Moreover, many health care professionals find that the practice of yoga enables them to overcome the effects of stress and function with more energy, focus, and empathy.

CONCLUSION

Although more clinical studies using modern methodologies are needed, at this time there is sufficient evidence to consider pranayama and asanas as taught in SKY and other yoga disciplines to be useful adjunctive treatments for stress, anxiety, PTSD, depression, stress-related medical illnesses, obsessive-compulsive disorder, substance abuse, and rehabilitation of criminal offenders. In addition, yoga programs can benefit children with anxiety, depression, ADHD, and behavior disorders. In normal populations, yogic techniques enhance well-being, mood, attention, mental focus, socialization, and stress resilience. Proper training by a skilled teacher is essential to ensuring the safe and appropriate use of yoga practices. The major challenge for yoga practitioners is that they must maintain a daily practice to maximize the benefits. Programs that provide weekly follow-up sessions and group support will improve compliance. Active encouragement and reinforcement by doctors and therapists are critical in sustaining patient involvement in yoga.

REFERENCES

Arnold LE: Alternative treatments for adults with attention-deficit hyperactivity disorder (ADHD). Ann N Y Acad Sci 931:310–341, 2001

Balzamo E, Gayan-Ramirez G, Jammes Y: Quantitative EEG changes under various conditions of hyperventilation in the sensorimotor cortex of the anaesthetized cat. Electroencephalogr Clin Neurophysiol 78:159–165, 1991

Bazhenova OV, Plonskaia O, Porges SW: Vagal reactivity and affective adjustment in infants during interaction challenges. Child Dev 72:1314–1326, 2001

Beauchaine T: Vagal tone, development, and Gray's motivational theory: toward an integrated model of autonomic nervous system functioning in psychopathology. Dev Psychopathol 13:183–214, 2001

Beauchaine TP, Katkin ES, Strassberg Z, et al: Disinhibitory psychopathology in male adolescents: discriminating conduct disorder from attention-deficit/hyperactivity disorder through concurrent assessment of multiple autonomic states. J Abnorm Psychol 110:610–624, 2001

Becker I: Uses of yoga in psychiatry and medicine, in Complementary and Alternative Medicine and Psychiatry. Edited by Muskin PR (Review of Psychiatry Series, Vol 19; Oldham JM and Riba MB, series eds). Washington, DC, American Psychiatric Press, 2000, pp 107–146

Berger BG, Owen DR: Mood alteration with yoga and swimming: aerobic exercise may not be necessary. Percept Mot Skills 75:1331–1343, 1992

Bernardi L, Spadacini G, Bellwon J, et al: Effect of breathing rate on oxygen saturation and exercise performance in chronic heart failure. Lancet 351:1308–1311, 1998

Bhatia M: EEG during Sudarshan Kriya: a quantitative analysis. Paper presented at the Science of Breath International Symposium on Sudarshan Kriya, Pranayam and Consciousness. New Delhi, All India Institute of Medical Sciences, March 2–3, 2002, pp 23–25

Bhatia M, Kumar A, Pandev RM, et al: Electrophysiological Evaluation of Sudarshan Kriya: an EEG, Baer, P300 Study. Paper presented at the Science of Breath International Symposium on Sudarshan Kriya, Pranayam and Consciousness. New Delhi, All India Institute of Medical Sciences, March 2–3, 2002, p 30

Biswas S: Indian stress-busters target Iraq. BBC News online BBCMMIV 14 January 2004. Available at: http://newsvote.bbc.co.uk/1/hi/world/south_asia/3393327. stm. Accessed September 3, 2004.

Block RA, Arnott DP, Quigley B, et al: Unilateral nostril breathing influences lateralized cognitive performance. Brain Cogn 9:181–190, 1989

Bowman AJ, Clayton RH, Murray A, et al: Effects of aerobic exercise training and yoga on the baroreflex in healthy elderly persons. Eur J Clin Invest 27:443–449, 1997

Boyce WT, Quas J, Alkon A, et al: Autonomic reactivity and psychopathology in middle childhood. Br J Psychiatry 179:144–150, 2001

Brown RP, Gerbarg PL, Muskin PR: Complementary and alternative treatments in psychiatry, in Psychiatry, 2nd Edition, Vol 2. Edited by Tasman A, Kay J, Lieberman J. West Sussex, UK, Wiley, 2003, pp 2147–2183

Calabrese P, Perrault H, Dinh TP, et al: Cardiorespiratory interactions during resistive load breathing. Am J Physiol 279:R2208–R2213, 2000

Cappo BM, Holmes DS: The utility of prolonged respiratory exhalation for reducing physiological and psychological arousal in non-threatening and threatening situations. J Psychosom Res 28:265–273, 1984

Carbon M, Wubbeler G, Trahms L, et al: Hyperventilation-induced human cerebral magnetic fields non-invasively monitored by multichannel "direct current" magnetoencephalography. Neurosci Lett 287:227–230, 2000

Carney RM, Saunders RD, Freedland KE, et al: Association of depression with reduced heart rate variability in coronary artery disease. Am J Cardiol 76:562–564, 1995

Chaudhary PK: Process of change in Bihar is on, says Sri Sri Ravishankar. The Times of India, February 26, 2004, pp 1–4

Clark KB, Smith DC, Hassert DL, et al: Posttraining electrical stimulation of vagal afferents with concomitant vagal efferent inactivation enhances memory storage processes in the rat. Neurobiol Learn Mem 70:364–373, 1998

Clark KB, Naritoku DK, Smith DC, et al: Enhanced recognition memory following vagus nerve stimulation in human subjects. Nat Neurosci 2:94–98, 1999

Cummins C: Prescription for pranayama. Yoga Journal 166:108–188, 2002

Descilo T, Vedamurthachar A, Gerbarg PL, et al: Comparison of a yoga breath-based program and a client-centered exposure therapy for relief of PTSD and depression in survivors of tsunami disaster. Proceedings World Conference Expanding Paradigms: Science Consciousness and Spirituality. New Delhi, India, AIIMS [All India Institute of Medical Sciences], 2006, pp 64–78

Feuerstein G: The Yoga Tradition: Its History, Literature, Philosophy, and Practice. Prescott, AZ, Hohm Press, 1998

Fokkema DS: The psychobiology of strained breathing and its cardiovascular implications: a functional system review. Psychophysiology 36:164–175, 1999

Fox CA, Fox B: Blood pressure and respiratory patterns during human coitus. J Reprod Fertil 19:405–415, 1969

Freud S: Civilization and its discontents (1930[1929]/1961), in The Standard Edition of the Complete Psychological Works of Sigmund Freud, Vol 21. Translated and edited by Strachey J. London, Hogarth Press, 1961, pp 72–73

Friedman BH, Thayer JF: Autonomic balance revisited: panic anxiety and heart rate variability. J Psychosom Res 44:133–151, 1998

Friedman EH, Coats AJ: Neurobiology of exaggerated heart oscillations during two meditative techniques (letter). Int J Cardiol 73:199, 2000

Gangadhar BN, Janakiramaiah N, Sudarshan B, et al: Stress-related biochemical effects of Sudarshan Kriya Yoga in depressed patients. Study no 6, presented at the Conference on Biological Psychiatry, United Nations NGO Mental Health Committee, May 2000

Gerbarg PL, Brown RP: Yoga: a breath of relief for Hurricane Katrina refugees. Current Psychiatry 4:55–67, 2005

Gozal D, Omidvar O, Konrad AT, et al: Identification of human brain regions underlying responses to resistive inspiratory loading with functional magnetic resonance imaging. Proc Natl Acad Sci U S A 92:6607–6611, 1995

Gupta A: The Great Gujarat Earthquake 2001: Lessons Learnt. 22nd Asian Conference on Remote Sensing. Singapore, National University Singapore, 2001

Heilman KM, Voeller KK, Nadeau SE: A possible pathophysiological substrate of attention deficit hyperactivity disorder. J Child Neurol 6 (suppl):S76–S81, 1991

Helping New Yorkers take a deep breath: from trauma workshops to food; Art of Living volunteers bring relief (press release). Santa Barbara, CA, Art of Living Foundation, 2001

Higashi M: Pranayama as a psychiatric regimen (letter). Lancet 14:1177–1178, 1964

Janakiramaiah N, Gangadhar BN, Naga Venkatesha Murthy PJ, et al: Therapeutic efficacy of Sudarshan Kriya Yoga (SKY) in dysthymic disorder. NIMHANS Journal January:21–28, 1998

Janakiramaiah N, Gangadhar BN, Naga Venkatesha Murthy PJ, et al: Antidepressant efficacy of Sudarshan Kriya Yoga (SKY) in melancholia: a randomized comparison with electroconvulsive therapy (ECT) and imipramine. J Affect Disord 57:255–259, 2000

Jella SA, Shannahoff-Khalsa DS: The effects of unilateral forced nostril breathing on cognitive performance. Int J Neurosci 73:61–68, 1993

Jensen PS, Kenny DT: The effects of yoga on the attention and behavior of boys with attention deficit hyperactivity disorder (ADHD). J Atten Disord 7:205–216, 2004

Jordan N: Psychotherapy with expressive technics in psychotic patients. Acta Psiquiatr Psicol Am Lat 35:55–60, 1989

Joseph J: Indian doves fly high in Iraq. The Times of India Online. August 4, 2004. Available at: http://timesofindia.indiatimes.com/articleshow/msid-802624,prtpage-1.cms. Accessed September 4, 2004

Kawachi I, Sparrow D, Vokonas PS, et al: Decreased heart rate variability in men with phobic anxiety. Am J Cardiol 75:882–885, 1995

Klein R, Pilon DPS, Shannahoff-Khalsa D: Nasal airflow asymmetries and human performance. Biol Psychol 23:127–137, 1986

Kwon JS, O'Donnell BF, Wallenstein GV, et al: Gamma frequency-range abnormalities to auditory stimulation in schizophrenia. Arch Gen Psychiatry 56:1001–1005, 1999

Lehofer M, Moser M, Hoehn-Saric R, et al: Major depression and cardiac autonomic control. Biol Psychiatry 42:914–919, 1997

Lehrer P, Sasaki Y, Saito Y: Zazen and cardiac variability. Psychosom Med 61:812–821, 1999

Luedemann W: Rebuilding war-torn Kosovo. Oppenau, Germany, Art of Living Europe, 2004. Available from the author via e-mail: IntAOLEurope.Luedemann@t-online.de

Malathi A, Damodaran A: Stress due to exams in medical students: role of yoga. Indian J Physiol Pharmacol 43:218–224, 1999

Mezzacappa E, Tremblay RE, Kindlon D, et al: Anxiety, antisocial behavior, and heart rate regulation in adolescent males. J Child Psychol Psychiatry 38:457–469, 1997

Miller JJ, Fletcher K, Kabat-Zinn J: Three-year follow-up and clinical implications of a mindfulness-based stress reduction intervention in the treatment of anxiety disorders. Gen Hosp Psychiatry 17:192–200, 1995

Monk C, Kovelenko P, Ellman LM, et al: Enhanced stress reactivity in paediatric anxiety disorders: implications for future cardiovascular health. Int J Neuropsychopharmacol 4:199–206, 2001

Morris K: Meditating on yogic science. Lancet 351:1038, 1998

Mukherjee A: Meditation classes for Tihar inmates. The Times of India, July 1, 2004. Available at: http://timesofindia.indiatimes.com/articleshow/msid-761499,prtpage-1.cms. Accessed September 4, 2004.

Muskin PM: Spiritual leader to guide psychiatrists from the head to the heart. Psychiatric News, March 19, 2004, p 36

Naga Venkatesha Murthy PJ, Gangadhar BN, Janakiramaiah N, et al: Normalization of P300 amplitude following treatment in dysthymia. Biol Psychiatry 42:740–743, 1997

Naga Venkatesha Murthy PJ, Janakiramaiah N, Gangadhar BN, et al: P300 amplitude and antidepressant response to Sudarshan Kriya Yoga (SKY). J Affect Disord 50:45–48, 1998

Nagendra HR, Nagarathna R: An integrated approach of yoga therapy for bronchial asthma: a 3–54 month prospective study. J Asthma 23:123–137, 1986

Naveen KV, Nagarathna R, Nagendra HR, et al: Yoga breathing through a particular nostril increases spatial memory scores without lateralizing effects. Psychol Rep 81:555–561, 1997

Porges SW: The polyvagal theory: phylogenetic substrates of a social nervous system. Int J Psychophysiol 42:123–146, 2001

Porges SW: The vagus: a mediator of behavioral and physiologic features associated with autism, in The Neurobiology of Autism, 2nd Edition. Edited by Bauman ML, Kemper TL. Baltimore, MD, Johns Hopkins University Press, 2004, pp 65–78

Posse S, Dager SR, Richards TL, et al: In vivo measurement of regional brain metabolic response to hyperventilation using magnetic resonance: proton echo planar spectroscopic imaging (PEPSI). Magn Reson Med 37:858–865, 1997a

Posse S, Olthoff U, Weckesser M, et al: Regional dynamic signal changes during controlled hyperventilation assessed with blood oxygen level-dependent functional MR imaging. AJNR Am J Neuroradiol 18:1763–1770, 1997b

Prevett MC, Duncan JS, Jones T, et al: Demonstration of thalamic activation during typical absence seizures using H2(15)O and PET. Neurology 45:1396–1402, 1995

Rama S: The Royal Path Practical Lessons on Yoga. Honesdale, PA, The Himalayan Institute Press, 1998

Rama S, Ballentine R, Hymes A: Science of Breath: A Practical Guide. Honesdale, PA, The Himalayan Institute Press, 1998

Raub JA: Psychophysiological effects of hatha yoga on musculoskeletal and cardiopulmonary function: a literature review. J Altern Complement Med 8:797–812, 2002

Restructuring Gujarat with human values and grassroots (press release). Santa Barbara, CA, Art of Living Foundation, 2001

Roldan E, Dostalek C: Description of an EEG pattern evoked in central-parietal areas by the Hathayogic exercise Agnisara. Act Nerv Super (Praha) 25:241–246, 1983

Roldan E, Dostalek C: EEG patterns suggestive of shifted levels of excitation effected by hathayogic exercises. Act Nerv Super (Praha) 27:81–88, 1985

Sackeim HA, Keilp JG, Rush AJ, et al: The effects of vagus nerve stimulation on cognitive performance in patients with treatment-resistant depression. Neuropsychiatry Neuropsychol Behav Neurol 14:53–62, 2001

Sageman S: How SK can treat the cognitive, psychodynamic, and neuropsychiatric problems of post traumatic stress disorder. Paper presented at the International Symposium on Sudarshan Kriya, Pranayam and Consciousness, New Delhi, India, March 2–3, 2002

Sageman S: Breaking through the despair: spiritually oriented group therapy as a means of healing women with severe mental illness. J Am Acad Psychoanal Dyn Psychiatry 32:125–141, 2004

Sahar T, Shalev AY, Porges SW: Vagal modulation of responses to mental challenge in posttraumatic stress disorder. Biol Psychiatry 49:637–643, 2001

Sakakibara M, Hayano J: Effect of slowed respiration on cardiac parasympathetic response to threat. Psychosom Med 58:32–37, 1996

Sargunaraj D, Lehrer PM, Hochron SM, et al: Cardiac rhythm effects of .125-Hz paced breathing through a resistive load: implications for paced breathing therapy and the polyvagal theory. Biofeedback Self Regul 21:131–147, 1996

Satyanarayana M, Rajeswari KR, Jhansi Rani N, et al: Effect of Santhi Kriya on certain psychophysiological parameters: a preliminary study. Indian J Physiol Pharmacol 36:88–92, 1992

Schachter SC, Saper CB: Vagus nerve stimulation. Epilepsia 39:677–686, 1998

Schiff BB, Rump SA: Asymmetrical hemispheric activation and emotion: the effects of unilateral forced nostril breathing. Brain Cogn 29:217–231, 1995

Shaffer HJ, LaSalvia TA, Stein JP: Original research: comparing hatha yoga with dynamic group psychotherapy for enhancing methadone maintenance treatment: a randomized trial. Altern Ther Health Med 3:57–67, 1997

Shannahoff-Khalsa DS: Kundalini yoga meditation techniques for the treatment of obsessive-compulsive and OC spectrum disorders. Grief Treatment and Crisis Intervention 3:369–382, 2003

Shannahoff-Khalsa DS, Ray LE, Levine S, et al: Randomized controlled trial of yogic meditation techniques for patients with obsessive-compulsive disorder. CNS Spectr 4:34–47, 1999

Singh V, Wisniewski A, Britton J, et al: Effect of yoga breathing exercises (*pranayama*) on airway reactivity in subjects with asthma. Lancet 335:1381–1383, 1990

Sjogren MJ, Hellstrom PT, Jonsson MA, et al: Cognition-enhancing effect of vagus nerve stimulation in patients with Alzheimer's disease: a pilot study. J Clin Psychiatry 63:972–980, 2002

Sovik R: The science of breathing: the yogic view. Prog Brain Res 122:491–505, 2000

Spicuzza L, Gabutti A, Porta C, et al: Yoga and chemoreflex response to hypoxia and hypercapnia. Lancet 356:1495–1496, 2000

Stancak A Jr, Kuna M: EEG changes during forced alternate nostril breathing. Int J Psychophysiol 18:75–79, 1994

Suarez V: Anxiety study at Lance Alternative Program. Paper presented at the Science of Breath International Symposium on Sudarshan Kriya, Pranayam and Consciousness. New Delhi, All India Institute of Medical Sciences, March 2–3, 2002

Taneja I, Deepak K, Poojary G, et al: Yoga versus conventional treatment in diarrhea-prone irritable bowel syndrome: a randomized control study. Appl Psychophysiol Biofeedback 29:19–33, 2004

Tang JS: Transforming the terrorists and healing the traumatized: the Art of Living's multi-faceted approach to restoring peace in Bihar, India, and the Balkans. Damocles: A Newsletter, 2003. Available at: http://gseweb.harvard.edu/~t656_web/peace/Articles_Spring_2003/Tang_Julia_ArtOfLivingBiharIndiaBalkans.htm. Accessed September 4, 2004.

Telles S, Desiraju T: Oxygen consumption during pranayamic type of very slow-rate breathing. Indian J Med Res 94:357–363, 1991

Telles S, Desiraju T: Heart rate alterations in different types of pranayamas. Indian J Physiol Pharmacol 36:287–288, 1992

Telles S, Hanumanthaiah BH, Nagarathna R, et al: Plasticity of motor control systems demonstrated by yoga training. Indian J Physiol Pharmacol 38:143–144, 1994

Thayer JF, Friedman BH, Borkovec TD: Autonomic characteristics of generalized anxiety disorder and worry. Biol Psychiatry 39:255–266, 1996

Vedamurthachar A: Biological effects of Sudarshan Kriya on alcoholics. Dissertation, National Institute of Mental Health and Neurosciences and Mangalore University, Bangalore, India, 2002

Vedamurthachar A, Janakiramaiah N, Jayaram Hedge M, et al: Effects of Sudarshan Kriya on alcohol dependent patients (abstract). Science of Breath International Symposium on Sudarshan Kriya, Pranayam and Consciousness. New Delhi, All India Institute of Medical Sciences, March 2–3, 2002

Waelde LC, Thompson L, Gallagher-Thompson D: A pilot study of yoga and meditation intervention for dementia caregiver stress. J Clin Psychol 60:677–687, 2004

Werntz DA, Bickford RG, Bloom FE, et al: Alternating cerebral hemispheric activity and the lateralization of autonomic nervous function. Hum Neurobiol 2:39–43, 1983

Werntz DA, Bickford RG, Shannahoff-Khalsa D: Selective hemispheric stimulation by unilateral forced nostril breathing. Hum Neurobiol 6:165–171, 1987

Wood C: Mood change and perceptions of vitality: a comparison of the effects of relaxation, visualization and yoga. J R Soc Med 86:254–258, 1993

Woolery A, Meyers H, Sternlieb B, et al: A yoga intervention for young adults with elevated symptoms of depression. Altern Ther Health Med 10:60–63, 2004

Zametkin AJ, Nordahl TE, Gross M, et al: Cerebral glucose metabolism in adults with hyperactivity of childhood onset. N Engl J Med 323:1361–1366, 1990

17

Qigong

Carolyn Coker Ross, M.D., M.P.H.

For more than 3,000 years, qi-related exercises have been practiced in ancient China. These practices date back before the Shang dynasty (16th–11th centuries B.C.E.) and have been known by many names: *daoyin* (directing extremities), *tuna* (exhalation and inhalation), and *lianqi* (training of vital energy). Those living in the Imperial court were the first to practice qi-related exercises. The first recorded use of the term *qigong* was in 1956 by Liu Gui Zhen (Ng 1999). On mainland China, it is estimated that not less than 5% of the population practices various forms of qigong daily to prevent illness, promote health, and increase longevity (Lake 2002; Ng 1999). Worldwide there are an estimated 100 million practitioners of qigong.

Qigong (also spelled Ch'i Kung and pronounced "chee gung") is philosophically linked to traditional Chinese medicine as one of four main modalities: acupuncture therapy, herbal remedies, Chinese massage (*tuina*), and medical qigong. Medical qigong is the oldest of these branches and forms the energetic basis for the other therapies. Although most Westerners think of qigong as the series of exercises done by practitioners for the purpose of improving their own health and well-being and reaching spiritual transcendence, medical qigong involves externally emitted energy by a skilled medical qigong master for the purpose of healing others.

The author is grateful for the assistance of Kenneth M. Sancier and Alex Holland, L.Ac., who provided resources that contributed to this chapter.

HISTORICAL OVERVIEW

There are notations about the benefits of qigong in many ancient Chinese medical texts. For example, in *The Yellow Emperor's Classic of Internal Medicine,* qigong is thought to be effective by 1) eliminating worries from the mind, 2) controlling and focusing thoughts, 3) participating in breathing exercises, and 4) toning the muscles. Reference to qigong was also made by a renowned physician of the later Han dynasty (206 B.C.E. to 25 C.E.), Zhang Zong Jing. In his *Synopsis of the Golden Cabinet,* he argued in favor of the practice of daoyin and massage: "As soon as the limbs feel heavy and sluggish, resort to such treatments as daoyin, tuna, acupuncture and massage by rubbing with ointment so as to allow the orifices to close up" (quoted from Ng 1999, p. 198). In the Sui dynasty (589–618 C.E.), Cao Yuanfang recorded many daoyin activities in his *Treatise on the Etiology and Symptomatology of Diseases.* During the Tang dynasty, in *Documents of Yimen,* Sun Simiao (581–682 C.E.) composed a "Song of Hygiene" that detailed the benefits of breathing exercises. Zhu Danxi of the Yuan dynasty (1281–1358) suggested "seeking quietness by getting rid of desires" as the mechanism underlying breath work.

In the first half of the twentieth century, traditional medicine was banned in China in favor of Westernized modern medicine. Recognizing the power that traditional practices had in the Chinese culture, on his ascent to power in the 1940s, Mao Zedong instituted research into "the storehouse of treasures." However, during the 10 years of the Cultural Revolution, the Chinese government suppressed all activities even remotely connected to ancient customs. Practicing qigong openly could lead to harassment and even death at the hands of the Maoist Red Guards.

Following this period, qigong again emerged but was attacked as being based on religion and superstition. To counter these attacks, from the late 1970s onward, the Chinese government funded studies into the essence of qigong. This resulted in the formation of the China Research Society for Qigong Science in 1986 and the start of annual world conferences beginning in 1987, at which qigong scientific research was discussed. International conferences held all over the world have led to qigong gaining international recognition (Ng 1999). Currently there are three main schools of qigong practice in China: 1) medical schools that train doctors and other healers in the practice of medical qigong, which includes both externally and internally applied qigong for the purpose of health maintenance, longevity, prevention of disease, and diagnosis and treatment of disease; 2) martial arts schools that use qigong to train martial artists; and 3) spiritual schools that train those who seek spiritual transcendence (Johnson et al. 2000).

BASIC PRINCIPLES OF QIGONG

Modern laws of physics now support the interchangeable nature of matter and energy and may eventually provide a scientific explanation for the putative energetic mechanism of action associated with qi. *Qi* means "vital energy," or life force, and *gong* means "skill." So *qigong* is the "skillful practice of gathering, circulating and applying life-force energy." The ancient Chinese believed that all things in life, nature, and the universe were connected energetically and that all people are symbiotically one with the universe through the system of qi or vital life energy.

Qi is stored in the human body in reservoirs and flows through the body in mapped pathways or channels (also called *meridians*). Qi can be divided into the five manifestations of matter and energy: mineral, plant, animal, human, and divine. The five manifestations of qi can be subdivided into the two equal and opposite aspects of *yin* and *yang* (Johnson et al. 2000). Yin and yang expressions of qi include the wilds of nature such as wind, rain, and the cosmic influences of the moon and the stars as well as interpersonal energies at play in families and communities. The medical application of this concept in traditional Chinese medicine evolved to mean that good health involves a balance of the yin and yang aspects of qi. As well, all other aspects of the practice of traditional Chinese medicine—each sign or symptom of the disease process, the treatment plan the physician develops, and the type of treatment chosen—involve yin and yang aspects. A traditional Chinese medicine diagnosis requires an analysis of qi, as qi reflects the delicate balance or imbalance of yin and yang (Holland 1997). Medical qigong views illness as a disturbance in one of the fundamental types of energy:

> *Qi* is one of three fundamental kinds of energy that are the basis of health and healing. The other two, *Shen* (spiritual energy) and *Jing* (sexual energy), are considered the yang (ascending, bright, active, etc.) and yin (descending, dark, passive, etc.) aspects of qi, respectively. More abstractly, Jing, Qi, and Shen can be translated into body, mind and spirit....Chinese medical theory posits that qi derives from three basic sources: food, breath, and the body's genetic constitution. Food and breath combine to form the "nutritive qi," which is the kind of qi that is believed to flow through the meridians and is altered or manipulated during acupuncture treatments. In contrast, the inherited constitution of the physical body is called "original qi." Jing has been translated numerous ways, but is perhaps most accurately rendered as "essence," or "the original source of life and growth." There are many kinds of Jing energy, but *yuan jing,* or "original essence," which comes from the parents and generates new life, is most important. The "original essence" is the source of both qi and shen.
>
> Just as the body is conceptualized as the interaction of subtle energies and matter, health and disease are likewise regarded as manifestations of the relative strength, state of balance or imbalance between these presumed energies, and complex biological structures and physiological processes. According to the theory, an external field of "protective energy," or *wei qi,* emanates from all living things. Internal stresses (including psychological traits and strong emotions) and external "stresses" or "pathogenic" factors (including disease-causing organisms or toxic substances) can damage this protective field, eventually resulting in illness if not corrected. Disruption of the wei qi may predispose the individual to retaining "toxic energy" or experiencing "depletion" of desirable energy, manifesting

as physical, emotional or psychosomatic illness. Emotional stress and neglect of one's physical health typically result in diminished qi. (Lake 2002, p. 185)

MEDICAL QIGONG

Medical qigong, which includes externally applied qigong therapy (EQT) as well as prescribed qigong exercises, involves the manipulation of qi for therapeutic purposes. The practitioners of this therapy are able to become aware of qi, use their minds or intent (*yi*) to manipulate and stimulate the qi of the patient without actually touching the patient, and guide the qi toward desired places in the body. The practice involves the emission of qi, the use of yi (consciousness or intent), or a combination of both. The practitioner uses techniques to rid patients of toxic pathogens or stores of old, painful emotions that cause mental and physical illness. Techniques taught to patients include breathing with movement techniques, creative visualization, and spiritual intention to improve health and regain personal power and control of one's health (Johnson et al. 2000). Most hospitals in China have qigong departments as well as herbal and acupuncture departments (Holland 1997).

No controlled trials have substantiated claims that EQT is effective, even in China. The official position of the Chinese Ministry of Public Health since 1989 has been "not to publicize and not to deny." There has also been a tightening of regulations governing the practice of medical qigong to protect the public against financial loss, quell superstitions regarding qigong in the community, and exercise more control over qigong masters (K.C. Tang 1994).

QIGONG AS A SELF-HEALING EXERCISE

The philosophy of qigong as a self-healing exercise also involves bringing intention (*yi*) to direct the movement of qi, or vital life energy, in the body. Good health requires balance, and balance derives from the proper movement and distribution of qi. The purpose of qi exercises is to strengthen the body's qi and remove blockages to the flow of qi that may be the result of emotions, injury, poor diet, or illness (Sancier and Holman 2004). Blockage of qi flow is thought to cause imbalance and disease or lack of harmony in the body and mind.

PRACTICE OF QIGONG

The practice of qigong includes postures, movement, self-massage, and breathing techniques. There is both an exercise and a meditative aspect to qigong. The ancient Chinese believed that the six healing sounds used in qigong correlate with specific meridians (channels along which qi flows) and organ systems, which are nourished and healed by the sounds. The qigong movements can be done in standing, seated, or supine positions, making them accessible to a wide range of ability levels (Ng 1999).

The two main qigong exercise techniques are *neigong* (internal exercise) and *waigong* (external exercise). Neigong is practiced in a meditative state with the practitioner focusing attention on the *dan tien* (elixir field) while inhaling, exhaling, and holding the breath to stimulate qi and blood and strengthen the constitution. The dan tien are regarded as the three primary storage sites of jing, qi, and shen. Qigong exercises are designed to correct imbalances in one or more of the dan tien, thereby restoring the body to a state of optimum balance and health. Waigong involves qigong exercises, an example of which is *Tai Ji Quan* (traditional Chinese shadow boxing), which "seeks quiescence within mobility" (Lake 2002; Ng 1999). Although qigong is considered a health exercise that forms the basis of traditional Chinese medicine, *tai chi, tai chi chuan,* and *taiji* originated from the martial arts. Tai chi is now practiced as an exercise for health maintenance but maintains many of the original martial arts moves. Although tai chi may have many self-healing benefits, it is not comparable with the medical form of qigong discussed above.

RESEARCH ON QIGONG

Research into the health benefits of qigong is complicated by the differences in worldviews between Western biomedicine and traditional Chinese medicine and therefore understandings of what mind–body therapy involves. There is no correlate in Western medicine to the notion of qi, nor does the flow of qi through the meridians or specific pathways correspond to any anatomical teaching in the West. For example, the Chinese notion of the mind is an "awareness flowing about the body," whereas the Western model of the mind involves a "nonphysical consciousness that is translated into physical reality by the brain" (Kerr 2002).

The philosophical underpinnings of Western medicine also include a division of labor with regard to patients. Physicians are entrusted with the treatment of physical conditions, and their realm is the body of the patient. Other aspects of illness—those that involve emotions, social relationships, or spiritual matters—are seen as discrete entities and are attended to by psychologists, social workers, and pastoral counselors, respectively. As noted above, Eastern philosophies of healing such as Buddhism, Taoism, and traditional Chinese medicine espouse a more holistic conceptualization of the individual:

> In this view, health is perceived as a harmonious equilibrium that exists between the interplay of "yin" and "yang": the five internal elements (metal, wood, water, fire and earth), the six environmental conditions (dry, wet, hot, cold, wind and flame), other external sources of harm (physical injury, insect bites, poison, overeat and overwork), and the seven emotions (joy, sorrow, anger, worry, panic, anxiety and fear). (Chan et al. 2001, pp. 261–262)

The Chinese Classification of Mental Disorders Version 3 (CCMD-3) reflects these differences in philosophy and eschews the Western psychiatric adherence to the mind–body dichotomy and primary reliance on symptoms in the diagnostic process. The inclusion in the classification of such culture-specific diagnoses as "traveling psychosis, neurasthenia, qigong-induced mental disorder, and dysfunctional homosexuality" reflect China's unique sociomoral and cultural viewpoint of illness (S. Lee 2001).

According to Lake (2002), the traditional Chinese medical understanding of psychiatric diseases, including psychosis, anxiety, and depression, stem from imbalances in shen energy (yang aspect of qi energy: consciousness or spirit):

> The yuan shen represents the innate or "inherited spiritual pattern of the individual and his or her connection to the divine energy of the universe." In contrast, the zhi shen corresponds to beneficial or toxic thought patterns acquired following birth. The yuan shen is believed to reside in the brain, while the zhi shen resides in the heart. In the natural state, the yuan shen (mind) rules over the zhi shen (heart) and imbalances or distortions of yuan shen and zhi shen manifest as various psychological or emotional symptoms. Failure to resolve intense emotions is believed to cause blockage of optimum qi circulation, resulting in relative deficiency of qi or accumulation of "toxic energy." (Lake 2002, p. 187)

Chinese doctors also classify diseases, including psychological diseases, by three causative factors: external causes, internal causes, and neither external nor internal causes. External disease causes apply to the six environmental excesses (wind, cold, heat, summer heat, dampness, and dryness) and pestilential or epidemic qi. Chinese physicians have come to emphasize neither external nor internal causes of disease. The internal causes apply to the seven affects: joy, thought, anxiety, sorrow, fear, fright, and anger. These affects are integrally related to the flow of qi:

> Joy leads to slackening (slowing in its flow) of qi, anger leads to rising qi, thought leads to binding of the qi, sorrow leads to scattering of the qi, fear leads to descending of the qi, and fright leads to chaos of the qi. In actual fact, anger and rising qi are one and the same thing. When we say we feel angry, we are feeling a physical sensation of rising qi.... The names of these affects or emotions are just abstract labels for felt, physical sensations of the flow of qi. (Flaws and Lake 2001, p. 19)

The final category of disease causation involves causes that are neither external nor internal: faulty diet, lack of regulation between activity and stillness, excessive sexual or reproductive activity, iatrogenesis, drug addiction, and parasites. Many of these causes have become the focus of preventive medical care in Western medicine, including a focus on improving diet, living a balanced lifestyle with moderate activity and time for reflection, curbing excesses in sexual activity, and, of course, avoiding addictions.

Research on qigong has focused on three main areas: 1) proving the existence of qi, 2) examining the physiological mechanism to explain the health benefits of qigong or EQT (e.g., the effect of qi on cortisol levels), and 3) demonstrating the potential of qigong or EQT as a healing modality.

Evaluating the Existence of Qi

Most studies use externally applied qi, usually from a qigong master. Fukushima et al. (2001) tested for evidence of qigong energy being applied to phosphate-buffered saline to determine if externally applied qi would increase the phagocytic activity of polymorphonuclear cells. The study was rigorously controlled and well designed and used both masking and randomization. The authors interpreted the results of this study as offering evidence that qi exists and can affect an electrolyte solution and its biological action. In an animal study (Chen et al. 2002), the effect of externally applied qi was measured on in vivo growth of transplantable murine lymphoma cells in mice. The mice were injected with the lymphoma cells and then randomized to three groups: qigong treatment administered by a qigong healer, sham treatment, and no treatment as the control condition. The sham treatment was a qigong treatment mimicked by someone without training in qigong. After the intervention, tumor growth in lymph nodes was assessed and found to be significantly smaller in the qigong-treated group ($P<0.05$) than either the control or sham treatment group, suggesting the ability of qigong to arrest the growth of this aggressive tumor. This study was repeated with the same design and with the same results, but the effects did not reach statistical significance, possibly because of the increased variance throughout the second study, which may be due to differences in the tumor cell preparation or in the effectiveness of qigong treatment between the two studies.

An excellent review of studies from the qigong database (Qigong Institute) examined more than 3,500 abstracts, published articles, and accessible publications in Chinese, including conference proceedings on the effects of externally applied qi, or external qi therapy (EQT). EQT was defined by the Chinese Society of Qigong Science as "the distant and directional effects produced by a well trained qigong practitioner under the qigong state." Most studies did not meet the academic standards set in Western medicine. Studies that did not have a systematic data collection system or did not use the above definition of EQT and those whose findings could not be generalized to offer new perspectives were not considered in the review. Studies were classified into five categories according to their method of measuring external qi: 1) physical signal detectors (e.g., light, electricity, heat, sound, magnetism, far-infrared detectors), 2) testing the effects of external qi on chemical reactions, 3) detectors using biological materials, 4) detectors using living sensors, and 5) measuring the effects of external qi on human bodies. Despite the limitations in study design, lack of compatible control groups, and, in some cases, deliberate deception by qigong healers or special interest groups, the external effects of qi were detected in many studies.

However, none of the studies could answer the question *What is qi, and how does external qi work?* Significant lessons learned in this review and other analyses of the available literature on qigong included the following: 1) not all qigong healers can effectively emit external qi, for this is apparently a specialized talent that can require years of study to master; 2) repeated studies with a better study design are needed to replicate and validate previous research; and 3) previous studies suggest that the external qi effect may consist of one or more of the following: matter, bioenergy, and information (Chen 2004).

Defining external qi does not necessarily explain how qigong works and why. Perhaps the focus of future research should be on understanding the process of self-healing from qigong exercises and external qi emission and how they can be applied in medicine.

Physiological Mechanism for the Health Effects of Qigong

Qigong Directly Increases Type 1 Cytokines and Reduces Cortisol Levels

Many theories have been examined to explain the anecdotal and historical health benefits of external qi and the self-healing practice of qigong. Qigong has been likened to generalized relaxation therapy with stress–reduction benefits similar to those described in Benson's classic work on "the relaxation response" (cited in Kerr 2002). In support of this, Jones (2001) tested cytokine and cortisol levels in 19 healthy volunteers with a mean age of 43.9 ± 7.8 years who received daily 2-hour instruction in Guolin-style qigong over a 14-week period. Cytokines are pro- and anti-inflammatory regulators of immune system responses. Type 1 cytokines are involved with cell-mediated immunity, and type 2 cytokines favor humoral immune responses. An overabundance of type 1 cytokines is associated with organ-specific autoimmune diseases, and an overabundance of type 2 cytokines may lead to allergies, systemic autoimmunity, and depressed responses to viruses and cancer. A balance between these types of cytokines is required for good health. The results of this small, nonrandomized, uncontrolled study showed that Guolin qigong changed the production of cytokines in the direction of type 1 responses. The number of interleukin (IL)-4– and IL-12–secreting cells did not change. IL-6 levels increased at week 7, and tumor necrosis factor-α increased at weeks 3 and 7. γ-Interferon–secreting cells increased and IL-10 levels decreased. The question of whether this relative increase in type 1 cytokines is beneficial could not be answered in this small, nonrandomized, uncontrolled study. There was also a decrease in cortisol levels ($P < 0.05$) at weeks 3 and 14. Cortisol is a known inhibitor of type 1 cytokine production.

Numerous studies have demonstrated the effect of cortisol levels on mood. For example, cortisol levels are indirectly related to State-Trait Anxiety Inventory scores (Rondo et al. 2004), and patients with schizophrenia and with de-pression have elevated cortisol levels compared with control subjects (Muck-Seler 2004). Elevated cortisol/dehydroepiandrosterone (DHEA) and cortisol/DHEA-S levels in schizophrenic patients versus healthy control subjects corre-lated with higher scores for anxiety, anger, depression, and hostility but were in-dependent of severity of psychopathology and antipsychotic treatment (Ritsner et al. 2004).

In a study presented by Higuchi and colleagues at the 1995 International Conference on Qigong, six healthy men only one of whom was trained in qigong, had blood samples taken at rest, immediately after receiving EQT from a qigong master, and 1 hour after treatment (Higuchi et al. 1995). Cortisol levels decreased during the resting period by between 20% and 30%. Adrenaline also decreased, returning to normal after 1 hour. No changes were observed in nor-adrenaline, dopamine, and beta-endorphin levels. During qi mobilization by the qigong master, the same results as during rest were seen, except that dopamine and beta-endorphin levels increased by about 20% in the one participant who had trained in qigong previously. These results suggest that decreases in these neurohormones are similar to the relaxation or stress-reduction response, with an enhancement of this response with qi mobilization, as demonstrated by the changes in beta-endorphin and dopamine release.

Changes in Beta-Endorphins May Predict Beneficial Changes in Mood Associated With Qigong Practice

Ryu et al. (1996) observed the effects of qigong training on levels of stress hor-mones (adrenocorticotropic hormone [ACTH], cortisol, DHEA-S), human en-dogenous opioids, and beta-endorphins in a group of ChunDoSunBup qigong trainees. The theory behind this study related to the known activation of the hypothalamic-pituitary-adrenal axis in response to exercise. It is postulated that changes in the axis may also modulate immune function. This study also in-cluded healthy volunteers ($n=20$) who were already involved in qi training. Hormone levels were measured 10 minutes before the start of exercise and 40 and 70 minutes after training. The results showed no change in plasma cortisol and DHEA-S levels. Beta-endorphin levels were increased ($P<0.05$) and ACTH levels had declined slightly at the mid- and posttraining measurements.

Qigong State Is Associated With Slowed Alpha-1 Wave Activity

Effects of qigong on the brain have been studied using modern technology, in-cluding electroencephalogram (EEG) and evoked potential studies. In one study, three groups were evaluated: 10 qigong masters with more than 10 years of prac-tice of qigong, 10 beginning qigong students with 2–3 years' experience, and 10 control subjects without any qigong experience. During qigong, the EEGs of qigong masters showed primarily alpha-1 activity in the anterior half of the brain with a slowed peak frequency. EEGs during the qigong state appear different from those in the resting state and from EEG changes described by Wallace (1970) during transcendental meditation or those reported for yoga states in which there is an increase in alpha and theta activity in the posterior brain regions. EEG alpha waves are associated with lowered anxiety, peak performance in sports, and increased creativity. An increase in alpha activity is generally associated with decreased depressed mood and better stress adaptation. It is theorized that increased alpha activity can also facilitate emotional cleansing or release of blocked emotions. The ratio of alpha activity in the right compared with the left side of the brain may also have clinical significance. A normal right-to-left ratio is approximately 1.05–1.10. In anxiety neuroses, the right-to-left ratio is 0.93, and in paranoid schizophrenia, it may be as low as 0.5–0.6. Based on EEG findings, qigong is described as a unique state of wakeful consciousness. The small number of individuals enrolled in these studies—the smallest included only two people—limits the significance of findings (Litscher et al. 2001; Zhang et al. 1988).

RESEARCH EXAMINING QIGONG AS A TREATMENT FOR MENTAL ILLNESS

Numerous studies have demonstrated psychological benefits from the consistent practice of qigong. Most studies done on qigong or tai chi have been conducted in China. Some have been published in Chinese medical journals, but many have been reported at qigong conferences and never subsequently published. Many studies are small and poorly designed, showing preliminary findings that need validation with larger, better-designed studies. Other issues that interfere with efforts to study qigong have to do with difficulties inherent in adapting the traditional Chinese medical concept of qigong to the Western research model, including the problem of identifying suitable sham treatments or sham qigong masters who cannot be distinguished by study participants from actual qigong masters.

Below is a summary reported by Lake (2002) of some studies presented at conferences in China that were never published.

Depression

Three studies have examined qigong as a treatment of depression. The first of these (C. Tang et al. 1990), which was presented at the Third International Conference on Qigong in 1990, was a double-blind study that showed evidence of efficacy. In this study, 122 elderly qigong practitioners and 55 participants who practiced Taijiquan (*tai chi chuan*) were compared with 90 age-matched control subjects who practiced neither qigong nor Taijiquan. The results demonstrated an improvement in mood, reduction in anxiety, and better "quality of sleep" in the intervention group. Two other studies showed significant findings and were presented at the Second World Conference and Academic Exchange on Medical Qigong. Wang (1993) found that improvements in baseline psychological and emotional state correlated with the duration of practice of qigong, and Schwartzman (1998) reported that 9 of 13 patients achieved some benefit from qigong, with a 25%–50% improvement in their depressed mood from before treatment. Both of these studies yielded promising prospective data with significant trends that require verification through future double-blind, controlled studies.

Anxiety

Lake (2002) identified five studies of qigong used to treat anxiety, three of which are reviewed here. Of these, only one reported promising evidence of a significant therapeutic effect. This open prospective study by L. Li et al. (1989) compared 35 qigong practitioners with age- and sex-matched control subjects who received biofeedback using electromyography; all participants had been diagnosed with anxiety, neurosis, and headaches. The authors found that after subjects received 2 weeks of the intervention, their overall measures of frequency and intensity of subjective stress indicators were decreased in male qigong practitioners as compared with the group receiving biofeedback. There were no significant differences among female practitioners. In a prospective open study by Kato (1992) in Japan, 13 subjects who underwent 20 minutes of combined passive and active qigong exercises reported a decrease in subjective feelings of anxiety. In a similar study (Shan et al. 1989), eight participants practiced the Fang Song Gong style of qigong 15 minutes per day for 1 month. All met DSM-III (American Psychiatric Association 1980) criteria for generalized anxiety disorders. Findings included increased amplitude in alpha wave frequency of EEG; decreases in heart rate, blood pressure, and oxygen consumption; and significant decreases in anxiety as measured by the Hamilton Anxiety Scale. This study was limited by its small sample size, short study period, lack of long-term follow-up, and lack of a control group. A final study by Hutton et al. (1996) compared progressive muscle relaxation with tai chi for treatment of generalized anxiety symptoms in war veterans diagnosed with posttraumatic stress disorder. Eight war veterans were randomly assigned to the two intervention groups. The results included significant decreases in subjective distress in the tai chi group with a trend toward lowered heart rate in the tai chi group. Bias may have occurred from the greater compliance in the tai chi group.

Aggression, Attention, and Restlessness

An unpublished study conducted in 1999 looked at the effects of qigong practice in elementary school-age children (C. Cousins, "Research Findings of the Qigong for Children Project" [unpublished data], 1999). Qigong practice was conducted every Monday for 2 months. The teachers rated most children as less restless and more attentive during class on the day of qigong practice but not on subsequent days. Many of the children reported feeling "full of energy." This study was limited by the lack of a control group and blind raters and the failure to measure pre- and poststudy changes in attention and aggression. There was also no effort to diagnose attention-deficit/hyperactivity disorder (ADHD) in children in the classroom before starting the study.

Addictions

A randomized study on the efficacy of qigong in treating withdrawal symptoms in heroin addicts was undertaken by M. Li et al. (2002). Participants were randomly assigned to qigong treatment ($n=34$), medication for detoxification ($n=26$), or a no-treatment control group ($n=26$). All participants were in a 1- to 3-month mandated treatment program. Participants in the qigong treatment group practiced the Pangu Gong style of qigong for 2 hours per day and received daily EQT. The medication group received lofexidine HCl by a 10-day gradual reduction method, and control subjects received only basic care and symptomatic treatment. Results of this study showed a more rapid reduction in withdrawal symptoms in the qigong group compared with the other groups, with the former showing lower mean symptoms ($P<0.01$). Anxiety scores in both the qigong and the medication groups were lower compared with the control group ($P<0.01$), with the qigong group having even lower anxiety than the medication group ($P<0.01$). The proposed physiological mechanism of action of qigong involves the ability of qigong to increase blood flow and bioelectric current in the brain. Qigong, like meditation, can also produce an overall sense of well-being that may reduce an individual's craving for drugs. The significance of the study results is limited by the lack of follow-up after termination of the study, the lack of completely compatible control and placebo treatments, and an inability to distinguish between the effects of EQT and qigong practice. The authors concluded that qigong therapy may be a good complement to medication for treatment of heroin addiction.

QIGONG AND GENERAL PSYCHOLOGICAL WELL-BEING

Many studies on qigong have been published in peer-reviewed journals. In one randomized clinical trial of a special form of qigong (the Eight Section Brocades), 50 geriatric patients in Hong Kong in subacute stages of chronic physical illnesses were assigned to 12 weeks of qigong practice versus traditional remedial rehabilitation activities. Results from the Perceived Benefits Questionnaire showed that participants in the qigong group reported improvements in physical health, psychological health, social relationships, and general health ($P<0.001$ for all variables listed). No significant differences were found between intervention and control groups on the Geriatric Depression Scale ($P=0.145$). Using qualitative feedback (individual comments), 75% reported improvement in psychosocial functioning after the 12-week qigong intervention, including feeling more relaxed and comfortable, sleeping better, and being more optimistic. The small number of participants may have limited the significance of the beneficial effects seen on standardized measures of depressed mood. It has been suggested that more prolonged qigong practice might result in increased mood benefits in future studies of elderly populations with chronic illnesses (Tsang et al. 2003). Szabo et al. (1998) found tai chi in combination with yoga to produce higher levels of tranquility compared with other forms of physical exercise (aerobic dance, weight training, martial arts, and music appreciation [control condition]) in 195 healthy volunteers.

QIGONG AND MOOD

Lee et al. (1997) investigated *ChunDoSunBup* (CDSB) qi training (a Korean form of qigong) in 13 trainees who were examined in the resting state (control condition), during CDSB qi training, and after training. All participants had 1–3 years of CDSB training. The mean age was 25 years, and none of the trainees had any psychiatric diagnoses. There were changes in state anxiety as measured on the State-Trait Anxiety Inventory XI in all but two subjects ($P<0.01$). EEG results showed a significant increase in alpha-wave power (ratio of alpha to alpha plus beta) during the sound exercise ($P<0.05$) and meditation ($P<0.05$) compared with in the resting/control state. These study findings replicated results from previous studies by the same authors using EEGs.

Jin (1989) conducted a multifactorial study of tai chi in 33 beginners and 33 practitioners to determine if the benefits of tai chi are dependent on experience and expertise The study was segmented by the following parameters: three phases (before, during, and after tai chi), experience (beginners versus practitioners), and time of tai chi practice (morning, afternoon, or evening). Heart rate was elevated for both beginners and experienced practitioners during tai chi, lending credibility to the claim that tai chi is similar to other forms of moderate exercise in stimulating cardiovascular responses. Catecholamine levels, which are usually triggered during exercise, were markedly increased during tai chi. Urinary dopamine and 5-hydroxytryptophan levels did not change from baseline during tai chi exercise. Salivary cortisol decreased compared with pre-exercise measures; this could be explained by either the meditation component of tai chi or the fact that the physical workload of tai chi is not greater than 50% peak O_2 consumption. Mood states were more positive with less tension, depression, anger, fatigue, confusion, and state anxiety reported during and 1 hour after tai chi.

Whether these mood changes were a result of selection bias or whether tai chi was a distraction from anxiety and other mood states could not be determined.

CAUTIONS AND TRAINING ISSUES

The few cases of "qigong-induced psychosis" reported in the Chinese medical literature were thought to be caused by the "inappropriate practice" of qigong. These psychological "aberrations" manifested as nervousness, insomnia and other sleep disturbances, frequent dreams, tachycardia, breathlessness, dry mouth, headaches, and giddiness. In more severe cases, altered states of consciousness may occur, including hallucinations and dissociative symptoms. Most cases of severe symptoms have been reported by individuals predisposed to psychiatric complications, including individuals diagnosed with personality disorders or schizophrenia. Individuals with qigong "deviations" generally score high on measures of hypochondriasis, depression, hysteria, and "psychopathic" symptoms. In these cases, qigong may "induce" preexisting predispositions or subclinical forms of mental illness. It is recommended that all students of qigong work with a qualified instructor and learn correct qigong techniques to minimize risks of "aberrant" reactions (Ng 1999).

Qigong training is offered in many schools of traditional Chinese medicine. In China, a certificate in qigong requires completion of a 3-year program followed by an internship. Western training programs are highly variable in content, level, and duration of instruction. There are no standard criteria for certification from either the National Qigong Association or the Qigong Institute (Johnson et al. 2000).

SUMMARY

As discussed above, practitioners of qigong and traditional Chinese medicine view illness as an energetic imbalance associated with physical and emotional symptoms. Most psychiatric disorders are thought to be a result of dysregulation of shen. Specific emission qigong protocols and self-directed qigong exercises can be prescribed for these imbalances. Qigong is also practiced by millions worldwide as a form of self-healing and for health maintenance and health promotion in general. Most studies conducted to date on the medical and psychiatric benefits of qigong are flawed by a lack of scientific rigor, and findings have limited significance because of small study sizes and the failure to use standardized outcome measures. These design problems are further complicated by problems inherent in all scientific investigations of phenomena that have no clear correlates to conventional Western concepts of illness and health. However, the long history of qigong as a treatment for both medical and psychological symptoms, strong anecdotal evidence supporting claims that qigong has general benefits for psychological well-being, its ease of use, and the absence of serious adverse effects warrant continuing research into this ancient healing art.

REFERENCES

American Psychiatric Association: Diagnostic and Statistical Manual of Mental Disorders, 3rd Edition. Washington, DC, American Psychiatric Association, 1980

Chan C, Ho PS, Chow E: A body-mind-spirit model in health: an Eastern approach. Soc Work Health Care 34:261–282, 2001

Chen KW: An analytic review of studies on measuring effects of external Q in China. Altern Ther 10:38–50, 2004

Chen KW, Shiflett SC, Ponzio NM, et al: A preliminary study of the effect of external qigong on lymphoma growth in mice. J Altern Complement Med 8:615–621, 2002

Flaws B, Lake J: Chinese Medical Psychiatry: A Textbook and Clinical Manual. Boulder, CO, Blue Poppy Press, 2001

Fukushima M, Kataoka T, Hamada C, et al: Evidence of Qi-gong energy and its biological effect on the enhancement of the phagocytic activity of human polymorphonuclear leukocytes. Am J Chin Med 29:1–16, 2001

Higuchi Y, Kotani Y, Kitagawa J, et al: Cortisol, catecholamines and beta-endorphin levels in plasma during and after qi mobilization in qigong. Fourth International Conference on Qigong, 1995, pp 3–4

Holland A: Voices of Qi: An Introductory Guide to Traditional Chinese Medicine. Berkeley, CA, North Atlantic Books, 1997

Hutton D, Liebling D, Leire R: Alternative relaxation training for combat PTSD veterans. Third World Conference for Academic Exchange of Medical Qigong, 1996

Jin P: Changes in heart rate, noradrenaline, cortisol and mood during tai chi. J Psychosom Res 33:197–206, 1989

Johnson JA, Stewart JM, Howell MH (eds): Chinese Medical Qigong Therapy: A Comprehensive Clinical Guide. Pacific Grove, CA, The International Institute of Medical Qigong, 2000

Jones BM: Changes in cytokine production in healthy subjects practicing Guolin Qigong: a pilot study. BMC Complement Altern Med 1:8, 2001

Kato T, Numata, Shirayama, et al: Physiological and psychological study of qigong. Japanese Mind-Body Science 1:29–38, 1992

Kerr C: Translating "mind-in-body": two models of patient experience underlying a randomized controlled trial of qigong. Cult Med Psychiatry 26:419–447, 2002

Lake J: Qigong, in Handbook of Complementary and Alternative Therapies in Mental Health. Edited by Shannon S. San Diego, CA, Academic Press, 2002, pp 183–207

Lee MS, Bae BH, Ryu H, et al: Changes in alpha wave and state anxiety during Chun-DoSunBup Qi-training in trainees with open eyes. Am J Chin Med 25:289–299, 1997

Lee S: From diversity to unity: the classification of mental disorders in 21st century China. Psychiatr Clin North Am 24:421–431, 2001

Li L, Qin C, Yang S, et al: A comparative study of qigong and biofeedback therapy. Second International Conference on Qigong, Xi'ian, China, 1989, p 88

Li M, Chen K, Mo Z: Use of qigong therapy in the detoxification of heroin addicts. Altern Ther 8:50–59, 2002

Litscher G, Wenzel G, Niederwieser G, et al: Effects of Qigong on brain function. Neurol Res 23:501–505, 2001

Muck-Seler D, Pivac N, Mustapic M, et al: Platelet serotonin and plasma prolactin and cortisol in healthy, depressed and schizophrenic women. Psychiatry Res 127:217–227, 2004

Ng B-Y: Qigong-induced mental disorders: a review. Aust N Z J Psychiatry 33:1440–1454, 1999

Ritsner M, Maayan R, Gibel A, et al: Elevation of cortisol/dehydroepiandrosterone ratio in schizophrenia patients. Eur Neuropsychopharmacol 14:267–273, 2004

Rondo PH, Vaz AF, Moraes F, et al: The relationship between salivary cortisol concentrations and anxiety in adolescent and non-adolescent pregnant women. Braz J Med Biol Res 37:1403–1409, 2004

Ryu I, Lee HS, Shin YS, et al: Acute effect of qigong training on stress hormonal levels in man. Am J Chin Med 24:193–198, 1996

Sancier K, Holman D: Multifaceted health benefits of qigong (commentary). J Altern Complement Med 10:163–165, 2004

Schwartzman L: Tai chi and Parkinson's disease. Paper presented at the Second World Congress on Qigong, San Francisco, CA, 1998

Shan H, Yan H, Sheng H, et al: A preliminary evaluation on Chinese qigong treatment of anxiety. Second International Conference on Qigong, Xi'ian, China, 1989, p 165

Szabo A, Mesko A, Caputo A, et al: Examination of exercise-induced feeling states in four modes of exercise. Int J Sport Psychol 29:376–390, 1998

Tang C, Lu Z, Wang J et al: Effects of qigong and Taijiquan on reversal of aging process and some psychological functions. Third National Academy Conference on Qigong, Kyoto, Japan, 1990

Tang KC: Qigong therapy: its effectiveness and regulation. Am J Chin Med 22:235–242, 1994

Tsang HWH, Mok CK, Au Yeung YT, et al: The effect of qigong on general and psychosocial health of elderly with chronic physical illnesses: a randomized clinical trial. Int J Geriatr Psychiatry 18:441–449, 2003

Wallace RK: Physiological effects of transcendental meditation. Science 167:1751–1754, 1970

Wang J: Role of qigong on mental health. Paper presented at the Second World Conference for Academic Exchange of Medical Qigong, Beijing, China, September 1993

Zhang JZ, Zhao J, He QN: EEG findings during special psychical state (QiGong state) by means of compressed spectral array and topographic mapping. Comput Biol Med 18:455–463, 1988

APPENDIX A

Supporting Evidence for Use of Complementary and Alternative Medicine in Mental Health Care

APPENDIX A. Supporting Evidence for Use of Complementary and Alternative Medicine (CAM) in Mental Health Care

Disorder or symptom treated	CAM treatment and supporting evidence	Evidence rating[a]	Comments and caveats
Depressed mood	Nutrition: ensure adequate intake of omega-3 EFAs (Chapter 7); optimize folate status (Chapter 11)	1	Omega-3 EFAs: Three positive double-blind placebo-controlled trials of adjunctive therapy (most effective dosage is 1.0–9.6 g/day); one negative study; amounts needed for therapeutic effect not established in all disorders
			Folate: Women may benefit more than men from folate supplementation, but folate supplementation is not effective as a monotherapy
	St. John's wort (Chapters 5 and 13)	1	For mild-to-moderate depression; conflicting data about effect on newborns of women taking this while breast-feeding
			Multiple drug and herb interactions: affects cytochrome P450; interacts with SSRIs, hormones, and oral contraceptives
			Cost and quality vary but cost considerably less than standard pharmaceuticals
			Low incidence of adverse effects (2.4% reported in study of 3,250 patients); most common are mild stomach discomfort, allergic skin rashes, tiredness, and restlessness (occurrence rate for all: 0.6% or less); reported manic and psychotic episodes, serotonin syndrome–like symptoms

APPENDIX A. Supporting Evidence for Use of Complementary and Alternative Medicine (CAM) in Mental Health Care *(continued)*

Disorder or symptom treated	CAM treatment and supporting evidence	Evidence rating[a]	Comments and caveats
Depressed mood *(continued)*	St. John's wort (Chapters 5 and 13) *(continued)*	1	Photosensitivity (hypericin known to cause photosensitivity reactions, especially in animals) in two case reports involving topical use of herb and one in which individual received intensive ultraviolet B therapy after oral use of herb; may be an increased risk of cataract occurrence due to hypericin photoactivation in lens of eye Concurrent use with an MAOI can lead to hypertensive crisis Has anticoagulant effects
	Ayurvedic herbs and polyherb formulas: *Withania somnifera, Mucuna pruriens, Convolvulus pluricaulis,* yogabalacurna,[b] Geriforte,[b] Mentat[b] (Chapter 10)	1	*W. somnifera* and *M. pruriens* are used together in "depressive neurosis"; *C. pluricaulis* is used in depressive neurosis; yogabalacurna is a traditional medhya rasayana; Geriforte is most promising in dysthymia; Mentat is used in depressive neurosis
	Omega–3 EFAs (Chapter 7)	1 (EPA or EPA + DHA); 2 for use in MDD, PPD	Protects against preterm delivery without adverse effect on fetal growth or course of labor

APPENDIX A. Supporting Evidence for Use of Complementary and Alternative Medicine (CAM) in Mental Health Care (*continued*)

Disorder or symptom treated	CAM treatment and supporting evidence	Evidence rating[a]	Comments and caveats
Depressed mood (*continued*)	SAMe (Chapter 13)	1, based on studies of men and women; 2 for PPD and postmenopausal depression	Costly, not covered by insurance; caution indicated in pregnant or lactating women; may lower prolactin levels May trigger hypomania/mania in some patients Butanedisulfonate salt more bioavailable and more stable than tosylate salt, making product selection extremely important
	Light therapy (Chapter 13)	1 for MDD; 2 for depression during pregnancy	May induce hypomania; warrants studies in postpartum depression
	Exercise, moderate, at least three times/week (Chapter 12); for MDD and PPD in women (Chapter 13)	2 for general population and women	Evidence more robust for mild-to-moderate depression Most data from epidemiological studies Intervention studies have been inconsistent Consult physician if pregnant
	Yoga (Chapter 16)	2	Double-blinding is not feasible in yoga studies

APPENDIX A. Supporting Evidence for Use of Complementary and Alternative Medicine (CAM) in Mental Health Care *(continued)*

Disorder or symptom treated	CAM treatment and supporting evidence	Evidence rating[a]	Comments and caveats
Depressed mood *(continued)*	Mindfulness–based cognitive therapy (MBCT) for relapse prevention (Chapter 14)	2	Only cognitive components of treatment studied; evidence suggests that MBCT is not helpful for people who have a history of two or fewer episodes of depression
	Qigong (Chapter 17)	3	Many unpublished studies in China, many case reports, three good studies, one double-blind study
			Reported cases of transient psychosis or agitation during qigong practice in patients diagnosed with personality disorders or schizophrenia
	Acupuncture (in women) (Chapter 13)	1	Caution in pregnancy; warrants further studies; pregnant patients should not have certain acupuncture points stimulated
	Acupuncture, electroacupuncture (Chapter 11)	3	Larger trial of acupuncture in the acute and maintenance phases of treatment warranted; depression associated with other disorders was not always differentiated

APPENDIX A. Supporting Evidence for Use of Complementary and Alternative Medicine (CAM) in Mental Health Care (*continued*)

Disorder or symptom treated	CAM treatment and supporting evidence	Evidence rating[a]	Comments and caveats
Depressed mood (*continued*)	Classical homeopathy (Chapter 9)	2	Many case reports, one small case series Large-magnitude placebo effect with drugs make small pilot studies less feasible Homeopathic remedies very safe; no toxic reactions reported in 200 years; FDA responsible for quality control of homeopathic remedies Patients may experience a "healing crisis" or "healing aggravation," a mild worsening of symptoms usually lasting only a few days
	Social religiosity and thankfulness for reduced risk of MDD (Chapter 15)	1	More than 80 studies
	Intercessory prayer and other forms of distant healing intention (Chapter 15)	1	More than three studies

APPENDIX A. Supporting Evidence for Use of Complementary and Alternative Medicine (CAM) in Mental Health Care *(continued)*

Disorder or symptom treated	CAM treatment and supporting evidence	Evidence rating[a]	Comments and caveats
Bipolar disorder	Nutrition: ensure adequate intake of omega-3 EFAs (Chapter 11)	2	Amounts needed for therapeutic effect not established. One double-blind, placebo-controlled trial found EPA + DHA adjunctive therapy to be superior to placebo; one study of EPA alone found no superiority over placebo in trial dosages of up to 9.6 g/day
	Ayurveda: *Rauwolfia serpentina* (Chapter 10)	1	May be useful in refractory mania
	Exercise (Chapter 12)	3	Studies compared "naturally active" individuals with those engaged in formula-based exercise
	Yoga (Chapter 16)	3	Caution in using with bipolar I patients or those with unstable rapid cycling
	Acupuncture (Chapter 8)	2	Study focused on depression associated with bipolar disorder; study of use in manic-depressive psychosis warranted
	Religious belief associated with improved self-management of bipolar symptoms (Chapter 15)	3	One large survey study

APPENDIX A. Supporting Evidence for Use of Complementary and Alternative Medicine (CAM) in Mental Health Care (*continued*)

Disorder or symptom treated	CAM treatment and supporting evidence	Evidence rating[a]	Comments and caveats
Anxiety disorders	Kava (Chapter 5); also reduction in perimenopausal and menopausal anxiety	1	More than three randomized clinical trials
			Moderate efficacy in treatment of anxiety
			Safe for short-term treatment (1–24 weeks); potential hepatotoxicity; heavy chronic use associated with renal dysfunction, hematological abnormalities, pulmonary hypertension, dermopathy, and choreathetosis (cited in case reports)
			Many drug interactions documented
			Germany, Switzerland, and England no longer permit public sales of kava products; American and Canadian governments are considering stopping sales of kava products
	St. John's wort (Chapter 5)	3; 2 for OCD	Only case reports; small, open, uncontrolled trials in OCD
	Ayurveda: *Bacopa monnieri* (Chapter 10)	1	Anxiety neurosis
			Healthy subjects
	Ayurveda: *Centella asiatica* (Chapter 10)	1	Anxiety neurosis
			Used with *C. pluricaulis*
			Healthy subjects

APPENDIX A. Supporting Evidence for Use of Complementary and Alternative Medicine (CAM) in Mental Health Care *(continued)*

Disorder or symptom treated	CAM treatment and supporting evidence	Evidence rating[a]	Comments and caveats
Anxiety disorders *(continued)*	Ayurveda: *Convolvulus pluricaulis* (Chapter 10)	1	Used with *C. asiatica*
	Ayurveda: *Withania somnifera* (Chapter 10)	1	Anxiety neurosis
	Ayurveda: Geriforte[b] (Chapter 10)	1	Anxiety neurosis, GAD, anxiety/depression
	Ayurveda: Mentat[b] (Chapter 10)	1	Healthy subjects
	Exercise: aerobic exercise, at least 20 minutes/session for a minimum of 10 weeks, maximum benefit after 40 minutes/session (Chapters 12 and 13)	2–3	Small number of studies support improvements in state and trait anxiety, postpartum women
	Yoga (Chapter 16)	2	Studies include several techniques combined

APPENDIX A. Supporting Evidence for Use of Complementary and Alternative Medicine (CAM) in Mental Health Care (*continued*)

Disorder or symptom treated	CAM treatment and supporting evidence	Evidence rating[a]	Comments and caveats
Anxiety disorders (*continued*)	Qigong (Chapter 17) for GAD	3	Five studies identified and one open prospective study reported promising evidence of a significant therapeutic effect; data significance limited by small sample size, short study period, lack of long-term follow-up, lack of control group
	Acupuncture, in women (Chapter 13)	2	Caution during pregnancy; warrants further studies
	Acupuncture, electroacupuncture (Chapter 8)	3	Mechanism of the effect on the cardiac autonomic nervous system was evaluated; most control groups received sham acupuncture that elicited some response
	Classical homeopathy for social phobia, GAD, panic disorder, PTSD (Chapter 9)	2 for panic disorder, GAD, social phobia; 3 for PTSD	Many case reports; one negative controlled study and one positive large observational study in GAD; one small case series in panic disorder; one small study in social phobia. No toxic reactions reported in 200 years of use
	Mindfulness meditation for GAD, panic disorder with or without agoraphobia (Chapter 14)	1	Nonrandomized, uncontrolled trials; positive results did appear to persist at 3-year follow-up

APPENDIX A. Supporting Evidence for Use of Complementary and Alternative Medicine (CAM) in Mental Health Care *(continued)*

Disorder or symptom treated	CAM treatment and supporting evidence	Evidence rating[a]	Comments and caveats
Anxiety disorders *(continued)*	Social religiosity and thankfulness associated with reduced risk for GAD and panic disorder (Chapter 15)	1	Many studies
Schizophrenia and other psychotic disorders	Nutrition: ensure adequate intake of omega-3 fatty acids (Chapter 11), avoid dairy and refined sugar	3	Amounts needed for therapeutic effect not established; trial dosages 2–3 g/day Four double-blind, placebo-controlled trials of adjunctive use (EPA alone) showed positive results
	St. John's wort (Chapter 5)	3	Lack of clear evidence for use Case reports of St. John's wort–induced psychosis; other case reports of relapsing schizophrenia (however, those patients had discontinued conventional therapy)

APPENDIX A. Supporting Evidence for Use of Complementary and Alternative Medicine (CAM) in Mental Health Care (*continued*)

Disorder or symptom treated	CAM treatment and supporting evidence	Evidence rating[a]	Comments and caveats
Schizophrenia and other psychotic disorders (*continued*)	*Ginkgo biloba:* may enhance effectiveness of haloperidol and possibly decrease its extrapyramidal side effects (Chapter 5)	2	Very few studies, more are warranted, case reports, pooled clinical trials of almost 10,000 people Ginkgo has anticoagulant action (decreases blood viscosity, antiplatelet activity); bleeding risk may be increased if used before surgery or labor/delivery Very few adverse effects documented; most common: gastrointestinal discomfort (21 cases), skin allergy, dizziness, headache; rare reports of subdural hematoma and hyphema, Stevens-Johnson syndrome, recurrent seizures in epilepsy patients with prior symptom control Cytotoxic and allergenic alkylphenols (e.g., ginkgolic acids) may be present in some extracts; possible product contamination problematic Ginkgo seeds rarely sold to the public (leaves used in most products); anti–vitamin B_6 neurotoxin (ginkgotoxin) in seeds; toxins removed from approved German products

APPENDIX A. Supporting Evidence for Use of Complementary and Alternative Medicine (CAM) in Mental Health Care (*continued*)

Disorder or symptom treated	CAM treatment and supporting evidence	Evidence rating[a]	Comments and caveats
Schizophrenia and other psychotic disorders (*continued*)	Ayurveda: *Rauwolfia serpentina* (Chapter 10)	3	Used in schizophrenia Crude plant extract has few side effects versus reserpine
	Ayurveda: Brahmyadiyoga[b] (Chapter 10)	2	Used in schizophrenia; crude *Rauwolfia* extract + five other herbs
	Ayurveda: smriti sagar rasa[b] (Chapter 10)	1	Residual schizophrenia
	Unmada gajakesari[b] (Chapter 10)	1	Residual schizophrenia
	Mentat[a] (Chapter 10)	1	Negative symptoms of schizophrenia
	Exercise (Chapter 12)	3	Single-intervention study
	Yoga (Chapter 16)	3	Modified nonstimulating yoga techniques used in supportive setting with skilled mental health professionals
	Acupuncture with herbal therapy and auricular acupuncture; acupressure (Chapter 8)	3, 2 (respectively)	One study focused on depression associated with a psychotic disorder; combination therapy used in traditional manner

APPENDIX A. Supporting Evidence for Use of Complementary and Alternative Medicine (CAM) in Mental Health Care (continued)

Disorder or symptom treated	CAM treatment and supporting evidence	Evidence rating[a]	Comments and caveats
Dementia and mild cognitive impairment	Nutrition: optimize B vitamin status (particularly folate, B_{12}, B_6); ensure adequate intake of omega-3 EFAs; optimize intake of antioxidant-rich foods; screen for and treat hyperhomocysteinemia (Chapter 11)	1 for B vitamin, 2 for omega-3 EFAs, 3 for antioxidant-rich foods	Amounts needed for therapeutic effect not established
	Ginkgo biloba: improves cognitive function and delays progress of dementia Chapter 5)	1	Based on many studies and reviews, but small sample sizes and some flawed research designs
	Bacopa monnieri[c] (Chapter 10)	1 for mental retardation, 2 for ADHD/AAMI	Mental retardation, ADHD, AAMI

APPENDIX A. Supporting Evidence for Use of Complementary and Alternative Medicine (CAM) in Mental Health Care *(continued)*

Disorder or symptom treated	CAM treatment and supporting evidence	Evidence rating[a]	Comments and caveats
Dementia and mild cognitive impairment *(continued)*	*Centella asiatica*[c] (Chapter 10)	2	Mental retardation
	Mentat[b,c] (Chapter 10)	3	ADHD
	Mentat[b,c] (Chapter 10)	2	Mental retardation
	Mentat[b,c] (Chapter 10)	1	Learning disability
	Memorin[b,c] (Chapter 10)	1	AAMI
	Exercise: walking and increased regularly performed daytime exercise (Chapter 12)	1–2	Epidemiological evidence supportive; intervention studies showed mixed results
	Classical homeopathy (Chapter 9)	3	Some case reports; animal studies suggest possible benefit of isopathic treatment with glutamate
	Acupuncture and inhalation herbal therapy (Chapter 8)	3	Study in hospital setting used combination therapies in the tradition of Chinese medicine

APPENDIX A. Supporting Evidence for Use of Complementary and Alternative Medicine (CAM) in Mental Health Care (continued)

Disorder or symptom treated	CAM treatment and supporting evidence	Evidence rating[a]	Comments and caveats
Substance and alcohol abuse	Ayurveda: Mentat[b] (Chapter 10)	1	Alcoholism
	Yoga (Chapter 16)	2	Studies included several techniques combined
	Qigong (Chapter 17)	3	Useful for withdrawal symptoms in heroin addicts, small group, some study limitations
	Acupuncture, auricular acupuncture (Chapter 8)	3, 2 (respectively)	Alcohol, narcotics, cocaine, and nicotine studied separately
	Classical homeopathy, for alcohol abuse) (Chapter 9)	3	Many case reports; animal studies suggest capacity to reduce alcohol-induced sleep time
	Social religiosity and thankfulness associated with reduced risk for alcohol and substance abuse (Chapter 15)	1	Many studies
Seasonal affective disorder	Light therapy (Chapter 13)	1	Light therapy may induce hypomania

APPENDIX A. Supporting Evidence for Use of Complementary and Alternative Medicine (CAM) in Mental Health Care *(continued)*

Disorder or symptom treated	CAM treatment and supporting evidence	Evidence rating[a]	Comments and caveats
Seasonal affective disorder *(continued)*	St. John's wort (Chapters 5 and 13)	2	Small open, uncontrolled trials Conflicts about effects on newborns of breast-feeding mothers Affects cytochrome P450; interacts with SSRIs, hormones, oral contraceptives
Somatoform disorders	Classical homeopathy (Chapter 9)	2	Many case reports; two positive controlled studies in fibromyalgia, one equivocal controlled study in chronic fatigue syndrome
Premenstrual dysphoric disorder	Classical homeopathy (Chapter 9)	2–3	Many case reports, one small study
Autism	St. John's wort (Chapter 5)	2	Small open, uncontrolled trials
	Classical homeopathy (Chapter 9)	3	Many case reports, no controlled studies
Traumatic brain injury	Classical homeopathy (Chapter 9)	2	Many case reports, one positive controlled study

APPENDIX A. Supporting Evidence for Use of Complementary and Alternative Medicine (CAM) in Mental Health Care *(continued)*

Disorder or symptom treated	CAM treatment and supporting evidence	Evidence rating[a]	Comments and caveats
Attention-deficit/ hyperactivity disorder (ADHD)	Yoga (Chapter 16)	2	Many case reports, one positive controlled study
	Classical homeopathy (Chapter 9)	2	Many case reports, one positive controlled study, one good observational study, some popular books
Epilepsy	Classical homeopathy (Chapter 9)	3	Many case reports
Stroke	Classical homeopathy (Chapter 9)	3	Some case reports; animal studies suggest possible benefit of isopathic treatment with glutamate (see Dementia and mild cognitive impairment)
Acute grief reaction	Classical homeopathy (Chapter 9)	3	Many case reports, no studies
Chronic headache	Classical homeopathy (Chapter 9)	3	Many case reports, one negative controlled study
Vertigo	Combination homeopathy (Chapter 9)	2	Many case reports, one positive controlled study

APPENDIX A. Supporting Evidence for Use of Complementary and Alternative Medicine (CAM) in Mental Health Care (*continued*)

Disorder or symptom treated	CAM treatment and supporting evidence	Evidence rating[a]	Comments and caveats
Insomnia	*Valeriana jatamansi*[c] (Chapter 10)	3	Studies used *Valeriana* species closely related to *V. jatamansi*
	Nardostachys jatamansi, Rauwolfia serpentina, Tinospora cordifoli (Chapter 10)	1	All three herbs used in combination
	Classical homeopathy (Chapter 9)	2	Many case reports, some animal studies, no clinical studies
Binge-eating disorder	Mindfulness meditation (Chapter 14)	1	One nonrandomized, uncontrolled pilot study
	Social religiosity and thankfulness associated with reduced risk for bulimia (Chapter 15)	1	Many studies
Borderline personality disorder	Nutrition: omega-3 EFAs (EPA alone) (Chapter 11)	2	One double-blind, placebo-controlled trial of monotherapy (dosage: 1 g/day)

APPENDIX A. Supporting Evidence for Use of Complementary and Alternative Medicine (CAM) in Mental Health Care (*continued*)

Disorder or symptom treated	CAM treatment and supporting evidence	Evidence rating[a]	Comments and caveats
Cognitive enhancement	*Ginkgo biloba*: may enhance short-term memory in healthy individuals (Chapter 5)	3	May need higher doses in healthy individuals
	Bacopa monnieri[c] (Chapter 10)	2	Healthy children and adults
	Centella asiatica[c] (Chapter 10)	1	Healthy children
	Withania somnifera[c] (Chapter 10)	1	Healthy adults
	Six-herb formula[b,c] (Chapter 10)	1	Healthy children
	Maharishi Amrit Kalash[b,c] (Chapter 10)	1	Healthy elderly individuals

APPENDIX A. Supporting Evidence for Use of Complementary and Alternative Medicine (CAM) in Mental Health Care *(continued)*

Disorder or symptom treated	CAM treatment and supporting evidence	Evidence rating[a]	Comments and caveats
Cognitive enhancement *(continued)*	Mentat[b,c] (Chapter 10)	2	Healthy children and adults
	Geriforte[b] (Chapter 10)	1	Healthy elderly individuals

Note. AAMI = age-associated memory impairment; DHA = docosahexanoic acid; EFA = essential fatty acid; EPA = eicosapentaenoic acid; GAD = generalized anxiety disorder; MAOI = monoamine oxidase inhibitor; MDD = major depressive disorder; PPD = postpartum depression; PTSD = posttraumatic stress disorder; OCD = obsessive–compulsive disorder; SAMe = S-adenosylmethionine; SSRI = selective serotonin reuptake inhibitor.

[a]Evidence-rating scale: 1—established use of specified modality supported by systematic review or three or more controlled, randomized, double-blind studies; 2—use of specified modality supported by consistent findings from open trials or fewer than three randomized, controlled trials; 3—use of modality supported by consistent anecdotal reports but few or no studies.

[b]Polyherb formulas, listed by traditional Sanskrit name or proprietary name, as appropriate.

[c]Herbs tested in randomized controlled trials.

APPENDIX B

Glossary of Key Terms in Complementary and Alternative Medicine

A

Acetylcholine A neurotransmitter that helps regulate learning and memory in the brain and control actions of skeletal and smooth muscles in the peripheral nervous system.

Acetyl-L-Carnitine (ALC) Modified form of L-carnitine made from lysine and methionine with the help of vitamin C that is synthesized in the brain, kidney, and liver. It readily crosses the blood-brain barrier to the brain, where it has two mechanisms of action. Structurally similar to acetylcholine, it has a cholinomimetic effect, increasing cholinergic neural transmission. This is the theoretical basis for the finding that ALC supplementation may partially correct cholinergic neurotransmission deficits characteristic of Alzheimer's disease and some cases of depressed mood.

Acupressure Ancient Chinese treatment in which pressure is applied to potent points to relieve pain.

Acupuncture Chinese treatment with tiny needles on specific acupuncture points to unblock energy pathways; based on the belief that energy (qi or chi) flows throughout the body in meridians. There is also a theory that inserted needles facilitate the release of neurotransmitters and endorphins.

Allopathy A Western medical treatment in which disease is cured by a means that has an effect opposite to that of the disease; uses drugs or surgery.

α-Linolenic acid (ALA) Essential polyunsaturated fatty acid that is elongated to form eicosapentaenoic acid and docosahexanoic acid.

Alternative medicine Nonconventional somatic, biological, mind–body, and/or energy healing practice of medicine.

Antioxidant Protects cells from a damaging effect of oxidation.

Asanas   Postures and stretching in yoga.

Ayurveda   Hindu system of healing that views health as the balance of body, mind, emotion, and spirit and uses yoga, meditation, diet, herbal medicine, and purification regimens to treat unbalances in these dimensions.

B

B vitamins   Vitamins (specifically folate, B_{12}, and B_6) that are integral to proper brain function, as they are participants in one-carbon metabolism reactions, resulting in the synthesis of thymidylate and purines (used for nucleic acid synthesis) and methionine (used for protein synthesis and biological methylations), which are believed to be a crucial part of the pathway for the health of the brain.

C

CCMD-3   Chinese Classification of Mental Disorders; reflects differences in philosophy from Western medicine and China's unique sociomoral and cultural viewpoint of illness.

Chromium   A trace mineral found in the diet that is an essential micronutrient. It is important in glucose and lipid metabolism and impacts monoamine neurotransmitter systems. By increasing the efficiency of insulin utilization, chromium increases insulin sensitivity and reverses impaired glucose tolerance. Chromium has been found in controlled studies to reduce depression.

Complementary medicine   The combining of traditional and alternative medicine therapies so as to enhance the effectiveness of treatment.

E

EMPowerPlus   A food supplement reportedly modeled after an agricultural treatment for aggressive behavior in farm animals (e.g., pigs who become violent and bite each other's ears and tails). The substance, which is recommended at high doses, contains 36 dietary nutrients, particularly chelated trace minerals.

Essential amino acids   Nine amino acids that must be obtained from the diet.

Essential substance   A necessary substance that comes from the diet and cannot be produced in the body.

F

Folate   A water-soluble B vitamin postulated to ameliorate depressive symptoms by increasing levels of *S*-adenosylmethionine; also may play a role in the synthesis of monoamines. There are no known adverse effects associated with folate.

Free radical   A molecule that chemically interacts with nearby molecules and causes cellular damage.

G

Ginkgo (*Ginkgo biloba*)   One of the oldest living tree species, originating in China, which has been used for many different medical conditions because of its neuroprotective, antioxidant, anti-inflammatory, vasodilatory, and anti–platelet-activating-factor activity.

H

Hahnemann, Samuel (1755–1843)   German physician who founded homeopathy.

"Health freedom" statutes   Laws that state that physicians may not be disciplined solely on the basis of incorporating complementary and alternative modalities.

Herbal medicine   System of healing and illness prevention that uses medicinal plants.

Holistic medicine   System that regards the body and mind as an integral entity and considers all aspects of person's health in treatment.

Homeopathy   A system of medicine that is one of the most popular forms of complementary and alternative medicine in the world. The name originates from the Greek words *homoios* ("same") and *pathos* ("suffering") and reflects one of homeopathy's cornerstones, the Law of Similars. In following the defining principle of "similar suffering," homeopaths prescribe medicines that act in concert with the patient's symptoms, thereby encouraging the patient's perturbed defenses to reestablish homeostasis (evoking self-healing). By contrast, the allopath (Hahnemann's term for physicians whose treatments produce suffering other than that related to the cause of illness) might suppress the patient's symptoms with antidepressants, antibiotics, or antipyretics, or use completely unrelated methods. *Classical homeopathy* is a controversial system of medicine developed more than 200 years ago by the German physician Samuel Hahnemann, a pioneer in the field of psychosomatic medicine.

Homocysteine   An endogenously produced, sulfur-containing amino acid; a precursor of the excitotoxic amino acids cysteine and homocysteic acid. Elevated levels of homocysteine are a risk factor for atherosclerosis and increased systemic inflammation.

Hormesis   A well-documented biological and chemical observation in the conventional field of pharmacology–toxicology that involves the interaction between an agent and host to stimulate homeostatic compensations in the host. As a result, nonlinear, often bidirectional, differential effects of the same substance can occur with variations in dosage.

5-Hydroxytryptophan (5-HTP)   A metabolite of L-tryptophan, which is an amino acid that is converted to serotonin and that is found in nuts, soybeans, dairy, eggs, poultry, and red meat

Hypnosis   Induced complex sleeplike state in which a person is receptive to suggestions from another person

I

Inositol   A precursor to the phosphatidylinositol cycle, an important intracellular second-messenger system.

Integrative medicine   Whole-person-oriented healing and preventive methods, including conventional and alternative medicine.

K

Kava-kava (*Piper methysticum*)   Plant with anesthetic, analgesic, sedative, anticonvulsive, antispasmodic, and antithrombotic effects used by Pacific Islanders for centuries.

L

Light therapy   A therapy using bright lights that in placebo-controlled trials has demonstrated effectiveness for treating seasonal and nonseasonal depression.

Limbs of yoga

Yama and Niyama   Ethical and moral standards such as honesty, nonviolence, patience, compassion, contentment with what one has (not being greedy), study of ancient wisdom to overcome dysfunctional habits, and devotion.

Svadhyaya   Study and learning ancient yoga scriptures and knowledge.

Asanas   Physical yoga postures used in meditation on the body to reexperience the self.

Pranayama   Yogic breathing techniques.

Pratyahara   Turning the attention away from the senses toward the inner world of self-experience.

Dharana   Concentration to focus attention.

Dyana   Meditation with mental clarity and total calmness.

Samadhi   Ecstasy or bliss that occurs when one is reunited with the true self, which is one and the same as universal energy or the divine.

Linoleic acid (LA)   Essential polyunsaturated fatty acid obtained from the diet; in the body is converted to arachidonic acid (AA).

Law of Similars   Principle of homeopathic medicine that states that a substance producing a characteristic set of symptoms in a healthy person can, when given in a small dose, cure an ill person suffering similar symptoms. Homeopaths view symptoms as manifestations of the organism's attempt to maintain health rather than as the problem itself. They prescribe medicines that encourage the patient's perturbed defenses to reestablish homeostasis (evoking self-healing).

M

Meditation   Technique of focused attention on a word or the breath to increase awareness and relaxation, reduce stress, and promote health.

Meridian   In traditional Chinese medicine, a channel that carries the vital *qi*.

Mindfulness meditation   A practice in which an individual attends to a wide range of changing objects of attention while maintaining moment-to-moment awareness rather than restricting his or her focus to a single object such as a mantra.

N

Naturopathy   A healing approach that uses natural substances and physical means.

National Acupuncture Detoxification Association (NADA)   Organization that has conducted successful training programs for physicians and related staff in using the technique and philosophy of traditional Chinese acupuncture.

O

Omega-3 essential fatty acids (EFAs)   Also known as omega-3 polyunsaturated fatty acids; include eicosapentaenoic acid, docosahexanoic acid, and linolenic acid, which are important components of the cell membrane structure and in the formation of prostaglandins and leukotrienes. Omega-3 EFAs are found in some fish and plant sources. They have anti-inflammatory and immunosuppressant effects; their beneficial action in depression occurs through suppression of serotonin signal transduction pathways. They may interact with anticoagulants and increase risk of bleeding.

P

Phosphatidylcholine   A component of lecithin.

Phosphatidylserine   A phospholipid derived from soy or cabbage.

Polyunsaturated fatty acids (PUFA)   The primary determinants of neuronal membrane structure and function (specifically, essential fatty acids).

Provings   A process in homeopathy in which the effect of specific substances is tested. Homeopaths conduct "provings" (*Prüfung* is the German word for "test") according to strict protocols. In this process, healthy individuals take an unknown substance and the homeopath carefully records every symptom ("side effect") the individual experiences, which forms the basis of a "drug picture" that guides homeopaths in using the now "proven" medicine ("remedy") for healing sick patients. The Greek physician Galen was the first to suggest using healthy people for such testing; the German physician Hahnemann was the first to rigorously conduct provings.

Q

Qigong   Also spelled *Ch'i Kung,* and pronounced "chee gung." Medical qigong involves externally emitted energy by a skilled medical qigong master for the purpose of healing others. *Qi* means "vital energy," or life force, and *gong* means "skill," so *qigong* is the "skillful practice of gathering, circulating, and applying life force energy." It involves a combination of exercises, breathing techniques, and postures to promote health and healing by improving an individual's qi.

S

Shen   In traditional Chinese medicine, the energetic principle embodied in spirit, mind, or consciousness.

St. John's wort (*Hypericum perforatum*) A perennial plant used in the treatment for many psychiatric conditions; its mechanism of action is based on in vitro inhibition of the reuptake of many neurotransmitters and may affect the hypothalamic–pituitary–adrenal axis. The herb affects the cytochrome P450 system and interacts with many medications.

Sudarshan Kriya yoga (**SKY**) A form of yoga developed by Sri Sri Ravi Shankar that combines ancient and modern pranayama with meditation, chanting, and yoga knowledge.

S-**Adenosylmethionine** (**SAMe**) A universal methyl donor active in a variety of reactions that are essential to normal brain function, including ones that produce nucleotides, phospholipids, and myelin. It has antidepressant properties, thought to be based on its role in the synthesis of catecholamines and other biogenic amines.

T

Traditional Chinese medicine A system of medicine founded on Daoist philosophy about 2,000 years ago that views the human body as a whole and in a mutual relationship with the environment; disease occurs when this harmony is disrupted.

Transcendental meditation An approach in which the meditator achieves a meditative state by repeating a word or phrase called a *mantra*.

Tryptophan The amino acid precursor to serotonin.

U

Unilateral forced nostril breathing (**UFNB**) A type of breathing in which a person gently compresses one side of the nasal ala with the tip of the thumb to occlude the nostril, thereby activating the contralateral cerebral hemisphere and the autonomic nervous system. Ancient yogis called right-nostril breathing *Surya Anuloma Viloma* (heat-generating) and left-nostril breathing *Chandra Anuloma Viloma* (heat-dissipating, or cooling).

Ujjayi A form of slow breathing (2–4 breath cycles per minute) in which a person, with the eyes closed, exhales through the nose against airway resistance and holds the breath at the end of inspiration and expiration, with the expiration longer than the inspiration; by so doing, the person increases vagal tone and improves oxygenation and exercise tolerance.

V

Vipassanâ   A Buddhist practice in which a person seeks insight into the nature of his or her own thoughts; the word is translated as "insight meditation" or "mindfulness."

Y

Yama   The moral discipline in yoga.

Yang   The ascending, bright, active aspect of *qi*.

Yin   The descending, dark, passive aspect of *qi*.

Yoga   A practice in which a person promotes the quality of life by uniting the individual life energy, *prâna,* with the universal energy, *Brahman,* through exercise practices, breath control, and self-observation. Yoga stimulates the parasympathetic nervous system through activation of vagal afferents.

APPENDIX C

Useful Resources for Complementary and Alternative Medicine

WEB SITES

CAM Information and Research

Alternative Health Dictionary: www.canoe.ca/AltmedDictionary/home.html

Alternative Health News Online: www.altmedicine.com/FrameSet.asp

Alternative Medicine Foundation, Inc.: www.amfoundation.org

Alternative Medicine Homepage, University of Pittsburgh: www.pitt.edu/~cbw/assoc.html

American Psychiatric Association: www.psych.org

American Psychiatric Association Caucus on Complementary, Alternative and Integrative Care: http://APACAM.org

Cochrane reviews: www.cochrane.org/index0.htm

Computer Retrieval of Information on Scientific Projects database: http://crisp.cit.nih.gov

Food and Nutrition Information Center: www.nal.usda.gov/fnic

Foundation for the Advancement of Innovative Medicine: www.faim.org/Default.htm

Health Index (MANTIS database): www.healthindex.com/Start.html

HealthWWWeb: www.healthwwweb.com/index.html

Medline Plus: www.nlm.nih.gov/medlineplus

National Center for Complementary and Alternative Medicine, search within complementary and alternative medicine subset of PubMed: www.nlm.nih.gov/nccam/camonpubmed.html

National Center for Complementary and Alternative Medicine Update eBulletin: www.nccaminfo.org/subscribenewsletter/addsubscriber.asp

National Institutes of Health Consensus Development Program: http://consensus.nih.gov

Office of Dietary Supplements, National Institutes of Health: http://dietary-supplements.info.nih.gov

Office of Extramural Research, National Institutes of Health: www.nih.gov/about/publicaccess/index.htm

PubMed database, National Institutes of Health and Library of Medicine: www.ncbi.nih.gov/entrez/query.fcgi

Ayurveda

BBC News report: "Lost city 'could rewrite history'": http://news.bbc.co.uk/1/hi/world/south_asia/1768109.stm

Marine Archaeology in the Gulf of Khambat: www.niot.res.in/m3/arch

World Health Organization Medicines Policy & Standards: www.who.int/medicines/en

Chinese Medicine

American Academy of Medical Acupuncture: www.medicalacupuncture.org

Doc Misha's Chicken Soup Chinese Medicine: www.docmisha.com/understanding/index.html

National Certification Commission for Acupuncture and Oriental Medicine: www.nccaom.org

Traditional Chinese Medicine Online: www.cintcm.com/index.htm

Exercise

Agency for Healthcare Research and Quality: www.ahrq.gov/clinic/uspstf/uspsphys.htm

Homeopathy

American Institute of Homeopathy: www.homeopathyusa.org

Homeopathic Academy of Naturopathic Physicians: www.hanp.net

Homeopathic Pharmacopoeia of the United States: www.hpus.com

Homeopathy Cured Cases: www.homeopathycuredcases.com

Homeopathy Online, A Journal of Homeopathic Medicine: www.lyghtforce.com/homeopathy online

National Center for Homeopathy: www.homeopathic.org

North American Society of Homeopaths: www.homeopathy.org

Legal Issues

American Medical Association Liability Insurance Requirements: www.ama-assn.org/ama/pub/category/print/4544.html

Federation of State Medical Boards: Model Guidelines for Physician Use of Complementary and Alternative Therapies in Medical Practice. April 2002. Available at: www.fsmb.org/pdf/2002_grpol_Complementary_Alternative_Therapies.pdf. Accessed February 5, 2004.

Law Offices of Michael Cohen, Esq.: www.michaelhcohen.com

National Center for Complementary and Alternative Medicine: www.nccam.nih.gov

Mind–Body Techniques/Yoga in Psychiatry

The Art of Living Foundation: www.artofliving.org (press releases available at www.artofliving.org/pressroom)

BBC News report: "Indian stress-busters target Iraq": http://newsvote.bbc.co.uk/1/hi/world/south_asia/3393327.stm

Therapy With Yoga program: www.therapywithyoga.com

The Times of India Online report, "Indian doves fly high in Iraq": http://timesofindia.indiatimes.com/articleshow/msid-802624,prtpage-1.cms

Nutrition

EPA Fish Advisories: www.epa.gov/waterscience/fish
"Fish for Your Health": http://fn.cfs.purdue.edu/anglingindiana
Food and Nutrition Information Center (lists Dietary Reference Intakes and Recommended Dietary Allowances): www.nal.usda.gov/fnic/etext/000105.html

Omega-3 Fatty Acids

National Institutes of Health clinical trials web site: www.clinicaltrials.gov

Safety

ConsumerLab.com: www.consumerlab.com
Health Notes: www.healthnotes.com
HealthGate: www.healthgate.com
iHerb.com: www.iherb.com
National Nutritional Foods Association: www.nnfa.org
Natural Medicines Comprehensive Database: www.naturaldatabase.com
NSF [National Sanitation Foundation] International: www.nsf.org
U.S. Department of Health and Human Services press release, "FDA Announces Major Initiatives for Dietary Supplements," December 30, 2003: www.hhs.gov/news/press/2003pres/20031230.html
U.S. Food and Drug Administration press release, "FDA Announces Major Initiatives for Dietary Supplements," November 4, 2004: www.fda.gov/bbs/topics/news/2004/NEW01130.html
U.S. Pharmacopoeia Dietary Supplement Validation Program: www.usp.org/USPVerified/dietarySupplements
Wolters Kluwer's Facts and Comparisons: www.factsandcomparisons.com

Western Herbal Medicines

National Institutes of Health clinical trials web site: www.clinicaltrials.gov
Natural Medicines Comprehensive Database: www.naturaldatabase.com
Natural Standard: www.naturalstandard.com

BOOKS AND PUBLICATIONS

Ayurveda

Arora UP (ed): *Graeco-Indica: India's Cultural Contacts With the Greek World.* New Delhi, India, Ramanand Vidya Bhavan, 1991
Charaka Samhita (Volumes I–VI). Translated from Sanskrit by Shree Gulab Kunverba Ayurvedic Society. Jamnagar, India, Shree Gulab Kunverba Ayurvedic Society, 1949
Choudhuri O, Singh RH: "Development of an Ayurvedic Regimen for the Management of Residual Schizophrenia." M.D. thesis (Kayachikitsa), Banaras Hindu University, Varanasi, India, 2001

Mookerji R: *Ancient Indian Education: Brahmanical and Buddhist.* London, Motilol Banarsidass, 1947

Possehl GL (ed): *Harappan Civilization: A Contemporary Perspective.* New Delhi, India, Oxford & IBH Publishing, 1982

Rajaram N, Frawley D: *Vedic Aryans and the Origins of Civilization.* St Hyacinthe, Canada, World Heritage Press, 1995

Rao SR: *Dawn and Devolution of the Indus Civilization.* Delhi, India, Aditya Prakashan Press, 1991

Singh B: *The Vedic Harappans.* Delhi, India, Aditya Prakashan Press, 1995

Singhal DP: *India and World Civilization.* Ann Arbor, Michigan University Press, 1969

Smith V: *The Early History of India.* Oxford, UK, Clarendon Press, 1924

Svoboda RE: *Ayurveda: Life, Health and Longevity.* New York, Arkana/Penguin Books, 1992

Svoboda R, Lade A: *Tao and Dharma: Chinese Medicine and Ayurveda.* Twin Lakes, WI, Lotus Press, 1995

Chinese Medicine

Chu ZYXJ: *Fundamentals of Chinese Medicine.* Translated by Wiseman N, Ellis A. Brookline, MA, Paradigm, 1995

Flaws B, Lake J: *Chinese Medical Psychiatry: A Textbook and Clinical Manual.* Boulder, CO, Blue Poppy Press, 2001

Kaptchuk T: *The Web That Has No Weaver.* Chicago, IL, Cogden & Weed, 1983

Ni M (transl): *The Yellow Emperor's Classic of Medicine.* Boston, MA, Shambala, 1995

Shanghai College of Traditional Medicine: *Acupuncture: A Comprehensive Text.* Seattle, WA, Eastland Press, 1981

Stux G, Berman B, Pomeranz B: *Basics of Acupuncture.* New York, Springer, 2003

Zheng-Cai L: *A Study of Daoist Acupuncture.* Boulder, CO, Blue Poppy Press, 1999

Exercise

U.S. Preventive Services Task Force: *Guide to Clinical Preventive Services,* 2nd Edition. Baltimore, MD, Lippincott Williams & Wilkins, 1996

Legal Issues

Cohen MH: *Legal Issues in Alternative Medicine.* Berne, NC, Trafford Publishing 2003

Gutheil TG, Appelbaum PS: *Malpractice and Other Forms of Liability,* 3rd Edition. Philadelphia, PA, Lippincott Williams & Wilkins, 2000

Ernst E: "Second thoughts about safety of St John's wort." Lancet 354:2014–2016, 1999

Cohen MH: *Beyond Complementary Medicine: Legal and Ethical Perspectives on Health Care and Human Evolution.* Ann Arbor, University of Michigan Press, 2000

Nutrition

Hendler SS, Rorvik D (eds): *PDR for Nutritional Supplements,* 1st Edition. Montvale, NJ, Thomson PDR, 2001

U.S. Preventive Services Task Force: *Guide to Clinical Preventive Services,* 2nd Edition. Baltimore, MD, Lippincott Williams & Wilkins, 1996

Safety

Bratman S, Girman AM: *Mosby's Handbook of Herbs and Supplements and Their Therapeutic Uses.* St. Louis, MO, Mosby, 2003

Brinker F: *Herb Contraindications and Drug Interactions,* 2nd Edition. Portland, OR, Eclectic Medical Publications, 1998 (Note: a somewhat subjective source)

Harkness R, Bratman S: *Mosby's Handbook of Drug–Herb and Drug–Supplement Interactions.* St. Louis, MO, Mosby, 2003

McGuffin M, Hobbs C, Upton R, et al: *Botanical Safety Handbook.* Boca Raton, FL, CRC Press, 1997

Western Herbal Medicines

Blumenthal M, Goldberg A, Brinckmann J (eds): *Herbal Medicine: Expanded Commission E Monographs.* Austin, TX, Integrative Medicine Communications, 2000

Bruneton J: *Pharmacognosy, Phytochemistry, Medicinal Plants,* 2nd Edition. Paris, France, Lavoisier, 1999

ORGANIZATIONS

Acupuncture and Oriental Medicine Alliance
Alternative Health Insurance Services
Alternative Medicine Foundation
American Academy of Medical Acupuncture
American Association for Health Freedom
American Association of Naturopathic Physicians
American Botanical Council
American Holistic Medical Association
American Psychiatric Association
British Columbia Naturopathic Association
British Holistic Medical Association
California Association of Naturopathic Physicians
Citizens for Health: The Voice of Natural Health Consumers
Cochrane Collaboration
Cochrane Complementary Medicine Field
European Herbal Practitioners Association
Food and Nutrition Information Center
Foundation for the Advancement of Innovative Medicine
Integrative Medical Alliance
International Food Information Council Foundation
National Center for Complementary and Alternative Medicine
National Center for Homeopathy
National Certification Commission for Acupuncture and Oriental Medicine

National Institute of Environmental Health Sciences
National Institute of Mental Health
National Library of Medicine
Office of Dietary Supplements
Oxford Health Plans Complementary and Alternative Medicine
Philanthropic Collaborative for Integrative Medicine
Qigong Association of America
Research Council for Complementary Medicine (United Kingdom)
U.S. Food and Drug Administration
Washington Association of Naturopathic Physicians
World Health Organization

JOURNALS

Advances in Mind–Body Medicine
Alternative Medicine Review: A Journal of Clinical Therapeutics
BMC Complementary and Alternative Medicine
Evidence-Based Complementary and Alternative Medicine
Homeopathy Online: Journal of Homeopathic Medicine
Integrative Medicine
Journal of Complementary and Alternative Medicine
Journal of Herbal Pharmacotherapy

Index

*Page numbers printed in **boldface** type refer to tables or figures.*